Macleod's Clinical Diagnosis

Macleod's Clinical Diagnosis

2nd Edition

Alan G Japp
MBChB(Hons) BSc(Hons) MRCP PhD
Consultant Cardiologist,
Royal Infirmary of Edinburgh;
Honorary Clinical Senior Lecturer,
University of Edinburgh
UK

Colin Robertson
BA(Hons) MBChB FRCPGlas FRCSEd
FICP(Hon) FSAScot
Honorary Professor of Accident and Emergency
   Medicine and Surgery,
University of Edinburgh
UK

Co-authors

Rohana J Wright
MBChB MD FRCPEd
Consultant Physician,
St John's Hospital,
Livingston, and Edinburgh Centre for Endocrinology
and Diabetes,
Edinburgh, UK

Matthew J Reed
MA(Cantab) MB BChir MRCS FCEM MD
Consultant and NRS Career Researcher Clinician in
   Emergency Medicine,
Royal Infirmary of Edinburgh;
Honorary Reader,
University of Edinburgh
UK

Andrew Robson
MA (Cantab) BM BCh FRCS PhD
Specialist Registrar in General Surgery,
Royal Infirmary of Edinburgh,
UK

ELSEVIER

Edinburgh   London   New York   Oxford   Philadelphia   St Louis   Sydney   2018

ELSEVIER

First edition 2013
Second edition 2018

ISBN   9780702069611
International ISBN   9780702069628

Notices

Practitioners and researchers must always rely on their own experience and knowledge in evaluating and using any information, methods, compounds or experiments described herein. Because of rapid advances in the medical sciences, in particular, independent verification of diagnoses and drug dosages should be made. To the fullest extent of the law, no responsibility is assumed by Elsevier, authors, editors or contributors for any injury and/or damage to persons or property as a matter of products liability, negligence or otherwise, or from any use or operation of any methods, products, instructions, or ideas contained in the material herein.

your source for books,
journals and multimedia
in the health sciences

www.elsevierhealth.com

 Working together
to grow libraries in
developing countries

www.elsevier.com • www.bookaid.org

The
publisher's
policy is to use
**paper manufactured
from sustainable forests**

Content Strategist: Laurence Hunter
Content Development Specialist: Helen Leng
Project Manager: Louisa Talbott
Designer: Miles Hitchen
Illustration Manager: Karen Giacomucci
Illustrator: Antbits

Printed in Poland
Last digit is the print number: 9   8   7   6   5   4   3   2   1

Contents

Preface

'Ninety per cent of diagnoses are made from the history.'
'Clinical examination is the cornerstone of assessment.'

These, or similar platitudes, will be familiar to most students in clinical training. Many, however, notice a 'disconnect' between the importance ascribed to basic clinical skills during teaching and the apparent reliance on sophisticated investigations in the parallel world of clinical practice. Modern diagnostics have radically altered the face of medical practice; clinical training is still catching up. We recognize that teachers and textbooks frequently fall into the trap of eulogizing clinical assessment rather than explaining its actual role in contemporary diagnosis.

Yet we come to praise the clinical assessment, not to bury it. The history may not, by itself, deliver the diagnosis in 90% of cases but it is essential in all cases to generate a logical differential diagnosis and to guide rational investigation and treatment. In many 'developed' countries, some so-called classical physical signs are rare and certain aspects of the clinical examination have been marginalized by novel imaging techniques and disease biomarkers. Nevertheless, a focused clinical examination is critical to recognizing the sick patient, raising red flags, identifying unsuspected problems and, in some cases, revealing signs that cannot be identified with tests (for example, the mental state examination).

Our aim is to show you how to use your core clinical skills to maximum advantage. We offer a grounded and realistic approach to clinical diagnosis with no bias towards any particular element of the assessment. Where appropriate, we acknowledge the limitations of the history and examination and direct you to the necessary investigation. We also highlight those instances where diagnosis is critically dependent on basic clinical assessment, thereby demonstrating its vital and enduring importance. We wish you every success in your training and practice, and hope that this book provides at least some small measure of assistance.

Alan Japp
Colin Robertson
Edinburgh, 2018

Acknowledgements

On behalf of the editors and authors, I would like to thank Laurence Hunter for encouraging and facilitating this new edition; and Helen Leng for once again providing the perfect blend of tolerance, support and discipline. We also thank everyone who volunteered suggestions and ideas for the 2nd edition, particularly Dr Vicky Tallentire, Dr Michael MacMahon and Dr Dean Kerslake. Finally we gratefully acknowledge a valuable contribution to individual chapters from Dr Mark Wright, Consultant Ophthalmologist, Edinburgh (Chapter 28, Red eye); Dr Lydia Ash, Specialty Registrar, Obstetrics & Gynaecology, Edinburgh (Chapter 33, Vaginal bleeding), Mr Andrew Duckworth, Specialty Registrar, Ortho-paedic Surgery, Edinburgh (Chapter 20, Joint swelling) and Mr Neil Maitra, Locum Consultant Urologist, Lanarkshire (Chapter 16, Haematuria) and everyone else who has volunteered ideas, comments, assistance or a friendly ear.

AJ

Abbreviations

Abbreviations that do not appear in this list are spelled out in the main text.

ABCDE	airway, breathing, circulation, disability, exposure	**DMARD**	disease-modifying anti-rheumatic drug
ABG	arterial blood gas	**ECG**	electrocardiogram/electrocardiography
ACE	angiotensin-converting enzyme	**EEG**	electroencephalogram/electroencephalography
ACPA	anti-citrullinated protein antibody		
ACTH	adrenocorticotrophic hormone	**ENA**	extractable nuclear antigen
AIDS	acquired immunodeficiency syndrome	**ENT**	ear, nose and throat
		ERCP	endoscopic retrograde cholangiopancreatography
ALP	alkaline phosphatase		
ALT	alanine aminotransferase	**ESR**	erythrocyte sedimentation rate
ANA	antinuclear antibody	**FBC**	full blood count
ANCA	antineutrophil cytoplasmic antibody	**FiO$_2$**	fraction of inspired oxygen
APTT	activated partial thromboplastin time	**GCS**	Glasgow Coma Scale (score)
ASMA	anti-smooth muscle antibody	**GFR**	glomerular filtration rate
ASO	anti-streptolysin O	**GGT**	gamma-glutamyl transferase
AST	aspartate aminotransferase	**GI**	gastrointestinal
AXR	abdominal X ray	**GP**	general practitioner
BMI	body mass index	**GU**	genitourinary
BP	blood pressure	**Hb**	haemoglobin
bpm	beats per minute	**hCG**	human chorionic gonadotrophin
BS	breath sound	**HIV**	human immunodeficiency virus
CBG	capillary blood glucose	**HR**	heart rate
CLO	*campylobacter*-like organism	**ICP**	intracranial pressure
CK	creatine kinase	**ICU**	intensive care unit
CKD	chronic kidney disease	**ID**	infectious disease
CNS	central nervous system	**IM**	intramuscular(ly)
COPD	chronic obstructive pulmonary disease	**INR**	international normalized ratio
		IV	intravenous(ly)
CPET	cardiopulmonary exercise test	**IVU**	intravenous urogram/urography
CRP	C-reactive protein	**JVP**	jugular venous pulse
CRT	capillary refill time	**LDH**	lactate dehydrogenase
CSF	cerebrospinal fluid	**LFT**	liver function test
CSU	catheter specimen of urine	**LIF**	left iliac fossa
CT	computed tomogram/tomography	**LKM**	liver kidney microsomal (antibodies)
CTPA	computed tomographic pulmonary angiography		
		LLQ	left lower quadrant
CVP	central venous pressure	**LP**	lumbar puncture
CXR	chest X-ray	**LUQ**	left upper quadrant
DC	direct current	**MRA**	magnetic resonance angiography

MRCP	magnetic resonance cholangiopancreatography	**RLQ**	right lower quadrant
		RR	respiratory rate
MRI	magnetic resonance imaging	**RUQ**	right upper quadrant
MSU	midstream urine (specimen)	**SaO$_2$**	oxygen saturation of arterial blood
NSAID	non-steroidal anti-inflammatory drug	**SC**	subcutaneous(ly)
PaCO$_2$	partial pressure of carbon dioxide in arterial blood	**SIRS**	systemic inflammatory response syndrome
PaO$_2$	partial pressure of oxygen in arterial blood	**SLE**	systemic lupus erythematosus
		SpO$_2$	peripheral (capillary) oxygen saturation
PCR	polymerase chain reaction		
PEFR	peak expiratory flow rate	**SSRI**	selective serotonin re-uptake inhibitor
PET	positron emission tomography		
PFTs	pulmonary function tests	**SVT**	supraventricular tachycardia
PR	per rectum	**TFT**	thyroid function test
PRN	pro re nata; whenever required	**TIA**	transient ischaemic attack
PSA	prostate-specific antigen	**TNF**	tumour necrosis factor
PT	prothrombin time	**TWI**	T wave inversion
PV	per vaginam	**U+E**	urea and electrolytes
qSOFA	quick Sepsis Related Organ Failure Assessment	**UGIE**	upper gastrointestinal endoscopy
		UMN	upper motor neuron
QTc	corrected QT interval	**USS**	ultrasound scan
RF	rheumatoid factor	**VT**	ventricular tachycardia
RIF	right iliac fossa	**WBC**	white blood count

Section 1

Principles of clinical assessment

From differential diagnosis to final diagnosis

A diagnosis is simply shorthand for a patient's condition or disease process. The ability to diagnose accurately is fundamental to clinical practice. Only with a correct diagnosis, or a short-list of possible diagnoses, can you:

- formulate an appropriate sequence of investigations
- begin correct treatment and assess its effectiveness
- give an informed prognosis and make follow-up arrangements.

Producing a *differential diagnosis* – a list of diagnoses, placed in order of likelihood, which may be causing the presentation – is a stepping-stone to the final diagnosis. This list may be lengthy at the outset of assessment but will become progressively shorter as you accumulate information about the patient's condition through your history-taking, examination and investigations. When one diagnosis begins to stand out from the rest as the most likely cause of the patient's presentation, it is often referred to as the *working diagnosis*. Investigations are then directed toward confirming (or refuting) this condition and thereby arriving at a *final diagnosis*. This entire process may happen very rapidly; for example, establishing a final diagnosis of acute ST segment elevation myocardial infarction in a patient presenting with acute chest pain should usually take less than 10 minutes.

Frequently, the identification of an abnormality is only the first step in the diagnostic process and additional assessment is required to characterize a condition in greater detail or search for an underlying cause. For example, in a middle-aged man presenting with fatigue, you might identify anaemia as the cause of his symptoms, but the diagnostic process would not stop there. The next step would be to establish the cause of the anaemia. If subsequent laboratory investigations revealed evidence of iron deficiency, you need to determine the cause. Gastrointestinal investigations might uncover a gastric tumour but, even then, further assessment would still be required to establish a tissue diagnosis and stage the tumour. The eventual 'final diagnosis' might be of iron-deficiency anaemia secondary to blood loss from a T3, N1, M1 gastric carcinoma with metastasis to liver and peritoneum. Clearly, the diagnosis of 'anaemia' would have been grossly inadequate.

Some conditions, especially functional disorders such as irritable bowel syndrome, lack a definitive confirmatory test; here diagnosis relies upon recognising characteristic clinical features and ruling out alternative diagnoses – especially serious or life-threatening conditions. Such disorders are often referred to as *diagnoses of exclusion*.

Probability and risk

Diagnostic tests are inherently imperfect, so regard diagnoses as statements of probability rather than hard facts. In practice, a disease is 'ruled in' when the probability of it being present is deemed to be sufficiently high, and 'ruled out' when the probability is sufficiently low. The degree of certainty required depends on factors such as the consequences of missing the particular diagnosis, the side-effects of treatment and the risks of further testing. Doctors must not become so 'paralysed' by the implications of missing a diagnosis that they admit the patient unnecessarily to hospital and/or investigate to levels that are not in the patient's best interests and are unacceptable because of time, expense and intrinsic risk, e.g. radiation exposure. On the other hand, a high threshold of certainty, i.e. very low probability, is required to exclude potentially life-threatening conditions. If the situation is explained appropriately, most patients will accept tests that yield a diagnostic accuracy of less than 1% for acute life-threatening conditions.

The current diagnostic approach to subarachnoid haemorrhage (SAH) illustrates this. For a middle-aged patient who presents, fully conscious, with a history of sudden (within a few seconds) onset of 'the worst headache ever', the chances of a diagnosis of SAH are approximately 10–12%. The presence of some clinical findings, e.g. photophobia, neck stiffness, cranial nerve palsies, subhyaloid haemorrhage – will increase these chances markedly but these features may take time to develop. Even if clinical examination is unequivocally normal, the chances of SAH are 8–10%. Currently, there is no simple bedside test for SAH and the initial investigation is normally a non-contrast CT scan. A positive scan will prompt appropriate treatment, possibly involving neurosurgical or neuroradiological intervention. A negative scan does not, however, exclude an SAH. The accuracy of CT scanning in detecting SAH depends upon the experience of the reporting individual, the nature of the scanner (principally, its resolution) and the time interval between the onset of symptoms and the scan (accuracy falls with time). A scan performed within 12 hours by most modern scanners and interpreted by a skilled radiologist has a diagnostic accuracy of approximately 98%. But, given the morbidity and mortality of unrecognized and untreated SAH, even this level of diagnostic accuracy is inadequate. For this reason, patients with a negative CT scan have a lumbar puncture. The CSF obtained must be examined by spectrophotometry in the laboratory for xanthochromia (direct visual inspection of the fluid is insufficiently accurate). Xanthochromia (produced from haemoglobin breakdown within the CSF) takes some time to develop and the sensitivity of this test peaks at about 12 hours after symptom onset. The combination of a negative CT scan performed within 12 hours of symptom onset and normal CSF findings at 12 hours reduces the chances of the patient's symptoms being caused by an SAH to well below 1% – a level of probability acceptable to most clinicians and, if appropriately explained, to their patient.

Special situations

Medically unexplained symptoms

Sometimes it is difficult to correlate patients' symptoms with a specific disease. This does not mean that the symptoms with which they present are factitious or that they are malingering – merely that we are unable to provide a physical cause for the symptoms. For patients in primary care, over 70% have symptoms that cannot be readily explained by a specific diagnosis. Nevertheless, the symptoms are very real to the patient and one of the major challenges, intellectually and practically, is to recognize which patients have physical disease.

Clusters of symptoms in recognisable patterns, in the absence of physical and investigational abnormalities, are called *functional syndromes* (Table 1.1).

In general, the greater the number of symptoms, the greater the likelihood that there is a psychological component to the presentation. Remember that patients with chronic disease are more likely to demonstrate psychological aspects of their condition, especially depression, which may, in turn, affect the mode of presentation. Avoiding excessive and inappropriate investigation

Table 1.1 Common functional syndromes[1]	
Syndrome	Symptoms
Chronic fatigue syndrome	Persistent fatigue[2]
Irritable bowel syndrome	Abdominal pain, altered bowel habit (diarrhoea or constipation) and abdominal bloating
Chronic pain syndrome	Persistent pain in one or more parts of the body, sometimes following injury but which outlasts the original trauma[2]
Fibromyalgia	Pain in the axial skeleton with trigger points (tender areas in the muscles)[2]
Chronic back pain	Pain, muscle tension or stiffness localized below the costal margin and above the inferior gluteal folds, with or without leg pain[2]

[1] In all cases, physical examination and investigation fail to reveal an underlying physical cause.
[2] Symptoms must have lasted more than 3 months.

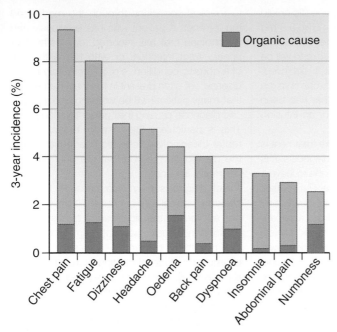

Fig. 1.1 Common symptoms and disease. (From Douglas JG, Nicol F, Robertson C. Macleod's Clinical Examination, 13th edn. Edinburgh: Churchill Livingstone, 2013.)

Box 1.1 Symptoms and their relationship to physical disease

More commonly

- Chest pain
- Breathlessness
- Syncope
- Abdominal pain

Less commonly

- Fatigue
- Back pain
- Headache
- Dizziness

---

to 'exclude' diagnoses is important, especially if patients have no specific 'red flags' in relation to their history, they are not in a recognized at-risk group, and there are no abnormalities on clinical examination and simple bedside tests (Fig. 1.1 and Box 1.1).

Treatment before diagnosis

Sometimes, accurate diagnosis depends upon the patient's response to treatment. In a few specific situations this may be life-saving as well as diagnostic. In any patient with altered consciousness or acute neurological dysfunction without a clearly identifiable cause, two conditions need to be excluded and treated immediately.

Hypoglycaemia can mimic conditions such as epilepsy and hemiplegia. Check the CBG. If the value is low, take a formal blood sample for laboratory blood glucose determination, but do not wait for this result before giving treatment – give glucose or glucagon immediately. If hypoglycaemia is the cause of the patient's symptoms, response will normally occur within 5–10 minutes (rarely, in cases where there has been severe, prolonged hypoglycaemia, this may take longer and residual neurological deficit may persist).

Opioid intoxication is usually associated with altered consciousness, reduced respiratory rate and depth, and small pupils. The diagnosis is rarely difficult in younger patients with a history or other features of illicit drug use. However, these features are not always present, and chronic opioid toxicity may develop over hours/days, particularly in elderly patients or those with renal impairment. Naloxone is a highly specific opioid antagonist with no agonist activity. Give 0.8 mg naloxone (SC, IM or IV) immediately. If there is any response, further doses of naloxone will be required until no further reversal is achieved. Remember that the half-life of naloxone is much shorter than that of the opioid that has been taken, so repeated stat. doses or an infusion are likely to be needed.

There is one other situation where treatment is necessary before, or to achieve, diagnosis. It is unnecessary, unhelpful and inhumane to leave a patient in pain from whatever cause. Put yourself in the patient's place. There is never any indication to withhold analgesia from a patient in pain. Concerns that you will 'mask' clinical signs, e.g. by giving opioids to a patient with an 'acute' abdomen, encourage opioid tolerance or addiction, and impair informed consent are completely unfounded. In fact, diagnostic accuracy is improved by making the patient more co-operative, aiding the performance of investigations such as ultrasound, and pain relief brings additional benefits in reducing catecholamine stimulation, improving respiratory and cardiovascular function. The 'pain ladder' approach is useful, but for patients in acute or severe pain, IV opioids titrated to the clinical response are usually needed.

The patient who comes with a diagnosis

Many patients have an idea of their own condition and, indeed, may begin the consultation by telling you their perceived diagnosis. In part this relates to improved education, greater exposure to medical conditions through the media and the Internet. A patient who has previously had a condition that has recurred, e.g. asthma or urinary tract infection, or who has a flare-up of a chronic condition, e.g. inflammatory bowel disease, will often present in this way. Remember that many patients will be worrying about a specific diagnosis causing their presenting complaint. This is particularly the case for breast lumps, rectal bleeding and chronic headache, where the perception may be that the only possible diagnosis is cancer.

Self-diagnosis may also cause a delay in seeking medical help because the patient does not appreciate the significance of a symptom or subconsciously may not want to consider the possibility of serious disease. Common examples include attributing ischaemic chest pain to 'indigestion' and assuming that rectal bleeding is due to haemorrhoids.

One way of initially handling patients who come with a diagnosis is to let them express this openly and then to acknowledge their concerns. You must respect these (indeed, the patient may well be right) while taking care not to miss a more likely diagnosis. In particular, do not take shortcuts with any of the components of history taking, examination and investigation that may be required.

Patients with rare or unusual diseases often know much more about their condition than you. Use this golden opportunity. There is no loss of face in admitting your ignorance. Patients will respect you for your honesty and you can learn much from them about the disease and its treatment and effects.

Assessing patients: a practical guide 2

Introduction

Before you can diagnose patients you must first obtain the necessary clinical and investigative information. Diagnostic success depends upon the accuracy and completeness of this initial data gathering so your history-taking and examination skills are crucial. During clinical training, you may have been taught a fairly idealized and rigid 'method' of patient assessment. However, in everyday practice, a more flexible, fluid approach is preferable; this will allow you to adapt to the clinical situation and acquire the essential information in the most efficient manner.

Traditionally, the assessment of patients has been divided into two distinct phases:

- *the clinical assessment:* history and physical examination
- *diagnostic investigations*.

At least in the hospital setting, this distinction is highly artificial due to the easy and real-time availability of basic tests such as ECG, CXR, glucose meter reading and ABG, and routine laboratory blood tests such as FBC, U+E and LFTs. Wherever appropriate, these simple tests should be carried out in tandem with the clinical assessment to form a 'routine patient work-up'. The information from all of these sources is combined to form a working or differential diagnosis. Where necessary, further targeted investigation can then be undertaken to confirm the suspected diagnosis, narrow the differential diagnosis, e.g. exclude high-risk conditions, inform prognosis and guide management.

Thus, in this book, we advocate the following system for patient evaluation:

- *the routine work-up:* history, physical examination and basic tests
- *targeted, supplementary investigations*.

The optimal approach to the routine work-up varies, depending on the stability and illness severity of the patient:

- acutely unwell patients require a rapid, targeted evaluation ('airway, breathing, circulation, disability, exposure [ABCDE] assessment') for life-threatening disorders and major derangements of physiology
- patients who are stable, including those initially assessed by the ABCDE approach, should have a full history and clinical examination, as outlined below ('full clinical assessment'), alongside basic tests relevant to the specific presentation
- the approach to frail, elderly patients may need to be modified to take account of differences in the nature of illness presentation, e.g. multi- versus single-organ pathology; significant functional decline secondary to minor illness.

Rapid assessment of the sick patient

The ABCDE assessment (see Clinical tool, p. 8) combines prompt identification of life-threatening pathology with immediate management of any abnormalities detected, prioritising those that are most rapidly fatal. Take an ABCDE approach if the patient:

- appears unwell or is unresponsive
- exhibits evidence of acute physiological derangement on basic observations (HR, RR, BP, arterial oxygen saturation [SpO$_2$], temperature)
- has features of a serious acute problem in any organ system.

Repeat the process to assess the effects of interventions or in the event of any further deterioration. Protect the spine at all times if there is any suspicion of recent trauma.

Routine assessment of the stable patient: the full clinical assessment

Use *Macleod's Clinical Examination* for a comprehensive guide to history taking and systems-based clinical examination. The following is an aide-mémoire with an emphasis on practical tips and avoidance of common pitfalls.

Clinical tool
The ABCDE assessment

What to look for	How to respond
A. Airway	
A1 **Ask 'How are you feeling?'** If patient can speak normally, airway is patent – move straight to B. A2 **Assess for airway obstruction** • Lack of airflow at the mouth (complete obstruction) • Throat or tongue swelling • Gurgling, snoring, choking, stridor • Paradoxical breathing (indrawing of chest with expansion of abdomen on inspiration; vice-versa on expiration) Only move to B once airway patent	If signs of obstruction: • Get help! • Try simple airway manoeuvres: head tilt/chin lift; jaw thrust (Fig. 2.1) • Remove foreign bodies/secretions from pharynx under direct vision • Insert Guedel or nasopharyngeal airway If obstruction persists: • Get expert assistance immediately • Consider laryngeal mask airway or tracheal intubation • In the context of anaphylaxis (see below), if throat or tongue swelling, give IM adrenaline (0.5 mg)
B. Breathing	
B1 **Give high concentration O_2 initially if hypoxaemic** B2 **Assess rate, depth and symmetry of breathing, noting:** • Poor respiratory effort: ↓↓RR, feeble, shallow Breaths • High respiratory effort: RR >20/min, use of Accessory muscles, visibly tiring • Asymmetrical chest expansion B3 **Check for tracheal deviation** B4 **Percuss and auscultate chest, noting:** • Dullness – suggesting pleural effusion, collapse, consolidation • ↓breath sounds – suggesting collapse pneumothorax, pleural effusion • Wheeze – suggesting bronchospasm • Crackles – suggesting pulmonary oedema, fibrosis, consolidation • Bronchial breathing suggesting consolidation B5 **Record SpO_2**	 If respiratory effort inadequate: • Get help! • Manually ventilate via bag-valve-mask • Consider a trial of naloxone, if any suspicion of opiate toxicity If severe respiratory distress and signs of tension pneumothorax (p. 264), perform immediate needle aspiration. If widespread wheeze, check for signs of anaphylaxis (see below). If present, manage as described; otherwise, give nebulized bronchodilator. If chronic type 2 respiratory failure or severe chronic obstructive pulmonary disease (COPD), titrate fraction of inspired oxygen (FiO_2) to patient's baseline SpO_2 (if known) or 90–92%. In all other critically ill patients, continue high FiO_2.

Clinical tool—cont'd
The ABCDE assessment

What to look for	How to respond
C. Circulation	
C1 **Check colour & temperature of hands** • Cold, clammy, blue, mottled? • Pink and warm?	In patients with evidence of shock, e.g. ↑CRT, cold peripheries, thready pulse, ↑HR, ↓BP: Secure IV access (large bore if possible) If ventricular tachycardia (VT), attempt defibrillation with a synchronized DC shock (ask anaesthetist to sedate if conscious).
C2 **Measure capillary refill time (CRT)** Press firmly over fingertip for 5 sec, release pressure then record time taken for skin to return to normal colour • ≤2 sec is normal • ≥2 sec suggests ↓peripheral perfusion	If bradycardia: • Give atropine 0.5–3 mg • if no response or HR <40/min, get expert help and consider IV adrenaline or transcutaneous pacing
C3 **Palpate radial and carotid pulse:** • Tachycardia: >100 bpm • Bradycardia: <60 bpm (or inappropriately slow for context) • Thready, weak – suggesting ↓cardiac output, e.g. hypovolaemia • Bounding – suggesting hyperdynamic circulation, e.g. early sepsis	If tongue/throat swelling, severe respiratory distress, widespread wheeze and/or a new rash, **assume anaphylaxis**: • Stop any potential trigger • Give 0.5 mg IM adrenaline (anterolateral aspect of middle 1/3 of the thigh) • Give fast IV fluids • Get immediate anaesthetic help Otherwise, give fluid challenge unless evidence of pulmonary oedema.
C4 **Measure blood pressure**	
C5 **Assess height of JVP at 45°**	
C6 **Auscultate the heart for:** • Murmurs • 3rd heart sound/gallop rhythm	
C7 **Attach ECG monitor and review rhythm:** • Regular broad complex tachycardia – likely ventricular tachycardia (VT) (p. 234) • Regular narrow complex tachycardia, e.g. sinus tachycardia, supraventricular tachycardia (SVT), a trial flutter (p. 232) • Irregular tachycardia – likely atrial fibrillation (p. 232) • Bradycardia ≤40 bpm, e.g. 2nd or 3rd degree atrioventricular (AV) block (p. 234)	
C8 **Perform a 12-lead ECG if chest pain or arrhythmia**	
D. Disability	
D1 **Check capillary blood glucose (CBG)**	If CBG <3 mmol/L: • Send blood for formal lab glucose measurement • Give immediate IV dextrose
D2 **Record Glasgow Coma Scale (p. 73)**	If ↓GCS • Perform an ABG if any suspicion of hypercapnia, e.g. chronic lung disease, depressed ventilation • Give 0.8–2 mg IV naloxone if ↓pupil size or no obvious cause • Assess response after 1 min and consider further doses if partial response

Clinical tool—cont'd The ABCDE assessment	
What to look for	How to respond
D3 **Take a '3D' history** **D**escription of symptoms **D**rugs and allergies **D**isorders/**D**isability prior to this illness	
D4 **Examine pupils with a pen torch:** • Bilateral pinpoint – suggests opioid intoxication or pontine lesion • Bilateral dilated – suggests cocaine/amphetamine or tricyclic antidepressant intoxication or atropine • Unilateral fixed, dilated suggests ↑intracranial pressure or 3rd nerve palsy	
E. Exposure	
E1 **Record body temperature** E2 **Fully expose the body (preserve dignity), looking for:** • Bleeding or injuries • Rashes • Jaundice • Medic alert bracelet E3 **Examine the abdomen for distension, tenderness, guarding, rigidity**	If temperature <34°C, confirm core temperature with a low-reading thermometer and start rewarming measures. Repeat the ABCDE assessment if a significant abnormality was noted at any stage. Refer to the relevant chapter for further assessment of specific presentations, e.g. dyspnoea, shock, chest pain, ↓GCS, abdominal pain, headache.

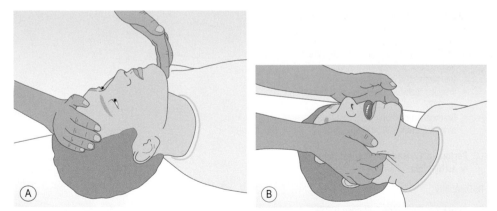

Fig. 2.1 Simple airway manoeuvres. A Head-tilt, chin-lift method. B Jaw-thrust method – preferred in patients with suspected neck injury. (From Douglas G, Nicol F, Robertson C. Macleod's Clinical Examination, 12th edn. Edinburgh: Churchill Livingstone, 2009.)

The history

Think of the history, not as a series of questions to be asked, but as a body of information that needs to be gathered using all available sources (Table 2.1 and Boxes 2.1–2.3). History taking is, usually, the single most important component in the diagnostic process. It is also the one area that many doctors perform inadequately. Let the patient tell their story (the presenting complaint) in their own words without interrupting. Use 'open'

questions initially and give the patient time. Only then should you move to more focused, 'closed' questions.

In particular, note:

- a supplementary account of the current problem is essential in patients presenting with confusion or transient loss of consciousness
- details of the past medical history are usually better established from the GP record and medical case notes than by simply asking the patient, particularly with respect to the outcome of previous investigations
- if available, use a repeat prescription or GP record to obtain the specific names and dosages of drugs, then ask patients if they are actually taking the medicines as prescribed. Ask about the use of any additional over-the-counter or herbal remedies. Also ask the patient about side-effects of any current or previous medications.

Box 2.1 Features of alcohol dependence in the history

- A strong, often overpowering, desire to take alcohol
- Inability to control starting or stopping drinking and the amount that is drunk
- Drinking alcohol in the morning
- Tolerance, where increased doses are needed to achieve the effects originally produced by lower doses
- Withdrawal state when drinking is stopped or reduced, including tremor, sweating, rapid heart rate, anxiety, insomnia and occasionally seizures, disorientation or hallucinations (delirium tremens). It is relieved by more alcohol
- Neglect of other pleasures and interests
- Continuing to drink in spite of being aware of the harmful consequences

The clinical examination

A routine 'screening' clinical examination (see Clinical tool, p. 12) is required in most patients. Some elements of the clinical examination that have traditionally been considered routine are only

Table 2.1 Key information required from the history

Information to be established	Specific details	Sources of information
Presenting complaint	Full details of recent symptoms and events	Patient, relatives, carers, witnesses, GP
Past history	Current and previous medical disorders Previous investigations and results Efficacy of previous treatments	Medical case notes, GP record, patient
Drugs and allergies	All prescribed and over-the-counter medications and doses; adherence to prescription; recent changes to medications; adverse drug reactions (what drug? what happened?)	Repeat prescription, GP record, patient, relatives, carers
Environmental risk factors	Smoking, alcohol (see Box 2.1), drug misuse[1] (see Box 2.2), travel, pets, sexual history[1] (see Box 2.3)	Patient, relatives
Impact and consequences of illness (if relevant)	Ability to mobilize, self-care, undertake activities (work, driving, hobbies) Effects on employment, family, finance, confidence	Patient, relatives, friends, carers, GP

[1] Only if appropriate.

Box 2.2 Non-prescribed drug history

- What drugs are you taking?
- How often and how much?
- How long have you been taking drugs?
- Any periods of abstinence? If so, when and why did you start using drugs again?
- What symptoms do you have if you cannot obtain drugs?
- Do you ever inject?
- Do you ever share needles, syringes or other drug paraphernalia?
- Do you see your drug use as a problem?
- Do you want to make changes in your life or change the way you use drugs?

Box 2.3 Sexual history questions

- Do you have a regular sexual partner at the moment?
- Is your partner male or female?
- Have you had any (other) sexual partners in the last 12 months?
- How many were male? How many female?
- Do you use barrier contraception – sometimes, always or never?
- Have you ever had a sexually transmitted infection?

Clinical tool
The 20-step clinical examination

1. Assess general demeanour, appearance, movements, odour, nutrition and hydration.
2. Record routine observations, including temperature, pulse, BP, RR and SpO₂.
3. Examine the hands: temperature, capillary refill, colour, nails, tremor, asterixis and joints.
4. Feel the radial and brachial pulses.
5. Inspect the face and eyes (Table 2.2).
6. Examine the mouth: dental hygiene, cyanosis, tonsillar inflammation, ulcers, blisters and candidiasis.

Position the patient at 45°

7. Assess the height and waveform of the JVP and feel the carotid pulse.
8. Inspect and palpate the trachea: check centrality and cricosternal distance.
9. Inspect and palpate the praecordium.
10. Auscultate the heart.
11. Examine the lung fields from the front.

Sit the patient up at 90°

12. Inspect the trunk (front and back) for rashes, moles, spider naevi, scars etc.
13. Palpate for lymphadenopathy and goitre; check for bony/renal angle tenderness, sacral oedema.
14. Examine the lung fields from the back.

Lay the patient flat

15. Examine the abdomen and hernial orifices.
16. Examine the legs.
    - Inspect for swelling, colour, rashes, skin changes.
    - Feel for pitting, temperature, pulses, capillary refill.
17. Perform a neurological examination of the legs.
    - Check tone, look for wasting, abnormal movements.
    - Assess power: flexion/extension of hips, knees, ankles.
    - Check reflexes: knees, ankle jerks, plantar response.

Clinical tool—cont'd
The 20-step clinical examination

- Test sensation: L2–S1 dermatomes (see Fig. 22.1, p. 200).
- Test coordination: heel–shin test (Fig. 2.2B).
- Assess transfer and gait (p. 215).

Sit the patient up

18. Perform a neurological examination of the arms.
    - Check tone, look for wasting, abnormal movements.
    - Assess power: abduction/adduction of shoulders, fingers; flexion/extension of elbows, wrists; grip strength.
    - Check reflexes: supinator, biceps, triceps.
    - Test sensation: C5–T1 dermatomes (see Fig. 22.1, p. 221).
    - Test coordination: rapid alternating movements and finger–nose test (Fig. 2.2A).

19. Screen for cranial nerve abnormalities.
    - Test visual acuity and pupillary reactions; check for homonymous field defects.
    - Check eye movements (characterize nystagmus) and hearing in each ear.
    - Test sensation above the upper lip and over the maxillae and eyelids.
    - Facial movements: raise eyebrows, show teeth, close eyes against resistance, blow out cheeks.
20. Perform urinalysis and bedside capillary blood glucose measurement.

Table 2.2 Characteristic faces and their features, including facial expression

Disorder	Appearance
Acromegaly	Coarsening with enlarged features, e.g. nose, lips, orbital ridges and jaw (prognathism)
Hypothyroidism	Pale, puffy skin with loss of lateral third of eyebrows
Hyperthyroidism	Startled appearance with lid retraction
Cushing's disease	'Moon face', plethoric complexion and buffalo hump over lower cervical–upper thoracic spine
Parkinsonism	Expressionless faces and drooling
Myasthenia gravis	Expressionless faces with bilateral ptosis
Myotonia dystrophica	Frontal baldness and bilateral ptosis
Superior vena caval obstruction	Plethoric, oedematous face and neck, chemosis of conjunctivae, prominent veins and venules
Malar flush	Dusky redness of cheeks seen in low cardiac output, e.g. mitral stenosis; also seen in myxoedema
Systemic lupus erythematosus	Rash over nose and cheeks – 'butterfly rash'
Progressive systemic sclerosis	Taut skin around mouth with 'beaking' of nose

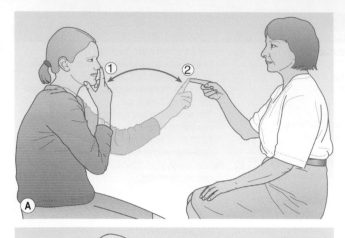

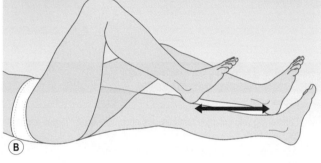

Fig. 2.2 Tests of coordination. A Finger–nose test. B Heel–shin test. (From Ford MJ, Hennessey I, Japp A. Introduction to Clinical Examination, 8th edn. Edinburgh: Churchill Livingstone, 2005.)

required in specific circumstances. These include examination of the fundi, rectum, genitalia, breasts and individual joints.

Additional steps

- You will gain an impression of higher mental function through taking the history. If you suspect impairment, perform an Abbreviated Mental Test (AMT; Box 2.4).
- If you detect a relevant abnormality on the routine examination, perform a detailed examination of the relevant system (see *Macleod's Clinical Examination*).
- Additional examination steps required for a specific presentation are described in the relevant chapters:
  - testicular examination (p. 258)
  - breast examination (p. 49)
  - examination for meningeal irritation (p. 169)
  - examination of lumbar spinal movements (p. 211)
  - 'confusion assessment method' for detection of delirium (p. 80)

Box 2.4 Abbreviated mental test

(Score 1 for each correct response)
- How old are you?
- What is the time just now?
- What year is it?
- What is the name of this place? (Where are we just now?)

Please memorize the following address: 42 West Street
- When is your birthday (date and month)?
- What year did the First World War begin?
- What is the name of the Queen?
- Can you recognize … ? Two people?
- Count backwards from 20 to 1
- Repeat the address that I gave you

Normal score: 8–10

Source: Hodkinson HM 1972. Evaluation of a mental test score for assessment of mental impairment in the elderly. Age Ageing. 1:233–238.

- assessment of gait (p. 215)
- head thrust test (p. 101)
- Dix–Hallpike manoeuvre (p. 103)
- jaw jerk (p. 109).

Basic investigations

The specific tests required for a routine work-up depend on the presenting problem. For example, an ECG is mandatory in patients with acute chest pain but not in those with chronic low back pain. The recommended tests for different clinical presentations are specified in the relevant chapters in Part 2. In several chapters we give detailed guidance on interpreting these tests, including:

- the ECG in chest pain (p. 54)
- arterial blood gases (p. 116)
- pulmonary function tests (p. 127)
- pleural tap and analysis of pleural fluid (p. 129)
- lumbar puncture and CSF analysis (p. 170)
- a septic screen (p. 142)
- anaemia (p. 136)
- renal failure (p. 230)
- hyponatraemia (p. 88).

Approach to the frail, elderly patient

Frail, elderly patients comprise a major proportion of acute medical and surgical admissions and are frequently challenging to assess and treat. They often present in a vague, non-specific way, and in many cases with acute delirium. This can result in difficulty identifying the specific culprit for the acute deterioration, especially as many will have a background of multiple chronic comorbidities and functional limitation. One unfortunate consequence of this is the tendency to categorize elderly patients into a small number of 'diagnostic dustbins'. Instead of a differential diagnosis, the impression at the end of the clerking may read 'Off legs', 'Mechanical fall', 'Social admission' or 'Collapse ?Cause'. Such impressions could be correct, but they are not diagnoses.

The challenges of acute assessment in the elderly are often compounded by a misconception that the process must always be painstaking and laborious. Comprehensive geriatric assessment does require time and input from multiple health professionals but it is often preferable to defer this for a period than to undertake it poorly in the midst of a busy acute admission. Where time and personnel are limited, use a focused approach to identify important problems rapidly and reliably, and to produce a useful list of differential diagnoses.

Chronological age is a poor marker for identifying who would benefit from a tailored 'geriatric' assessment. Some elderly patients present with a single specific acute pathology, e.g. the fit 90-year-old with an acute myocardial infarction. This patient may require rapid coronary revascularization rather than a comprehensive geriatric assessment. Conversely, a 59-year-old with multiple medical problems and medications, and an inability to mobilize may benefit greatly from a geriatric assessment. Frailty is the increased vulnerability in reserve and function across multiple physiological systems such that the ability to withstand acute stressors is compromised. Identification of frailty is difficult, and debate continues over robust criteria. Formal frailty scores such as the Edmonton Frailty Scale (www.nscphealth.co.uk/edmontonscale-pdf) can be used to grade the degree of frailty and various screening tools have been developed for use in acute settings to help identify patients most likely to benefit from comprehensive geriatric assessment. As a guide, the presence of two or more of these criteria suggests frailty:

- functional decline, e.g. inability to perform basic activities of daily living (ADLs)
- confusion (delirium, dementia)
- polypharmacy
- care home resident
- recent immobility or falls
- ≥1 unplanned admissions in the past 3 months
- difficulty in walking
- malnutrition
- incontinence.

Specific tips for assessment of the elderly/ frail patient

An accurate history is important in the frail, elderly patient, but may be significantly more difficult to obtain.

- Use open questions sparingly.
- Clarify vague terms, e.g. 'a while', and question inconsistencies, e.g. if patients cannot recall the details of their 'fall', how do they know that they did not black out?
- Wherever possible, complement the patient's history with collateral information

from witnesses, carers, relatives, other health professionals and previous notes.

Frail patients may tire easily during the history and examination:

- If necessary, perform the assessment in 'bite-sized' chunks.
- If there are multiple symptoms, address them in order of importance to the patient, unless they are 'red-flag'.
- If the list of established diagnoses is long, determine which problems are 'active' ('When did you last have angina?') and explore those relevant to the current presentation in detail.

Prioritize important and common problems in the systemic enquiry.

- How far can you walk?
- Can you manage a flight of stairs?
- What stops you?
- Do you have a cough?
- When did you last move your bowels?
- Do you have any difficulty passing urine?
- Have you been incontinent?
- Have you lost weight?
- Have you fallen or blacked out?
- Do you get dizzy?
- Do you have any weakness or numbness in your face or limbs?
- Are you forgetful?

An exhaustive 'social history' during the initial assessment is often unproductive.

- Establish the key information regarding functional status and social/care arrangements but avoid replicating work that will be undertaken by other health professionals, e.g. occupational therapist.
- Do not overlook specific issues in the social history, e.g. alcohol intake, driving.

Inspection

Certain aspects of the examination demand closer attention in the elderly.

- Observe carefully for evidence of dehydration, malnutrition, constipation, injuries and pressure sores in frail, dependent or demented patients.
- Consider a formal swallow test to exclude aspiration in patients with recurrent pneumonia.

Elderly patients with abdominal pathology may present 'atypically'.

- Consider perforation of a viscus or ischaemic bowel, even in the absence of abdominal rigidity – have a low threshold for imaging
- Percussion and palpation of the bladder may reveal 'asymptomatic' urinary retention in patients with non-specific deterioration.

Most elderly patients can follow the instructions required for a standard neurological examination

- Try to overcome sensory impairment with aids (put the hearing aid in!), repetition and demonstration
- If the patient struggles to cooperate, obtain equivalent information by observing movement, passive or provoked
- Pay close attention to muscle bulk, gait (p. 215), visual acuity and functional movements of the arms and hands
- Assess joint movements in conjunction with the neurological examination. Screening for cognitive impairment is an integral part of examination in the elderly: use objective tests, e.g. AMT (see Box 2.4) or 4AT (p. 80), rather than general impressions. Record the score, even if the patient appears to have intact cognition – documentation of a normal baseline may aid a subsequent diagnosis of delirium.

Depression is common in elderly hospitalized patients and is a well-recognized mimicker of dementia.

- Maintain a high index of suspicion but remember that low mood may be situational and appropriate ('stuck in hospital').
- Exclude organic disease before attributing 'biological symptoms' to depression.

Basic investigations have a higher yield in elderly patients due to the increased prevalence of disease and the frequent absence of characteristic clinical features.

- Perform FBC, U+E, ECG and CXR in any elderly patient with non-specific deterioration.
- Have a low threshold for considering additional tests such as CRP, LFTs, calcium or TFTs.

With time and practice, most trainees will acquire the skills necessary to take a history, perform a competent physical examination and interpret basic tests. The next stage is to translate the resulting raw clinical data into a diagnosis. The primary aim of this book is to show you how this can be achieved.

Diagnostic methods

The exact method by which a diagnosis is reached may seem mysterious to newcomers to clinical medicine. The best diagnosticians invariably use several complementary skills which have been honed through years or decades of experience; these are often applied subconsciously and hence are difficult to explain. Consequently, the diagnostic process may be taught poorly and, most often, is simply experienced at second hand, by observation.

As an inexperienced clinician you cannot expect to achieve diagnostic skills overnight, but this book aims to show you how to make a diagnosis in the great majority of the most commonly encountered and important clinical presentations. As a first step, it helps to consider two well-established, contrasting approaches to diagnosis: pattern recognition and probability analysis. These methods illustrate some fundamental principles of diagnostic reasoning but both have major drawbacks that limit their application in everyday practice.

Pattern recognition

The diagnosis is made by recognising characteristic features of the patient's illness that you have encountered previously in other patients with the same disorder. For most people, visual information is a strong prompt to memory recall, so the technique is particularly helpful for conditions with an obvious abnormality of appearance, e.g. skin conditions. Moving visual images are even more evocative. Ornithologists commonly describe how they recognize a bird by its 'jizz' – a combination of its appearance, movement and behaviour. Some medical conditions, e.g. Parkinsonism, are readily identified in a similar way.

Pattern recognition can be a powerful technique, particularly when employed by an experienced clinician. In theory, it requires you to have experienced an identical, or at least very similar, presentation previously, and so is less suited to the newcomer. However, the diagnostic method most commonly utilized by medical students and junior doctors is actually a variant of this approach. The major difference is that their 'database' of patterns corresponds to the descriptions of signs and symptoms provided in textbooks rather than previous real-life examples. This has several major disadvantages. Firstly, descriptions of physical signs from textbooks or lectures, e.g. pill-rolling tremor or festinating gait, are poor substitutes for experiencing them at first hand. Textbooks also tend to present an idealized account of the way in which illnesses present, emphasising classical signs and symptoms that are often relatively rare in everyday clinical practice. Similarly, a reliance on textbook learning does not allow you to appreciate the multiple subtle variations in presentation that exist for the same disorder. Pattern recognition may fail even the most experienced clinician when conditions present atypically or when characteristic features are masked, e.g. the patient with acute coronary syndrome who has sharp chest pain rather than crushing or heavy discomfort, or the diabetic patient who has no pain or discomfort at all because of coexistent autonomic neuropathy. This tendency is greatly amplified when these conditions have not been experienced repeatedly in the real world.

Probability analysis

For the great majority of conditions, no single symptom, sign or test will have sufficient power to enable you to rule in or rule out a diagnosis. However, each will alter the probability of the diagnosis to a greater or lesser extent. The diagnostic weighting of a particular symptom, sign or test can be expressed as a likelihood ratio (LR). The LR is the proportion of patients with the specific disease who exhibit the particular finding, divided by the proportion without the disease who also exhibit the same finding. Note that the finding may be positive, e.g. presence of a particular sign, or negative, e.g. absence of a particular sign.

If the LR value is >1, the chance of the disease is increased; the higher the value, the greater the likelihood of the disease. If the LR value is <1, the chance of the disease being present is reduced. For example, an LR of 5 increases the absolute probability of a disease by approximately 30% and an LR of −0.2 decreases it by 30%.

LRs are available for many clinical features and tests. In theory, this allows you to use the information derived from your assessment to calculate the probability of a disease. However, before you can do this, you need to know the pre-test probability of the patient having the disease in question – in other words, the prevalence of the disease in a population with similar baseline characteristics to your patient. Among other things, the pre-test probability may be influenced by a patient's age, sex, ethnic origin, occupation, social background and past history, as well as the clinical setting within which you work (rural versus urban environment, primary care versus secondary care). For example, the probability of *Plasmodium falciparum* malaria being the cause of headache, myalgia and fever in a previously fit, 19-year-old in the UK in the middle of a winter influenza epidemic is vanishingly small, but it will be very much higher for a similar individual returning from sub-Saharan Africa.

Another problem with using LRs to calculate probability lies in trying to combine information from multiple symptoms, physical signs and test results. This is hampered by a need for the findings to be independent of each other – an area of considerable uncertainty. In practice, it is not usually possible to combine more than two or three LRs outside a validated scoring system. For readers interested in using LRs to calculate diagnostic probabilities, we recommend *Evidence Based Physical Diagnosis*, by Steven McGee (4th edn, 2017, Elsevier).

In everyday practice, this approach has two major applications. Firstly, knowledge of LRs for different symptoms, risk factors or clinical signs allows you to identify those with the highest diagnostic value. As a rough rule of thumb, LR values between 0.5 and 2 are rarely helpful, whereas values ≥5 or ≤0.2 are usually clinically useful. Secondly, for some conditions, LRs have been used to develop and validate diagnostic algorithms that allow the condition to be ruled in or ruled out based on thresholds of probability. Examples are the Wells scores for deep vein thrombosis (p. 193) and pulmonary thromboembolism (p. 120).

A different approach: tailored diagnostic guides

For the inexperienced clinician, neither fuzzy pattern recognition nor rigid probability analysis offers a practical and satisfactory approach to diagnostic reasoning. We therefore advocate an alternative system that takes positive elements from both of these methods but is easy to apply in everyday practice and does not rely on vast amounts of clinical experience. We set out this system in the form of individual 'diagnostic guides' for all of the major presenting clinical problems. With experience, you will start to use your own unique methods but, at the outset, following an established framework may help to prevent crass, potentially damaging, errors.

Each chapter in Part 2 is a diagnostic guide or 'road-map' for a common clinical presentation. The purpose of the guides is not to tell you which questions to ask and which examination steps to perform – this was outlined in Chapter 2 and will be broadly similar for most presentations. Rather, it is to explain how to use the information you have extracted from the history, examination and initial tests to work toward a diagnosis.

To do this, we focus on the most valuable pieces of diagnostic data – those symptom characteristics, signs and test results with the greatest potential to narrow the differential diagnosis or to rule in/rule out suspected conditions.

The guides follow a logical and consistent approach designed to reflect contemporary medical practice. They provide a secure framework to work within but are *not* rigid protocols and allow ample scope for clinical judgement.

The highest priority is always given to immediately life-threatening problems. In some cases, this means focusing on aims of assessment other than diagnosis, e.g. gauging illness severity or determining resuscitation requirements. The next aim is, wherever necessary, to exclude major pathology; for each of the most serious potential disorders, the guides will identify those patients who require further investigation to rule in or rule out the diagnosis. Thereafter we prioritize diagnostic information with the highest yield whilst avoiding data that do not significantly alter probabilities or help to target investigation. In situations where the information obtained from the routine work-up is unlikely to yield a clear working diagnosis we may opt to provide a strategy for further investigation to help narrow the differential diagnosis.

How to use the diagnostic guides

The first step is to determine which guide, if any, is the most appropriate for the patient in front of you. Ensure that you have clarified the true nature of the problem; a patient who presents with a fall may have had a black out, whilst a patient who has had a 'funny turn' may have experienced focal limb weakness. In general, you should match the guide to the patient's predominant complaint. However, if the presentation entails two or more related symptoms, e.g. abdominal pain + dysphagia; dyspnoea + haemoptysis, we recommend choosing the symptom with the

narrower differential diagnosis (dysphagia or haemoptysis in the examples above).

After you have decided on which guide to use, the format is simple to follow:

- each begins with the *differential diagnosis*: a rundown of the important diagnoses to consider for the particular presenting problem
- we then present an *overview of assessment*: this is essentially a flowchart that lays out the route to diagnosis. It is vital that you understand the format of the overview, so an example is provided in Fig. 3.1 and is explained below
- each overview is accompanied by a *step-by-step assessment*. This is a textual companion to the overview that explains and expands on each individual step
- some chapters also contain details on further assessment of common disorders or abnormalities that may have been identified during the initial assessment.

The example in Fig. 3.1 shows the initial stages of the overview of assessment for jaundice (shown fully in Ch. 19).

- Blue boxes are stages of action – they contain the steps of assessment that you need to undertake. This will always include one of the two principal methods of clinical assessment outlined in Chapter 2 ('airway, breathing, circulation, disability, exposure [ABCDE]' or 'full clinical assessment') plus the essential basic tests, e.g. ECG, CXR and any necessary additional examination steps. Note: The diagnostic process that follows assumes that you have performed these steps and extracted the relevant clinical information.
- Yellow boxes are stages of diagnostic reasoning – they do not show 'what to do now' but rather 'what to think about now'. Each numbered step in the diagnostic process is accompanied by a detailed explanation in the step-by-step assessment section (see above).

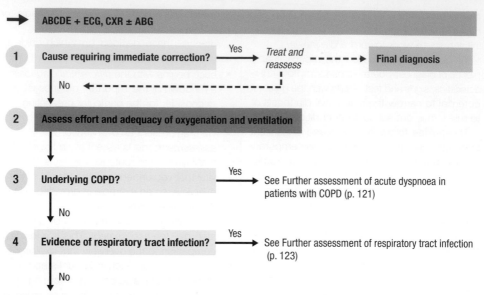

Fig. 3.1 A guide to using the 'overview of assessment'.

- Red boxes represent important elements of the assessment that are independent of the diagnostic process, e.g. evaluation of illness severity or resuscitation requirements.
- Green boxes represent the potential endpoints of the diagnostic process. As with the yellow boxes, explanatory text is provided in the accompanying step-by-step assessment. In some cases, further investigation may be required to confirm the diagnosis, refine it, assess severity or guide optimal management; if so, the necessary steps will be outlined in the text.

3

Section 2

Assessment of common presenting problems

Abdominal pain

Acute abdominal pain

Acute abdominal pain has a vast differential diagnosis. The spectrum of disease severity is also wide, ranging from the life-threatening to the innocuous. Effective assessment requires the rapid recognition of critically unwell patients and, where appropriate, targeted investigations. Causes of acute abdominal pain are listed below. The numbers in brackets correspond to the different regions of the abdomen, as displayed in Fig. 4.1, at which the pain is typically most prominent:

- cholecystitis/cholangitis (1)
- biliary colic (1, 2)
- hepatitis (1, 2)
- pneumonia (1 or 3)
- peptic ulcer disease/gastritis (2)
- acute coronary syndrome (2)
- pancreatitis (2, 5)
- ruptured abdominal aortic aneurysm (AAA) (2, 5)
- splenic rupture (3, diffuse)
- renal calculus (4, 7 or 6, 9)
- pyelonephritis (4 or 6)
- early appendicitis (5, diffuse)
- established appendicitis (7)
- terminal ileitis, e.g. Crohn's disease, Yersinia (7)
- mesenteric adenitis (7, diffuse)
- diverticulitis (7 or 9)
- colitis (7, 8, 9)
- ectopic pregnancy (7, 8, 9)
- pelvic inflammatory disease/endometriosis (7, 8, 9)
- ovarian torsion/cyst rupture (7, 8, 9)
- lower urinary tract infection (UTI)/cystitis (8)
- intestinal obstruction (diffuse)
- perforation (diffuse)
- mesenteric ischaemia (diffuse)
- gastroenteritis (diffuse mid-/upper-abdominal)
- diabetic ketoacidosis/hypercalcaemia/adrenal crisis (diffuse)
- functional abdominal pain (any region or diffuse).

Key questions

What are the characteristics of the pain?

An educated analysis of a patient's abdominal pain symptoms yields immeasurable information. The mnemonic 'SOCRATES' is often helpful: consider the Site, Onset, Character, Radiation, Associated features, Timing, Exacerbating factors and Severity of the pain. Based on these features, it should be possible to distinguish between most of the above causes of pain.

Visceral pain is conducted by autonomic nerve fibres, so its location corresponds to the embryological origin of the affected structure (Fig. 4.2). The pain may arise from distension or excessive contraction (spasm) of hollow organs. It also arises from tissue damage (inflammation), ischaemia or direct chemical stimulation of pain receptors in organs. It is typically dull and poorly localized and is not associated with abdominal guarding or rigidity. True 'colicky' pain reflects intermittent episodes of intense smooth muscle contraction that produce short-lived spasms of discomfort lasting seconds to minutes before subsiding. Some disorders are described as 'colic' but are actually pseudocolic, (e.g. renal or biliary colic). In these cases, the pain builds to a crescendo over several minutes before reaching a steady peak that may last for several hours before easing. Visceral pain may also be constant, for example in bowel ischaemia.

Somatic pain arises from irritation and inflammation of the parietal peritoneum and is conducted by somatic nerves. It is sharp, well localized, constant and often associated with local tenderness and guarding. Widespread inflammation of the parietal peritoneum produces generalized peritonitis.

Referred pain is perceived at a site remote from its source and arises due to convergence of nerve fibres at the same spinal cord level (Fig. 4.3).

Is there a systemic inflammatory response?

Many serious causes of acute abdominal pain either stem from or provoke an inflammatory process within the abdominal cavity. The presence of fever, ↑CRP or ↑WBC with neutrophilia suggests that the patient is mounting an acute systemic inflammatory response (Box 4.1) and

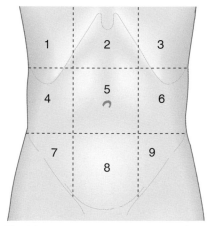

Fig. 4.1 Regions of the abdomen. See text for typical sites of pain. (From Ford MJ, Hennessey I, Japp A. Introduction to Clinical Examination, 8th edn. Edinburgh: Churchill Livingstone, 2005.)

may thereby contribute to the diagnostic process. In some patients, the presence of inflammatory features may assist the interpretation of uncertain physical signs, e.g. mild localized abdominal tenderness, reinforcing suspicion of local peritonitis. In patients without a clear cause for pain, these features may suggest the need for admission and further investigation. By the same token, the absence of these features can, when used correctly, help to exclude important inflammatory pathology. Finally, recognising and grading the presence of a systemic inflammatory response are central to the assessment of illness severity.

Note that the significance of an individual result depends on the clinical context, particularly with respect to CRP. In general, the higher the result, the greater the extent of systemic inflammation. A marginal rise in CRP, e.g. <30 mg/L, does not provide compelling evidence of a major inflammatory process. However, if the test is being used to help 'rule out' a condition, then it is safer to regard any limit above the upper range of normal as elevated.

4

Box 4.1 Indicators of systemic inflammation
• Fever (>38°C)
• ↑CRP (>10 mg/L)[1]
• WBC >11 × 10^9/L or <4 × 10^9/L
[1] The significance of the result depends on the clinical context – see text.

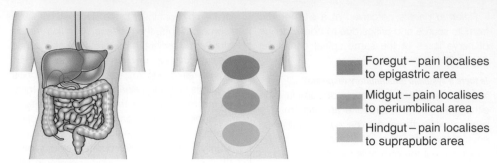

Foregut – pain localises to epigastric area

Midgut – pain localises to periumbilical area

Hindgut – pain localises to suprapubic area

Fig. 4.2 Abdominal pain. Perception of visceral pain is localized to the epigastric, umbilical or suprapubic region, according to the embryological origin of the affected organ. (From Douglas G, Nicol F, Robertson C. Macleod's Clinical Examination, 12th edn. Edinburgh: Churchill Livingstone, 2009.)

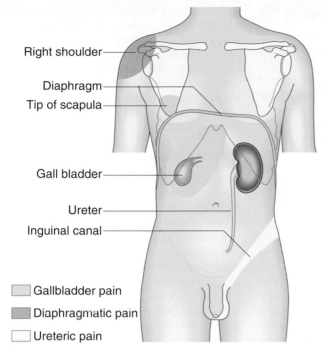

Right shoulder
Diaphragm
Tip of scapula

Gall bladder

Ureter
Inguinal canal

Gallbladder pain
Diaphragmatic pain
Ureteric pain

Fig. 4.3 Characteristic radiation of pain from the gallbladder, diaphragm and ureter. (From Douglas G, Nicol F, Robertson C. Macleod's Clinical Examination, 12th edn. Edinburgh: Churchill Livingstone, 2009.)

Chronic/episodic abdominal pain

Chronic abdominal pain is common and challenging to assess. Careful evaluation with targeted investigation is required to exclude organic pathology. Most younger patients will have a functional disorder, e.g. irritable bowel syndrome (IBS), but this should be a diagnosis of exclusion. In older patients with new, persistent abdominal pain, the priority is to exclude underlying malignancy.

Gastroduodenal disorders

Peptic ulcer disease is a common cause of chronic upper abdominal pain. Almost all duodenal ulcers and 70% of gastric ulcers are attributable to *H. pylori* infection. Typical features include recurrent episodes of burning or gnawing discomfort, relationship to food (variable), and associated dyspeptic symptoms, e.g. nausea, belching and relief with antacids. Classically, pain from gastric ulcers occurs several minutes after eating whereas pain from duodenal ulcers occur hours later and may be relieved by food.

Gastritis without frank ulceration may produce similar symptoms.

Gastric cancer occurs more frequently in patients >55 years. In addition to pain, associated symptoms include early satiety, unintentional weight loss and vomiting. All of the above disorders are best diagnosed by upper gastrointestinal endoscopy (UGIE).

Gallstones

Most gallstones are asymptomatic.

Biliary colic occurs when a gallstone obstructs the cystic duct, causing gallbladder distension. It tends to occur 1–6 hours after a meal, manifesting as intense, dull, RUQ or epigastric pain ± radiation to the back or scapula (see Fig. 4.3). The pain builds to a crescendo over minutes, and may last several hours before subsiding. It does not cause jaundice, deranged LFTs or abdominal signs. USS should confirm the presence of gallstones or, rarely, demonstrate pathological gallbladder changes. In *cholecystitis*, infection of the gallbladder due to gallstones obstructing the cystic duct occurs. The pain classically persists over time, is associated with a fever and there may be jaundice in cases of Mirizzi's syndrome (where a large gallstone and inflamed gallbladder wall causes extrinsic compression of the common hepatic duct).

Choledocholithiasis (stone in the common bile duct – CBD) causes cholestatic jaundice (see Ch. 19) with less severe upper abdominal pain, or indeed no pain. In *ascending cholangitis*, infection of the biliary tree occurs upstream from a blockage in the CBD (gallstone, tumour, liver fluke). Patients present with significant sepsis (pyrexia), jaundice and abdominal discomfort (Charcot's triad).

Pancreatic pain

Acute pancreatitis causes severe upper abdominal pain that radiates to the back, often with repeated vomiting. It is associated, depending on the severity, with a systemic inflammatory response and may progress to multiorgan failure. The majority of cases are caused by gallstones passing down the common bile duct and irritating the pancreas or by alcohol directly injuring the pancreas. *Chronic pancreatitis* develops in a subset of patients with recurrent episodes of acute pancreatitis. In some patients, it is constant and unremitting, while in others, episodes are provoked by drinking alcohol or eating. Associated features include weight loss, anorexia and, in advanced disease, diabetes mellitus (endocrine deficiency) and steatorrhoea (exocrine insufficiency). The majority of cases are due to chronic alcohol excess. Diagnosis is usually made by CT but endoscopic ultrasound with biopsy may be required to rule out malignancy. Unlike acute pancreatitis, serum amylase is usually unhelpful; ↓faecal elastase indicates pancreatic exocrine insufficiency.

Pancreatic cancer may cause severe, unrelenting pain in the upper abdomen that radiates to the back (50% patients), and is usually associated with cachexia ± cholestatic jaundice.

Mesenteric ischaemia

Chronic mesenteric ischaemia is a rare cause of chronic abdominal pain that tends to occur in patients with widespread severe atherosclerotic disease. Dull periumbilical or lower abdominal pain develops approximately 30 minutes after eating ('abdominal angina') and may be associated with bloody diarrhoea. This may lead to a fear of eating so weight loss is common. However, even the patient who eats 'normally' is often cachectic due to poor absorption. The diagnosis is made by CT mesenteric angiography.

Acute mesenteric ischaemia presents very differently: acute, agonizing, constant diffuse abdominal pain with minimal examination findings (poor localization, no peritonism), systemic upset and, usually, lactic acidosis. It is a surgical emergency with a high mortality. It is due either to mesenteric embolism 50% (patients may have atrial fibrillation), thrombosis in situ 25% (atherosclerotic disease), congestive venous infarction due to mesenteric vein thrombosis (5%) or due to non-occlusive causes (20%) such as cardiac failure or septic shock.

Inflammatory bowel disease

Colitis due to either Crohn's disease or ulcerative colitis may cause cramping lower abdominal pain, usually in association with bloody diarrhoea. Small bowel inflammation in Crohn's disease is often manifest by persistent cramping periumbilical or RLQ pain ± diarrhoea (non-bloody) and constitutional upset. Subacute small bowel obstruction due to oedema or fibrosis (strictures) may lead to colicky postprandial abdominal discomfort. Both disorders are also associated with a range of extraintestinal features (see Box 9.3, p. 91).

Colon cancer

This is a common cancer in men and women. In many countries, screening programmes detect tumours before they cause symptoms. However, patients may present with colicky lower abdominal pain (from partial or complete bowel obstruction). Other important features include a history of weight loss, change in bowel habit (alternating between constipation and diarrhoea as liquid faeces bypasses around firmer stool that is partially held up), rectal bleeding and iron deficiency anaemia. Tenesmus is a feature of low rectal tumours. Right-sided cancers present insidiously with vague pain and iron deficiency anaemia. This is because the proximal colon is more distensible and contains liquid faeces, so obstructive features are not seen and blood loss is occult. Diagnosis is usually made by colonoscopy. CT colonography may be used for frail patients who are unfit for endoscopic colonoscopy.

Functional disorders

These are extremely common, particularly in younger adults. Diagnosis is based on typical clinical features in the absence of apparent organic disease.

Non-ulcer dyspepsia causes symptoms that may be indistinguishable from peptic ulcer. UGIE and mucosal biopsies are normal.

IBS causes abdominal pain that is relieved by defecation or is associated with a change in bowel habit. Diagnostic criteria are shown in Box 9.1, page 90. Symptoms tend to follow a relapsing and remitting course, and are often exacerbated by psychosocial stress. It is essential to rule out other organic causes of these symptoms, including inflammatory bowel disease, malignancy, coeliac disease and tropical sprue.

Renal tract disorders

Infrequent, discrete attacks of severe loin pain radiating to the groin ± haematuria suggest renal stone disease. Chronic dull, aching or 'dragging' discomfort may be due to cancer, adult polycystic kidney disease (APKD), loin pain–haematuria syndrome or chronic obstruction/pyelonephritis. Patients with acute renal colic typically writhe in pain and are unable to find a comfortable position (in contrast to patients with peritonitis who lie very still).

Gynaecological conditions

Sudden onset lower abdominal pain in women of reproductive age may represent ovarian torsion (around a cyst) or ruptured ectopic pregnancy. Both are surgical emergencies. Recurrent episodes of acute lower abdominal pain that regularly occur midway through the menstrual cycle may be a manifestation of ovulation (mittelschmerz). The pain typically occurs suddenly, as the graafian follicle ruptures, and subsides over 24 hours.

An ovarian cancer or cyst may present with non-specific persistent lower abdominal discomfort ± evidence of a pelvic mass on abdominal/PV examination.

Endometriosis (endometrial tissue outside the uterus) and pelvic inflammatory disease (PID; infection of the upper reproductive tract) are common causes of chronic lower abdominal pain in women of reproductive age.

Other diagnostic possibilities

- Constipation.
- Hypercalcaemia.
- Small bowel ulcers/tumours.
- Acute intermittent porphyria.
- Giardiasis.
- Abdominal tuberculosis.
- Coeliac disease.

Acute abdominal pain: overview

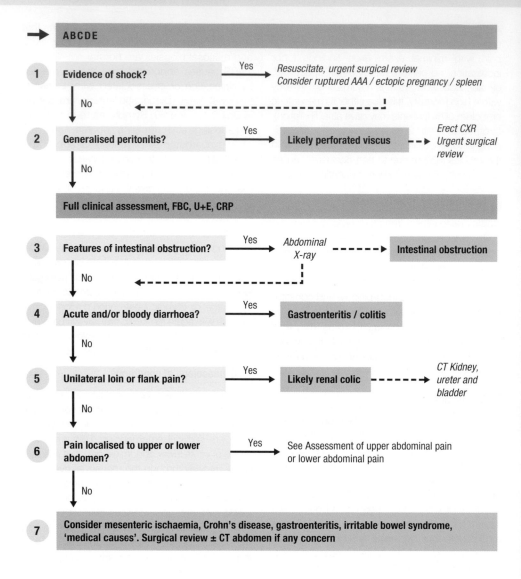

ABCDE

1 Evidence of shock? — Yes → *Resuscitate, urgent surgical review*
Consider ruptured AAA / ectopic pregnancy / spleen

No

2 Generalised peritonitis? — Yes → **Likely perforated viscus** - - ▸ *Erect CXR Urgent surgical review*

No

Full clinical assessment, FBC, U+E, CRP

3 Features of intestinal obstruction? — Yes → *Abdominal X-ray* - - - - → **Intestinal obstruction**

No

4 Acute and/or bloody diarrhoea? — Yes → **Gastroenteritis / colitis**

No

5 Unilateral loin or flank pain? — Yes → **Likely renal colic** - - - - - → *CT Kidney, ureter and bladder*

No

6 Pain localised to upper or lower abdomen? — Yes → See Assessment of upper abdominal pain or lower abdominal pain

No

7 Consider mesenteric ischaemia, Crohn's disease, gastroenteritis, irritable bowel syndrome, 'medical causes'. Surgical review ± CT abdomen if any concern

1 Evidence of shock?

Rapidly identify patients who are shocked with hypotension and evidence of tissue hypoperfusion (see Box 30.1, p. 267).

Remember that young, fit patients can often maintain BP in the face of major fluid losses; in these patients hypotension occurs late, so look carefully for early features such as ↑HR, ↑RR, narrow pulse pressure, anxiety, pallor, cold sweat or light-headedness on standing ± postural ↓BP.

If the patient has overt or incipient shock, secure two large-bore IV lines; send blood for cross-match, U+E, FBC, amylase and LFTs; and begin aggressive resuscitation.

The diagnoses to consider first are rupture of an AAA, ectopic pregnancy or other viscus, as these may require immediate surgical intervention.

- Suspect ruptured AAA in any patient with known AAA, a pulsatile abdominal mass or risk factors, e.g. male >60 years old, who experiences sudden-onset, severe abdominal/back or loin pain followed rapidly by haemodynamic compromise.
- Suspect ruptured ectopic pregnancy in any pregnant woman or woman of child-bearing age with recent-onset lower abdominal pain or PV bleeding; perform an immediate bedside pregnancy test.
- Consider splenic rupture in any shocked patient with abdominal pain who has a history of recent trauma, e.g. road traffic accident.

If any of these diagnoses is suspected, arrange immediate surgical review prior to imaging.

In the absence of these conditions, perform an ECG, CXR, urinalysis and ABG, continue to assess for an underlying cause, as described below, and refer for urgent surgical review. Other important diagnoses to consider include:

- perforated viscus
- acute mesenteric ischaemia
- acute inflammatory conditions, e.g. pancreatitis, colitis, cholangitis
- medical conditions, e.g. diabetic ketoacidosis, myocardial infarction, adrenal crisis, pneumonia
- any condition associated with repeated vomiting, e.g. intestinal obstruction, gastroenteritis.

2 Generalized peritonitis?

Generalized peritonitis is usually the manifestation of a perforated hollow viscus with inevitable spillage of enteric fluid, e.g. stomach, duodenum or colon. Suspect it if there is severe, non-colicky abdominal pain that is worse on movement, coughing or deep inspiration, and which is associated with inflammatory features and generalized abdominal rigidity. The patient will usually be lying still, taking shallow breaths, and will be in obvious distress or discomfort; reconsider the diagnosis if the patient appears well or is moving freely.

Patients require aggressive resuscitation, antibiotics and immediate surgical referral. Free air under the diaphragm on erect CXR (present in 50–75% of cases) confirms the diagnosis (Fig. 4.4); if CXR non-diagnostic consider CT with oral and IV contrast. A very high index of suspicion is required in the elderly and in patients taking systemic steroids; signs are often subtle, so reassess frequently.

Localized peritonitis (or peritonism) occurs where the parietal peritoneum is irritated, for example by an inflamed appendix or diverticular abscess. This results in focal abdominal rigidity over the area affected and may precede progression to generalized peritonitis should the patient's condition deteriorate.

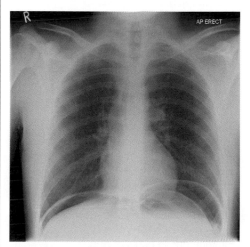

Fig. 4.4 Free air under the diaphragm.

③ Features of intestinal obstruction?

Suspect intestinal obstruction if abdominal pain is colicky and accompanied by vomiting, absolute constipation and/or abdominal distension. The predominant symptoms will vary, depending on the site of obstruction; in high small bowel obstruction vomiting and pain are pre-eminent, whereas in low colonic lesions constipation and distension are more pronounced. If any of these features are present, perform an abdominal X-ray (AXR) (Fig. 4.5) to confirm the diagnosis and estimate the level of the obstruction.

Examine for an incarcerated hernia in any patient with suspected bowel obstruction. Consider further imaging and rectal examination to confirm an obstructing lesion and differentiate from pseudo-obstruction in patients with large bowel obstruction.

Patients may be profoundly dehydrated – check U+E, provide adequate fluid resuscitation, insert a large-bore nasogastric tube and consider a urinary catheter. Refer to surgery for further assessment and management.

④ Acute and/or bloody diarrhoea?

Recent onset of acute diarrhoea with cramping abdominal pain ± vomiting suggests infective gastroenteritis. Suspect colitis (infective, inflammatory or ischaemic) if the patient has bloody diarrhoea with cramping lower abdominal pain ± tenesmus and features of systemic inflammation (see Box 4.1). Always consider the possibility of ischaemic colitis if the patient is elderly or has known vascular disease/atrial fibrillation; if ischaemic colitis is suspected, arrange a CT mesenteric angiogram. Otherwise, send stool for culture and assess as described in Chapter 9.

⑤ Unilateral loin or flank pain?

Suspect renal tract obstruction (usually due to a calculus) if there is severe, colicky loin pain (see above) that radiates to the groin ± testes/labia. Patients will typically writhe in pain, unable to find a comfortable position (in contrast to patients with peritonitis who lie very still). Visible (macroscopic) or dipstick (microscopic) haematuria is present in 90% of cases and vomiting is common during bouts of pain.

Distended loops of small bowel   Stomach

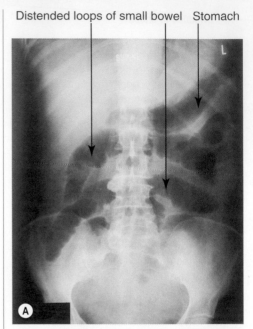

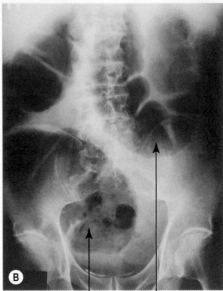

Very distended   Distended low-lying
caecum   transverse colon

Fig. 4.5 Intestinal obstruction. [A] Small bowel. [B] Large bowel. (From Begg JD. Abdominal X-rays Made Easy, 2nd edn. Edinburgh: Churchill Livingstone, 2006.)

Exclude an AAA if the patient is at high risk, e.g. male >60 years with vascular disease, or if the presentation is atypical, e.g. absence of haematuria/restlessness/radiation to groin: request an urgent USS and, if this confirms the presence of an AAA, arrange immediate surgical review. Otherwise, organize non-contrast abdominal CT (or IVU if CT is not available) to confirm the presence of a stone.

In patients with a confirmed stone, check renal function and look for features of infection proximal to the obstruction including ↑temperature/WBC/CRP or leucocytes/nitrites on urinalysis. If you suspect proximal infection, take urine and blood cultures, give IV antibiotics and refer urgently to urology.

Suspect pyelonephritis if flank pain is non-colicky and associated with inflammatory features (see Box 4.1), leucocytes and nitrites (produced by bacteria) on urine dipstick, or loin/renal angle tenderness ± lower urinary tract symptoms. Consider alternative diagnoses, e.g. acute cholecystitis, appendicitis, if there is prominent abdominal tenderness/guarding or if urinalysis is negative for both leucocytes and nitrites. Take blood and urine cultures, start IV antibiotics and arrange prompt renal USS to exclude a perinephric collection or renal obstruction.

6   Pain localized to upper or lower abdomen?

The localization of pain within the abdomen can be very helpful in narrowing the differential diagnosis (see Figs 4.1 and 4.2).

- If the patient has predominantly RUQ, LUQ, epigastric or generalized upper abdominal pain, proceed to *Acute upper abdominal pain* (p. 34).
- If the patient has RIF, LIF, suprapubic or bilateral lower abdominal pain, proceed to *Acute lower abdominal pain* (p. 38).

7   Consider other causes ± surgical review or further imaging if any concern

Organize CT angiography to look for features of mesenteric ischaemia in any patient with severe, diffuse pain, shock or unexplained lactic acidosis – especially if patients are elderly or have vascular disease/atrial fibrillation. The abdominal examination may be unremarkable until advanced stages.

Consider atypical presentations of common disorders such as acute appendicitis or inflammatory bowel disease. A retrocaecal appendix may present with flank pain while any area of the gut may develop a Crohn's inflammatory mass.

Both gastroenteritis and hypercalcaemia may cause abdominal discomfort with conspicuous vomiting and minimal abdominal signs – measure serum calcium and enquire about infectious contacts and recent ingestion of suspicious foodstuffs.

Functional disorders, e.g. IBS, are a frequent cause of acute abdominal pain. The diagnosis of IBS is discussed on page 90, but enquire about a background of longstanding intermittent abdominal pain with altered bowel habit and review the notes for previous similar admissions.

A period of observation with repeated clinical evaluation is very often the key to successful diagnosis; for example, abdominal pain that was originally central and non-specific may, on repeat examination, have migrated to the RIF, suggesting a diagnosis of acute appendicitis. Patients who remain systemically well and whose pain appears to be settling can usually be discharged safely, with outpatient review. Those with marked systemic upset or other features causing concern but no clear underlying cause require further investigation ± surgical review.

4

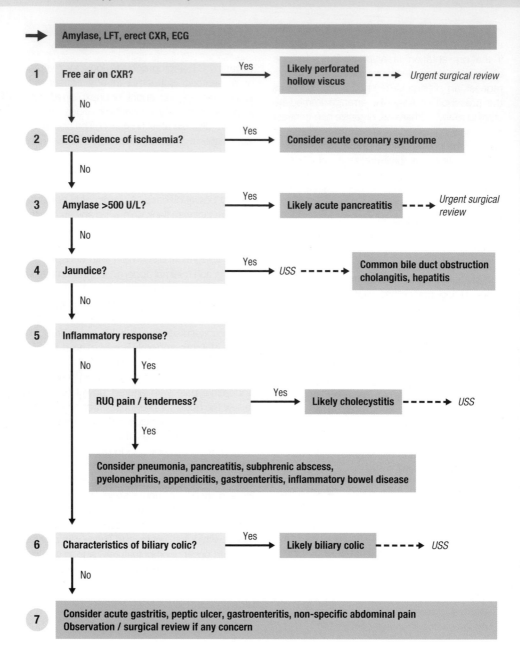

→ Amylase, LFT, erect CXR, ECG

1 Free air on CXR? — Yes → Likely perforated hollow viscus ---→ *Urgent surgical review*

No ↓

2 ECG evidence of ischaemia? — Yes → Consider acute coronary syndrome

No ↓

3 Amylase >500 U/L? — Yes → Likely acute pancreatitis ---→ *Urgent surgical review*

No ↓

4 Jaundice? — Yes → *USS* ---→ Common bile duct obstruction cholangitis, hepatitis

No ↓

5 Inflammatory response?

No ↓   Yes ↓

RUQ pain / tenderness? — Yes → Likely cholecystitis ---→ *USS*

Yes ↓

Consider pneumonia, pancreatitis, subphrenic abscess, pyelonephritis, appendicitis, gastroenteritis, inflammatory bowel disease

6 Characteristics of biliary colic? — Yes → Likely biliary colic ---→ *USS*

No ↓

7 Consider acute gastritis, peptic ulcer, gastroenteritis, non-specific abdominal pain Observation / surgical review if any concern

1   Free air on CXR?

Perform an erect CXR in all unwell patients with acute upper abdominal pain; the presence of free air under the diaphragm (see Fig. 4.4) indicates perforation of a hollow viscus. Secure IV access, cross-match for blood, resuscitate with IV fluids and refer immediately to surgery.

If the CXR fails to demonstrate free air or is equivocal but clinical suspicion is high, e.g. sudden-onset severe pain with epigastric tenderness and guarding, consider an abdominal CT, but first check amylase and ECG as described in steps 2 and 3.

2   ECG evidence of ischaemia?

Acute coronary syndromes, particularly inferior myocardial infarction (MI), may present atypically with epigastric pain. However, hypotension or severe bleeding in patients with acute abdominal pathology may provoke or exacerbate ischaemia in patients with stable coronary artery disease; in these circumstances, administration of powerful antithrombotic agents may have catastrophic consequences.

- Perform an ECG in all patients.
- Refer immediately to cardiology if there are features of an ST elevation MI (see Box 6.1, p. 51).
- In patients with ST depression, evaluate carefully for hypotension, sepsis, hypoxia and bleeding before attributing changes to an acute coronary event.
- In patients with non-specific T wave changes (see Box 6.1, p. 51), measure cardiac biomarkers to assist diagnosis and continue to search for alternative causes.
- Seek cardiology input if there is any diagnostic doubt.

3   Amylase >500 U/L?

Measure serum amylase in any patient with acute severe epigastric pain. Patients with an amylase >3x the reference range are 95% likely to have pancreatitis; levels >1000 U/L are considered diagnostic.

If amylase levels are normal or equivocal, continue to suspect the diagnosis if the history is characteristic and:

- there has been a delay in presentation OR
- there is a history of alcoholism – especially if the patient has had previous episodes of pancreatitis.

In these patients, consider CT with intravenous contrast (provided renal function is satisfactory) to look for evidence of pancreatic inflammation.

Once the diagnosis has been made, evaluate repeatedly for evidence of complications, e.g. shock, hypoxia (acute respiratory distress syndrome, ARDS), disseminated intravascular coagulation (DIC); calculate the Glasgow prognostic criteria score (Box 4.2) or other validated prognostic score; and monitor CRP.

Box 4.2 Modified Glasgow criteria[1] for assessing prognosis in acute pancreatitis

- Age >55 years
- PaO_2 <8 kPa (60 mmHg)
- WBC >15 × 10^9/L
- Albumin <32 g/L
- Serum calcium <2.00 mmol/L (8 mg/dL) (corrected)
- Glucose >10 mmol/L (180 mg/dL)
- Urea >16 mmol/L (45 mg/dL) (after rehydration)
- ALT >200 U/L
- LDH >600 U/L

[1]Severity and prognosis worsen as the number of these factors increases. More than three implies severe disease.

Manage all patients with severe or high-risk acute pancreatitis (shock, organ failure, Glasgow score ≥3 or peak CRP >210 mg/L) in a critical care unit.

Perform an abdominal USS to look for gallstones and an MRCP if there is jaundice or a dilated common bile duct (CBD) on USS. Rarely, those with severe pancreatitis may require urgent ERCP and stone extraction. Consider CT after five days to assess the extent of pancreatic injury and look for evidence of complications, e.g. infection, particularly in patients with persistent organ failure or a systemic inflammatory response. In cases of diagnostic uncertainty, an earlier CT may be helpful.

4   Jaundice?

Organize an urgent abdominal USS for all patients with acute upper abdominal pain and jaundice to look for evidence of biliary obstruction or hepatitis.

Assume biliary sepsis, at least initially, if the patient is unwell with high fever ± rigors or cholestatic jaundice (p. 176); give IV antibiotics and, if the USS confirms a dilated CBD, refer immediately to surgery for further investigation (MRCP) and biliary decompression (ERCP).

Assess as described in Chapter 19 if there are clinical or USS features of acute hepatitis.

5   Inflammatory response?

At this stage, use the presence or absence of a systemic inflammatory response (see Box 4.1) to narrow the differential diagnosis.

Arrange prompt abdominal USS to confirm or exclude acute cholecystitis in any patient with inflammatory features accompanied by any of the following:

- localized RUQ pain
- direct tenderness to palpation in the RUQ
- positive Murphy's sign (sudden arrest of inspiration while taking a deep breath during palpation of the gallbladder).

In the absence of acute cholecystitis, the USS may reveal an alternative cause for the presentation, e.g. pyelonephritis, hepatitis, subphrenic collection.

If none of these features is present, consider alternative disorders:

- basal pneumonia if there is clinical or CXR evidence of basal consolidation (see Figs 12.3 and 12.4, p. 118), especially if accompanied by productive cough or dyspnoea
- gastroenteritis in patients with an acute vomiting illness and no abdominal guarding or rigidity (reassess regularly)
- acute pyelonephritis if urinalysis is positive for leucocytes/nitrites.

Otherwise, consider USS/CT to exclude atypical presentations of acute appendicitis/pancreatitis/cholecystitis, Crohn's disease or other acute inflammatory pathology.

6   Characteristics of biliary colic?

Biliary colic is a common cause of acute severe upper abdominal pain in patients who are otherwise well and do not exhibit evidence of a systemic inflammatory response. Abdominal USS can assist the diagnosis by demonstrating the presence of gallstones. However, asymptomatic gallstones are very common and so the history is critical to making an accurate diagnosis.

Look for the following suggestive features:

- onset of pain a few hours after a meal (may waken the patient from sleep)
- duration ≤6 hours followed by complete resolution of symptoms
- the main site is the epigastrium or RUQ ± radiation to the back
- constant, vague, aching or cramping discomfort (it is not, strictly speaking, 'colicky')
- history of previous similar episodes.

Arrange abdominal USS only in patients with a suggestive history.

 7 | **Consider other causes ± observation/ surgical review if any concern**

Systemically well patients with an acute vomiting illness and recent infectious contact or

ingestion of suspicious foodstuffs are likely to have gastroenteritis.

Suspect acute gastritis if the patient reports new-onset gnawing, burning or vague epigastric discomfort ± mild tenderness – especially if this is associated with dyspeptic symptoms, e.g. nausea, belching, heartburn or a history of recent alcohol excess/NSAID use; consider peptic ulcer disease if there is a background history of similar symptoms.

In many cases, no definite diagnosis is reached. Admit for observation ± surgical review if symptoms are not improving or there are worrying features on examination. Otherwise, patients can usually be discharged, with further outpatient assessment if symptoms recur or persist.

4

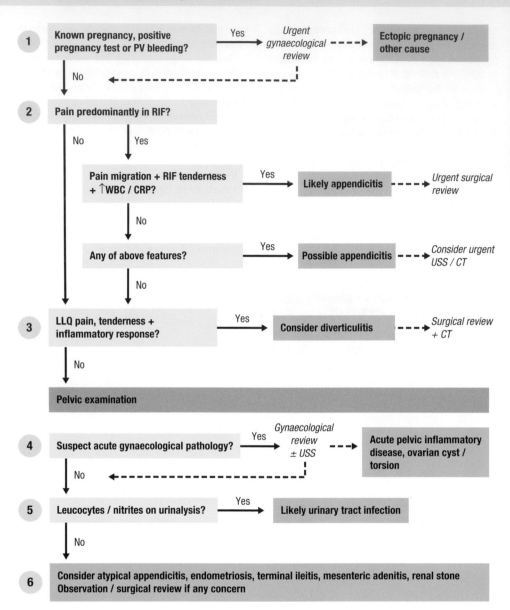

1 Known pregnancy, positive pregnancy test or PV bleeding? — Yes → *Urgent gynaecological review* - - - - ► Ectopic pregnancy / other cause

No

2 Pain predominantly in RIF?

No / Yes

Pain migration + RIF tenderness + ↑WBC / CRP? — Yes → Likely appendicitis - - - - ► *Urgent surgical review*

No

Any of above features? — Yes → Possible appendicitis - - - ► *Consider urgent USS / CT*

No

3 LLQ pain, tenderness + inflammatory response? — Yes → Consider diverticulitis - - - ► *Surgical review + CT*

No

Pelvic examination

4 Suspect acute gynaecological pathology? — Yes → *Gynaecological review ± USS* - - ► Acute pelvic inflammatory disease, ovarian cyst / torsion

No

5 Leucocytes / nitrites on urinalysis? — Yes → Likely urinary tract infection

No

6 Consider atypical appendicitis, endometriosis, terminal ileitis, mesenteric adenitis, renal stone
Observation / surgical review if any concern

1 Known pregnancy, positive pregnancy test or PV bleeding?

Perform a bedside pregnancy test in any pre or peri-menopausal woman with acute lower abdominal pain. If positive or the patient has vaginal bleeding, request an urgent gynaecological review with transabdominal ± transvaginal USS to exclude ectopic pregnancy. If the pregnancy test is negative but there is ongoing suspicion of pregnancy, e.g. missed period, vaginal bleeding, send blood for formal laboratory measurement of beta-human chorionic gonadotrophin.

Request a gynaecological review for assessment of pregnancy-related complications in any woman with known intra-uterine pregnancy who develops acute lower abdominal pain, but consider alternative diagnoses, including acute appendicitis.

2 Pain predominantly in RIF?

The two most helpful clinical characteristics of acute appendicitis are:

- migration of pain from the periumbilical region to the RLQ
- RLQ tenderness or signs of local peritonism.

In the absence of previous appendectomy, acute appendicitis is highly likely if both of these features are present, alongside mild fever or an ↑WBC or ↑CRP. In these circumstances, imaging is unlikely to contribute to the diagnosis and patients should be referred immediately to the on-call surgeon.

An ↑WBC and ↑CRP are not specific for appendicitis but the diagnosis is unlikely if both are within normal limits. Nevertheless, a surgical review is mandatory if the presentation is otherwise typical – especially if <12 hours from onset of symptoms.

Maintain a high index of suspicion for appendicitis in any patient with RLQ pain. Request prompt surgical review and consider urgent imaging to assist diagnosis if pain is accompanied by either of the two clinical features listed above or an ↑WBC/↑CRP.

Abdominal USS may help to confirm the diagnosis rapidly or, in females, identify pelvic pathology, e.g. ovarian cyst/torsion.

CT offers greater diagnostic accuracy and may be considered in males or if diagnostic uncertainty persists after USS.

3 LLQ pain, tenderness + inflammatory response?

Exclude sigmoid diverticulitis in any patient with acute LLQ pain and tenderness (± guarding) with evidence of systemic inflammation (see Box 4.1) – especially if >40 years. Even in the absence of overt tenderness or inflammatory features, maintain a high degree of suspicion if the patient is elderly or has known diverticular disease. Arrange urgent CT to confirm the diagnosis and identify complications, e.g. abscess, or to seek an alternative cause for the presentation.

4 Suspect acute gynaecological pathology?

Have a high index of suspicion for acute gynaecological pathology in any woman of child-bearing age with acute pelvic or lower abdominal pain.

Organize an urgent USS if there is a history of abrupt-onset, severe, unilateral pelvic or lower abdominal pain with any of the following features:

- associated nausea and vomiting
- unilateral tenderness
- adnexal tenderness or palpable adnexal mass
- age <35 years.

The principal aim of USS is to look for evidence of ovarian torsion but it may reveal an alternative diagnosis, e.g. ovarian cyst. Request a gynaecology review if you have a strong clinical suspicion of torsion or the USS result is equivocal.

In the absence of features suggesting ovarian torsion, consider acute pelvic inflammatory disease (PID). Suspect the diagnosis if there is bilateral lower abdominal pain and tenderness ± fever associated with any of the following features:

- abnormal vaginal or cervical discharge
- tenderness on moving the cervix during bimanual vaginal examination ('cervical excitation')
- adnexal tenderness on bimanual vaginal examination.

The diagnosis is often one of exclusion and, in the emergency setting, it is prudent to seek formal gynaecological input; in difficult cases, diagnostic laparoscopy may be required. Whenever the diagnosis is considered, take endocervical swabs for chlamydia and gonorrhoea, and treat in all cases if positive.

5 Leucocytes/nitrites on urinalysis?

Suprapubic pain/tenderness is common in UTI but the absence of nitrites and leucocytes on urinalysis makes the diagnosis unlikely.

Acute appendicitis may cause dysuria, frequency and urgency with positive urinalysis, e.g. haematuria, leucocytes, if the inflamed appendix lies adjacent to the bladder or ureter; always consider this possibility, particularly in males (in whom cystitis is rare). However, in the absence of other worrying features, a positive urinalysis for both leucocytes and nitrites, especially in women, suggests UTI; send an MSU and start empirical treatment.

6 **Consider other causes ± observation/ surgical review if any concern**

Consider atypical presentations of appendicitis resulting from variations in the position of the appendix; for example, an inflamed appendix that lies within the pelvis may only be tender on rectal examination. Alternative diagnoses in patients with inflammatory features include terminal ileitis and mesenteric adenitis. Seek a formal surgical opinion if the diagnosis is uncertain.

Consider mesenteric ischaemia in any patient who appears unwell or has an unexplained lactic acidosis – especially if they have known vascular disease or atrial fibrillation.

An obstructed renal stone most commonly presents with loin pain but, once descended to the ureter, may cause more localized tenderness in the RLQ or LLQ; suspect this if the pain radiates to the testes/labia or is associated with visible/dipstick haematuria.

The diagnosis of acute urinary retention is usually obvious but should be excluded in confused patients with lower abdominal tenderness and distress. Clinical examination should be diagnostic but a bladder scan may be helpful.

In female patients, consider the possibility of alternative pelvic pathology, e.g. endometriosis or mittelschmerz (recurrent episodes of lower abdominal pain that regularly occur midway through the menstrual cycle), especially if there is a background of previous similar episodes at the midpoint of their menstrual cycle.

In many patients, a precise diagnosis remains elusive and, as with upper and generalized abdominal pain, functional disorders are a common cause.

4

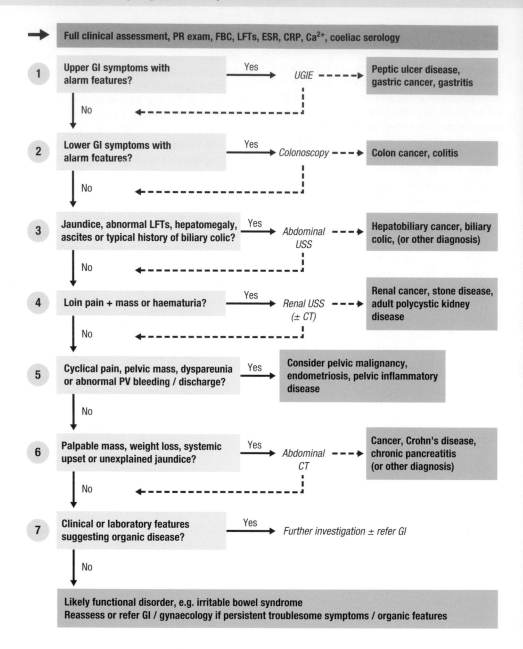

1 Upper GI symptoms with alarm features?

Arrange prompt UGIE if there is upper abdominal discomfort ± other dyspeptic symptoms with any of the following:

- weight loss
- dysphagia
- persistent vomiting or early satiety
- abdominal distension
- haematemesis or iron deficiency anaemia
- ≥55 years with new-onset persistent symptoms.

If a gastric ulcer is identified, ensure that a biopsy is sent to exclude malignancy, prescribe *H. pylori* eradication therapy if the CLO test is positive, recheck the history for NSAID use, and consider an interval UGIE to ensure satisfactory healing.

Eradicate *H. pylori* in any patient with a duodenal ulcer and confirm successful eradication with a urea breath test.

In patients with macroscopic appearances of an upper GI tumour, obtain the formal biopsy result and consider a staging CT scan.

2 Lower GI symptoms with alarm features?

Arrange urgent lower GI endoscopy in any patient with:

- rectal bleeding
- a palpable rectal mass
- iron deficiency anaemia
- change in bowel habit and >45 years or recent weight loss.

Consider flexible sigmoidoscopy as the first-line investigation in patients <45 years, colonoscopy if >45 years. Obtain the biopsy results of any suspicious lesions or sections of GI mucosa.

3 Jaundice, abnormal LFTs, hepatomegaly, ascites or typical history of biliary colic?

The combination of new-onset jaundice and persistent/recurrent abdominal discomfort suggests hepatitis, choledocholithiasis or, most frequently, malignancy, e.g. biliary, ampullary, pancreatic or hepatocellular cancer or hepatic metastases. USS may reveal the cause but, if inconclusive, further investigation, e.g. CT or MRCP, is mandatory.

4

Arrange USS and perform a diagnostic ascitic tap in any patient with ascites (send for biochemistry, microbiology and cytology). If the ascites is exudative and USS fails to reveal an underlying cause, organize an abdominal CT scan.

The features of biliary colic are described above. If present, arrange USS to look for gallstones. Note that gallstones are a very frequent finding in asymptomatic patients so, unless the history is typical or there is evidence of a complication, e.g. dilated CBD, chronic cholecystitis, they are unlikely to explain the presentation.

Refer to a GI specialist if there is a convincing history of biliary pain in the absence of gallstones, especially if associated with abnormal LFTs or a dilated CBD.

4 Loin pain + mass or haematuria?

You must exclude upper renal tract cancer in any patient presenting with persistent loin pain associated with a mass or haematuria (visible or dipstick). Renal USS is a first-line investigation and may reveal alternative causes, e.g. APKD or chronic hydronephrosis. Consider CT ± urology referral if the cause remains unclear, especially in patients >40 years.

5 Cyclical pain, pelvic mass, dyspareunia or abnormal PV bleeding/discharge?

Organize a pelvic USS in any patient with a pelvic mass or any postmenopausal patient with PV bleeding or recent-onset, persistent lower abdominal pain. The features of PID are described above; if present, take endocervical or vaginal swabs for gonorrhoea and chlamydia – treat if positive.

Consider endometriosis in any woman of reproductive age with severe dysmenorrhoea, or chronic lower abdominal pain and any of the following features:

- variation with menstrual cycle
- deep dyspareunia
- other prominent cyclical or perimenstrual symptoms.

Establishing a definitive diagnosis of endometriosis may be challenging – refer to a gynaecologist for further assessment, e.g. laparoscopy if symptoms are severe.

6 Palpable mass, weight loss, systemic upset or unexplained jaundice?

At this stage, organize an abdominal CT if the patient has any of the above features. Patients with a palpable mass may have been investigated with other modalities in steps 1–5 above but CT is more likely to identify certain masses, e.g. pancreas, small bowel, renal tract and omental, and should be performed if the cause remains uncertain. In patients with abdominal pain and significant weight loss or other major constitutional upset, e.g. fevers, night sweats or ↑↑ESR, CT may reveal evidence of lymphoma, solid organ malignancy or inflammatory disease, e.g. chronic pancreatitis, abscess, Crohn's disease.

7 Clinical or laboratory features suggest organic disease?

Further investigation is usually required if the patient is >45 years with recent-onset symptoms, weight loss, constitutional upset or abnormal screening investigations. Important organic causes of pain that may easily be missed include chronic pancreatitis, chronic mesenteric ischaemia and Crohn's disease.

Consider chronic pancreatitis in any patient with a background of chronic alcohol excess or steatorrhoea. Check faecal elastase, perform an abdominal CT and consider specialist referral for further assessment.

Exclude mesenteric ischaemia (CT mesenteric angiography) if there is a close relationship between eating and the onset of pain, especially if evidence of vascular disease elsewhere, e.g. angina, intermittent claudication.

Assess any patient with associated diarrhoea. Even in the absence of diarrhoea, consider further investigation for small bowel Crohn's disease, e.g. enteroscopy, barium follow-through or small bowel MRI in a young patient with unexplained mouth ulcers, ↑ESR/CRP, extraintestinal manifestations (see Box 9.3, p. 91) or persistent RLQ tenderness.

If none of the above is present, a functional cause, e.g. IBS, is likely – particularly when typical symptoms are present (see Box 9.1, p. 90). However, patients with persistent, troublesome symptoms may require specialist assessment and investigation to exclude organic disease.

4

5 Breast lump

Breast lump is the most common presenting feature of breast cancer. All breast lumps must be referred to a specialist breast service for evaluation by triple assessment, comprising clinical, radiological and pathological evaluation. The majority of referrals to breast services are benign. Results of malignant lumps should be managed in a multidisciplinary team setting.

USS is the imaging modality of choice in women <35 years due to the high density of breast tissue. MRI scanning is suitable for selected patients. Older women should have mammography ± USS. Pathological assessment is undertaken by ultrasound-guided core biopsy, fine needle aspiration (for cystic lesions) or occasionally excision biopsy.

Breast cancer

The breast is the most common site of cancer in women; 1 in 9 women in the UK are affected by breast cancer in their lifetime. The risk increases with age and the mean age at diagnosis is 60 years. Risk factors are shown in Box 5.1. Features of a breast lump that suggest cancer are shown in Box 5.2. However, it is not possible to exclude cancer by clinical examination alone and all palpable masses should be regarded as potentially malignant until proven otherwise.

Breast abscess

The lump usually develops rapidly and is tender. There is often overlying erythema; there may be fever and evidence of a systemic inflammatory response.

In lactating women, breast abscesses occur most frequently in the first 12 weeks post-partum; painful, cracked nipples are common. It may be difficult to distinguish an abscess if breast tissue is grossly indurated due to mastitis; in these cases referral should be made for further assessment and ultrasound imaging.

In non-lactating women, abscesses are uncommon and an underlying inflammatory cancer should be excluded. Subareolar abscesses are the most common form, typically associated with a periductal mastitis; there is a strong association with smoking.

Fibroadenoma

Fibroadenoma is a common benign neoplasm that occurs after puberty in younger women, usually <30 years. It typically presents as a discrete, mobile, non-tender mass with a rubbery consistency. The diagnosis should be confirmed by triple assessment.

Fibrocystic change

Fibrocystic change is a benign condition associated with tender, lumpy breasts that may affect up to 50% of women between 20 and 50 years but is

---

Box 5.1 Risk factors for breast cancer

- Previous breast cancer
- Increasing age
- Family history
- Oral contraceptive pill
- Hormone replacement therapy
- Early menarche
- Late menopause
- Nulliparity
- First pregnancy >35 years
- Current smoker

Box 5.2 Suspicious features of breast lump

- Hardness
- Immobility
- Skin tethering/puckering
- Skin changes (peau d'orange, eczema)
- Nipple retraction
- Lymphadenopathy
- Bloody nipple discharge

rare after menopause. Features often vary over the course of the menstrual cycle due to hormone fluctuations. Areas of firm, lumpy breast tissue without a discrete mass are often termed nodular breast tissue; if this is localized or asymmetrical and persists throughout the cycle, referral should be made to exclude underlying cancer. Breast cysts are firm, smooth, well-defined lumps which may cause discomfort if enlarging. USS confirms their cystic nature. If needle aspiration yields bloody fluid, this should be sent for cytological examination.

Fat necrosis

Fat necrosis is a benign condition that arises after trauma or surgery. It may present as a firm, irregular mass with tethering to overlying skin, making it difficult to distinguish from malignancy. Irrespective of recent trauma, all lumps with suspicious features should be regarded as potentially malignant and evaluated urgently by triple assessment.

Other causes

Skin and subcutaneous lesions, such as epidermoid cysts and lipomata, may occur on the breast. Phylloides tumours are rare and share many clinical features with fibroadenomas but are typically more aggressive; metastasis is rare but can occur. Superficial thrombophlebitis (spontaneous thrombosis of superficial breast veins) presents with palpable, erythematous linear nodules, and resolves over weeks. Galactocoele is a rare cystic lesion of the breast. It contains milk and most commonly occurs in lactating women; occurrence in non-lactating women requires further endocrine investigation.

Nipple lesions

These must be investigated (triple assessment) to rule out an underlying cancer. Causes include Paget's disease of the nipple (95% association with cancer), nipple adenoma, eczema of the nipple, basal cell carcinoma, melanoma and Bowen's disease.

Male breast disease

Breast lumps in men are rare. Gynaecomastia most commonly presents as a rubbery button of tissue, concentric to the areola. It occurs frequently at puberty and necessitates careful testicular examination and assessment of sexual development. Around 25% are idiopathic. Other causes include drugs (~20%), e.g. spironolactone, anabolic steroids, liver cirrhosis (decreased metabolism of oestrogen, <10%), gonadal failure (decreased androgens, <10%) and testicular tumours (increased oestrogen production, ~3%). Male breast cancer (1% of all breast cancers) typically presents as a hard, fixed lesion, sometimes with overlying skin involvement, and is usually eccentric to the areola.

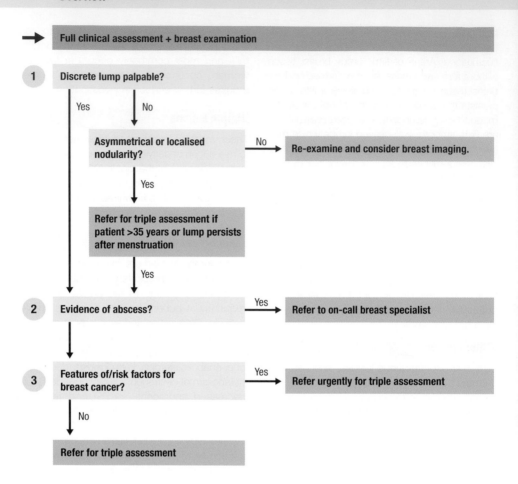

➡ Full clinical assessment + breast examination

1 Discrete lump palpable?

Yes / No

Asymmetrical or localised nodularity? — No → Re-examine and consider breast imaging.

Yes

Refer for triple assessment if patient >35 years or lump persists after menstruation

Yes

2 Evidence of abscess? — Yes → Refer to on-call breast specialist

3 Features of/risk factors for breast cancer? — Yes → Refer urgently for triple assessment

No

Refer for triple assessment

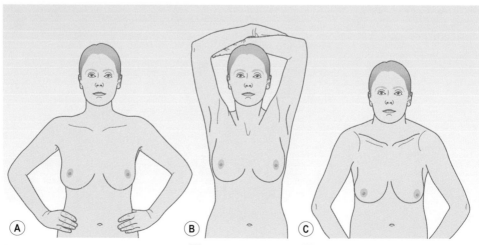

Fig. 5.1 **Positions for inspecting the breast.** A Hands pressed into hips. B Hands above head. C Leaning forward. (From Ford MJ, Hennessey I, Japp A. Introduction to Clinical Examination, 8th edn. Edinburgh: Churchill Livingstone, 2005.)

1 Discrete lump palpable?

If you are unable to locate a lump, ask the patient to attempt to find it and examine in different positions, e.g. supine and upright. In the absence of a discrete lump, assess carefully for nodularity.

Refer any patient >35 years old with a localized area of nodularity or discrete lump for urgent triple assessment. If the patient is <35 years, refer for triple assessment if the localized nodularity persists at review after menstruation.

If no lump or nodularity is detected, consider ultrasound or mammography as appropriate to exclude underlying impalpable pathology.

2 Evidence of abscess?

Suspect breast infection if there is an acute, painful swelling with overlying erythema, fever or a systemic inflammatory response; start antibiotic treatment and refer as an emergency to the breast/surgical team. Refer to a breast specialist to exclude an abscess in any breast-feeding woman with gross mastitis and induration.

3 Features of/risk factors for breast cancer?

Refer any patient with a palpable breast lump for specialist triple assessment to exclude breast cancer.

Request urgent review if:

- patient has risk factors for breast cancer (Box 5.1)
- lump is rapidly enlarging
- lump has features of breast cancer (Box 5.2)
- patient ≥30 years with a new discrete lump
- patient <30 years with a major risk factor, e.g. personal or family history of breast cancer.

5

Clinical tool
Breast examination

- Obtain consent and offer a chaperone; ensure privacy and a warm room.
- Enquire whether the patient has noticed any breast lumps and ask her to point them out.
- With the patient sitting comfortably, hands resting on the thighs, inspect for asymmetry, local swelling, skin changes, e.g. dimpling, redness and nipple inversion or discharge.
- Repeat the inspection (Fig. 5.1) with the patient's hands pressed against her hips (contracting the pectoral muscles), raised above her head (stretching the pectoral muscles) and sitting forward with the breasts dependent.
- With the patient supine, and hands under the head, palpate each breast: compress the breast tissue against the chest wall using the palmar surface of the fingers held flat on the surface of the breast. Palpate clockwise to cover all of the breast tissue, including under the nipple.
- Record the size, position, attachments, mobility, surface, edge and consistency of any lumps and look for associated signs of inflammation (tenderness, warmth, redness).
- Palpate for axillary lymph nodes. Ask the patient to sit facing you and support the full weight of her arm at the wrist with your opposite hand. After warning of possible discomfort, use your other hand to palpate all around the axilla, compressing its contents against the chest wall. Repeat on the other side.

Chest pain is one of the most common presentations encountered in both emergency medicine and medical outpatient clinics. The diagnostic approach to acute chest pain is different from that of intermittent chest pain and they should be considered as distinct clinical entities.

Acute chest pain

The primary aim is to identify acute coronary syndromes (ACSs) and other life-threatening causes, such as aortic dissection and pulmonary embolism (PE). ECG analysis, CXR and biomarkers, e.g. troponin, D-dimer, play a central role in evaluation and are intimately linked with the clinical assessment. Pleuritic chest pain has a sharp or stabbing character and varies with respiration (worse on inspiration); it should be differentiated from non-pleuritic pain at an early stage, as it suggests a different range of possible diagnoses.

Acute coronary syndromes

Acute thrombus formation in a ruptured or eroded atheromatous coronary artery plaque causes an ACS. Sudden total occlusion of a major vessel causes ischaemia of a full-thickness segment of myocardium resulting in acute ST elevation myocardial infarction (STEMI). The mainstay of treatment in these patients is immediate reperfusion by primary angioplasty or fibrinolytic therapy.

With incomplete occlusion or a good collateral blood supply there is less extensive ischaemia, which is usually associated with a degree of cardiomyocyte necrosis (non-ST elevation myocardial infarction; NSTEMI). Less frequently, myocardial ischaemia can occur without cell loss (unstable angina). The introduction of high-sensitivity cardiac troponin measurements (with gender-specific cut-offs) has resulted in an increase in the detection of MI (~4% absolute and 20% relative increase) and a decrease in the diagnosis of unstable angina.

Unstable angina or NSTEMI may also occur in the absence of acute plaque rupture if hypoxaemia, anaemia, tachyarrhythmia or hypotension is superimposed upon stable coronary artery disease (CAD).

The pain of myocardial ischaemia is described below (see 'angina pectoris').

- In unstable angina, the pain:
  - is of new onset and severe
  - occurs at rest or
  - occurs with increasing frequency, duration or intensity.
- In STEMI, the pain is typically severe, with an abrupt onset, and is persistent, unrelieved by glyceryl trinitrate (GTN) spray and accompanied by autonomic upset (sweating, nausea and vomiting).
- The presentation of NSTEMI may lie anywhere between these two extremes; it is distinguished from unstable angina by biochemical evidence of infarction (↑troponin), and from STEMI by ECG features (Boxes 6.1 and 6.2).
- Certain groups of patients, e.g. elderly or diabetic, may have no or minimal pain.

Aortic dissection

This is a tear in the wall of the aorta. It typically causes sudden-onset, intense, unrelenting chest pain that radiates to the back, between the shoulder blades (this may be the main site of pain). The character of the pain is often described as 'ripping', 'tearing' or, most frequently, 'sharp'. Autonomic upset is common; syncope or focal neurological deficit may occur. Mortality is high (1% per hour in the initial phase). Aortic dissection must be suspected in any patient presenting with coexisting cardiovascular and neurological symptoms or signs.

Box 6.1 ECG abnormalities in acute coronary syndromes

ECG abnormalities in STEMI

1. ≥1 mm ST elevation in at least 2 adjacent limb leads, e.g. II and III; I and aVL *OR*
2. ≥2 mm ST elevation in at least 2 adjacent praecordial leads, e.g. V_2 and V_3; V_5 and V_6 *OR*
3. Left bundle branch block of new onset

Major ischaemic ECG changes (strongly suggestive of myocardial ischaemia)

1. ST changes that vary with onset and offset of pain ('dynamic' changes)
2. ≥1 mm horizontal ST depression in ≥2 adjacent leads
3. Deep symmetrical T wave inversion

Minor ischaemic ECG changes (less specific for myocardial ischaemia)

1. <1 mm horizontal ST depression
2. New or evolving T wave inversion or flattening

Box 6.2 Universal definition of myocardial infarction

Outside the context of sudden death, percutaneous coronary intervention or coronary surgery, acute myocardial infarction (MI) should be used when there is evidence of myocardial necrosis in a clinical setting consistent with acute myocardial ischaemia. Under these conditions any one of the following criteria meets the diagnosis for MI.

- Detection of a rise and/or fall of cardiac biomarker values (preferably cardiac troponin [cTn]) with at least one value above the 99th percentile upper reference limit (URL) and with at least one of the following:
  - symptoms of ischemia
  - new or presumed new significant ST-segment–T wave (ST–T) changes or new left bundle branch block (LBBB)
  - development of pathological Q waves in the ECG
  - imaging evidence of new loss of viable myocardium or new regional wall motion abnormality
  - identification of an intracoronary thrombus by angiography or autopsy.

Source: Thygesen K, Alpert JS, Jaffe AS et al. 2012. Universal definition of myocardial infarction. Eur Heart J. 33:2551–2567.

Pulmonary embolism

Pain due to PE depends on the site and size of the embolism. Small emboli commonly produce pleuritic symptoms due to distal pulmonary infarction and may produce few other clinical signs; large emboli may produce severe, sudden-onset, central chest pain that mimics MI due to central pulmonary occlusion. Most patients with large emboli are dyspnoeic and have other features such as haemoptysis, syncope or shock. The majority of emboli arise from lower limb deep vein thrombosis (DVT), but clinical features of DVT are inconsistent and often absent.

Acute pericarditis

This typically causes constant retrosternal pain with a sharp, stabbing character that may radiate to the shoulders, arm or trapezius ridge. It is usually more localized than ischaemic pain and may be accompanied by a rub on auscultation. Pain is often, but not invariably, worsened by inspiration, lying down, with movement or during swallowing, and eased by sitting forward.

Gastro-oesophageal disorders

Oesophageal spasm can cause severe retrosternal discomfort that mimics cardiac pain. Gastro-oesophageal reflux disease (GORD) usually presents with 'heartburn': a hot or burning retrosternal discomfort that radiates upwards; some patients experience severe episodes of pain that mimic cardiac pain, possibly due to reflux-induced spasm. Important clues include onset after eating, aggravation of symptoms by lying supine or bending over, and, often, a history of recent weight gain. Oesophageal rupture is often diagnosed late and carries a high mortality. It should be suspected in any patient who develops chest pain after vomiting.

Pneumothorax

Pneumothorax causes unilateral, sudden-onset pleuritic chest pain, often associated with breathlessness. In large pneumothoraces there may be ↓breath sounds and hyper-resonance to percussion. Diagnosis is usually confirmed on CXR.

Pneumonia

This may cause pleuritic pain, usually accompanied by other clinical features such as fever, cough, purulent sputum and breathlessness.

Musculoskeletal problems

A common cause of chest discomfort with a wide variety of presentations. The pain often varies with posture or movement, and may be reproduced or exacerbated by local palpation. Rib fracture typically causes severe pain following trauma but most cases are due to minor soft tissue injuries. Even these can be symptomatic for up to 6 weeks. Malignant chest wall invasion produces constant, unremitting, localized pain that is not related to respiration and may disturb sleep.

Anxiety

A common cause of chest pain. Occasionally, presentations are dramatic, with patients reporting intense symptoms. Associated features may include breathlessness with 'inability to take enough air' and tingling around the mouth; the onset of symptoms may coincide with stressful situations or emotional distress.

Other causes

- Intrathoracic malignancy or connective tissue disorders, e.g. systemic lupus erythematosus, rheumatoid arthritis, may involve the pleura and present with pleuritic pain ± pleural effusion.
- Subdiaphragmatic inflammatory pathology, e.g. abscess, can mimic pneumonia (pleuritic pain, fever, small pleural effusion).
- Mediastinal masses, e.g. thymoma or lymphoma, tend to cause a dull, constant, progressive retrosternal pain that disturbs sleep.
- Herpes zoster may cause severe pain, sometimes preceded by tingling or burning, followed by development of a vesicular rash in a dermatomal distribution. The rash has often not manifested at the time of presentation, making diagnosis difficult.

Intermittent chest pain

Angina pectoris

Angina is the symptomatic manifestation of myocardial ischaemia. It tends to be perceived as a diffuse retrosternal discomfort that may radiate to the left (or right) shoulder/arm, throat, jaw or back. Typical descriptions include 'tightness',

---

Box 6.3 Estimating the likelihood of coronary artery disease[1]

High risk

- Previously documented CAD or other vascular disease, e.g. stroke, peripheral arterial disease
- Male >60 years *OR* >50 years with ≥2 risk factors *OR* >40 years with ≥3 risk factors
- Female >60 years with ≥3 risk factors

Moderate risk

- All patients not in high-risk or low-risk group

Low risk

- Age <30 years
- Female <40 years with no risk factors

[1] *Risk factors: cigarette smoking, diabetes mellitus, hypertension, hypercholesterolaemia (total cholesterol ≥6.5 mmol/L), family history of premature CAD.*

'pressure' and 'heaviness' but many others, e.g. 'burning' are recognized. Many patients do not perceive angina as painful but most feel a sense of 'discomfort' – if you only ask about 'pain', you may miss the diagnosis.

Stable angina is almost always due to atherosclerotic narrowing in one or more coronary arteries. In considering the likelihood of angina, it is therefore important to consider the underlying risk of CAD (Box 6.3). Myocardial blood flow is adequate under resting conditions but is insufficient to meet metabolic demands during periods of increased cardiac work. Consequently, episodes of angina tend to be precipitated by a predictable degree of exertion and rapidly relieved by rest and/or GTN spray, with episodes typically lasting <10 minutes. Less commonly, angina may result from tachyarrhythmias (especially on a background of significant coronary narrowing) or transient coronary artery spasm.

Gastro-oesophageal disorders

Gastro-oesophageal reflux typically causes a hot, burning retrosternal discomfort which radiates upwards; it is often provoked by bending or lying flat, e.g. in bed, and there may be a relationship with food. Symptoms are relieved by antacids. Oesophageal spasm can cause severe retrosternal discomfort that closely mimics cardiac pain and may be worsened by exertion and relieved by nitrates. There is often an associated history of dysphagia, dyspepsia or typical heartburn.

Musculoskeletal disorders

These are a common cause of chest discomfort with a wide variety of presentations; most are due to minor soft tissue injuries. The pain typically varies with posture or movement and may respond to NSAIDs. In costochondritis, there is well-localized tenderness of the costochondral junctions that is exacerbated by local pressure.

Asthma

Patients with asthma may describe exertional chest 'tightness' on account of bronchospasm, which may be difficult to distinguish from angina. There is usually an associated history of wheeze, breathlessness and cough, and precipitants other than exertion may be apparent, e.g. common allergens, viral upper RTI.

Anxiety

Emotional distress is a very common cause of chest pain and many suspected angina attacks are actually 'panic attacks'. Presentations are often quite dramatic, with patients reporting throat tightness, a 'choking' sensation and/or difficulty taking a breath. There may be evidence of hyperventilation with tingling around the mouth and extremities, and $\downarrow PaCO_2$ on ABG. Episodes tend to arise in the context of stress rather than exertion.

6

Clinical tool
ECG abnormalities in chest pain

The ECG in STEMI

Acute transmural ischaemia produces ST elevation in leads that 'look at' the affected region of myocardium:
- in anterior MI (Fig. 6.1), V_2–V_5
- in lateral MI, V_5, V_6, I and aVL
- in inferior MI (Fig. 6.2), II, III and aVF.

There may be associated ST depression in the opposing leads ('reciprocal change'). Posterior MI (Fig. 6.3) is recognized by reciprocal anterior ST depression and a dominant R wave (reciprocal Q wave) in V_1. Further ECG changes occur as the infarct progresses (Fig. 6.4): loss of the R wave, followed by development of Q waves and T wave inversion (TWI). ST segments typically return to baseline; persistent ST elevation may indicate the development of a left ventricular aneurysm. Extensive anteroseptal infarction may cause new left bundle branch block (Fig. 6.5) rather than ST elevation.

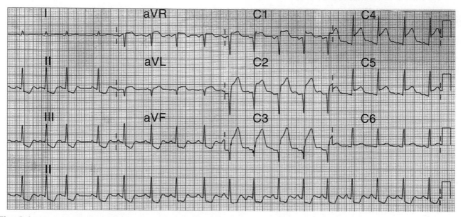

Fig. 6.1 Acute anterior ST elevation myocardial infarction. (From Douglas G, Nicol F, Robertson C. Macleod's Clinical Examination, 12th edn. Edinburgh: Churchill Livingstone, 2009.)

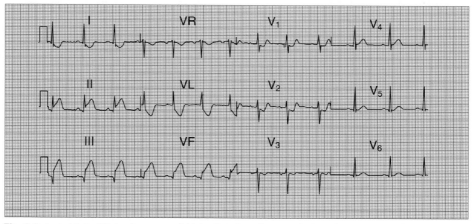

Fig. 6.2 Acute inferior ST elevation myocardial infarction. (From Hampton JR. The ECG in Practice, 5th edn. Edinburgh: Churchill Livingstone, 2008.)

Clinical tool—cont'd
ECG abnormalities in chest pain

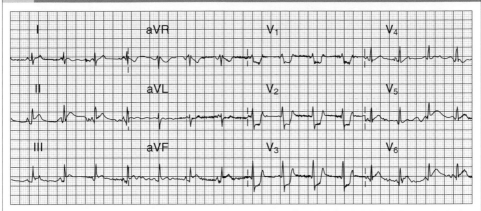

Fig. 6.3 Acute inferoposterior ST elevation myocardial infarction. (From Grubb NR, Newby DE. Churchill's Pocketbooks Cardiology, 2nd edn. Edinburgh: Churchill Livingstone, 2006.)

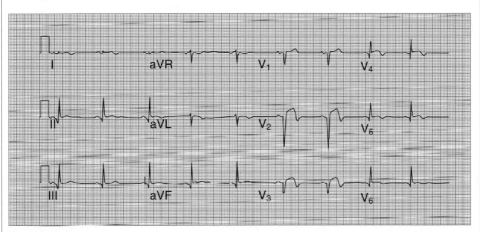

Fig. 6.4 Evolving anterior ST elevation myocardial infarction.

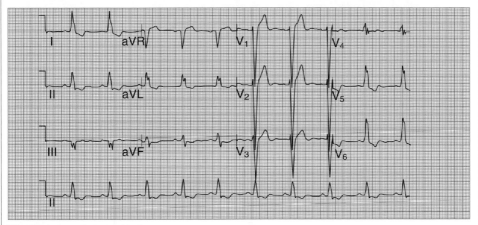

Fig. 6.5 Left bundle branch block.

Continued

Clinical tool—cont'd
ECG abnormalities in chest pain

ST elevation in leads V_2–V_5 can be a normal finding ('high take-off') and, in the absence of a previous ECG, may cause diagnostic confusion. With high take-off, the ST elevation is typically concave and frequently associated with notching in the terminal portion of the QRS complex (Fig. 6.6). Appearances remain stable over time and there are no reciprocal changes. ECG features that favour acute pericarditis from STEMI include: widespread ST elevation (not corresponding to the territory of a single coronary artery); PR depression; the absence of reciprocal changes, Q wave formation or R wave loss; and TWI only after normalization of ST segments.

The ECG in unstable angina/NSTEMI

New horizontal ST depression suggests active ischaemia (Fig. 6.7); the extent and depth of depression correlate with severity of ischaemia and risk of adverse outcomes. 'Dynamic' ST segment changes – those that coincide with pain and normalize with resolution of pain – strongly suggest ischaemia. It is therefore important to compare the presenting hospital ECG with that obtained by the pre-hospital ambulance service. On the other hand, slight ST depression, especially if up-sloping, may be normal.

TWI may be the only ECG evidence of ischaemia. Biphasic TWI in leads V2–V3 (Fig. 6.8) or deep symmetrical TWI in these leads +/– other praecordial leads (Fig. 6.9) suggests critical obstruction of the left anterior descending artery (Wellens' syndrome). Other patterns of TWI are less specific. Lateral TWI, together with downward-sloping ST depression, is a common feature of left ventricular hypertrophy (Fig. 6.10) or digitalis treatment; comparison with previous ECGs is very helpful. TWI confined to leads V_1–V_3 (Fig. 6.11) suggests right heart strain and favours a diagnosis of PE over ACS. TWI also occurs with cardiomyopathies, pericarditis, myocarditis, cerebrovascular events (especially subarachnoid haemorrhage), electrolyte abnormalities and hyperventilation. However, in the appropriate clinical context, new or evolving TWI supports a diagnosis of ACS.

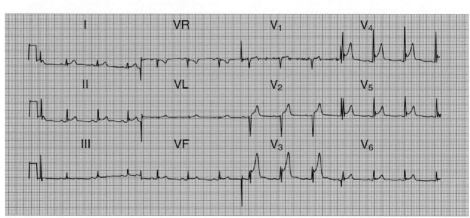

Fig. 6.6 'High take-off' ST segments. (From Hampton JR. The ECG Made Easy, 7th edn. Edinburgh: Churchill Livingstone, 2008.)

Clinical tool—cont'd
ECG abnormalities in chest pain

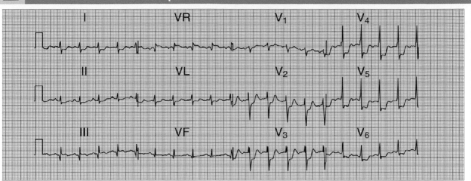

Fig. 6.7 Ischaemic anterolateral ST segment depression. (From Hampton JR. The ECG in Practice, 5th edn. Edinburgh: Churchill Livingstone, 2008.)

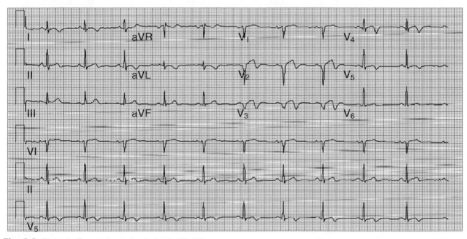

Fig. 6.8 Biphasic T wave inversion in leads V2–V3.

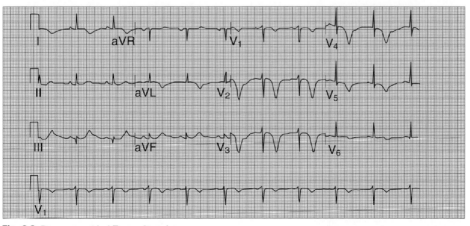

Fig. 6.9 Deep symmetrical T wave inversion.

Continued

6

Clinical tool—cont'd
ECG abnormalities in chest pain

The ECG in acute pericarditis

Acute pericarditis characteristically produces diffuse, concave (upward-sloping) ST elevation in most leads, with ST depression in aVR (Fig. 6.12). Associated PR segment depression (with PR elevation in aVR) is highly suggestive. Unlike STEMI, ST elevation typically persists for many days. T waves are upright during ST changes but subsequently invert.

The ECG in PE

In most cases, the ECG is normal or shows only sinus tachycardia. Specific abnormalities suggestive of PE include new right axis deviation, a dominant R wave in lead V_1, TWI in leads V_1–V_3 (Fig. 6.11) or right bundle branch block (Fig. 6.13). The 'classical' ECG finding of a deep, slurred S wave in I with a Q wave and TWI in III ('$S_1Q_3T_3$') is rare.

The ECG in aortic dissection

The ECG may be normal or show non-specific abnormalities. If the dissection flap involves the ostium of a coronary artery, there may be ECG changes of a STEMI (usually inferior). The ECG may change rapidly, i.e. changes of STEMI may resolve then recur, due to differential changes in blood pressure in the true and false aortic lumens.

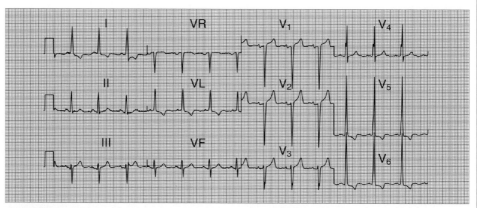

Fig. 6.10 Left ventricular hypertrophy. (From Hampton JR. The ECG Made Easy, 7th edn. Edinburgh: Churchill Livingstone, 2008.)

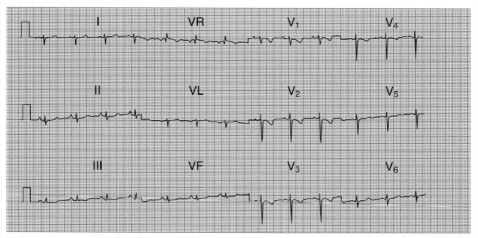

Fig. 6.11 Anterior T wave inversion due to acute right heart strain. (From Hampton JR. The ECG in Practice, 5th edn. Edinburgh: Churchill Livingstone, 2008.)

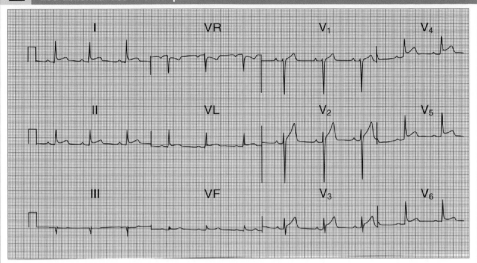

Fig. 6.12 Acute pericarditis. (From Hampton JR. 150 ECG Problems, 3rd edn. Edinburgh: Churchill Livingstone, 2008.)

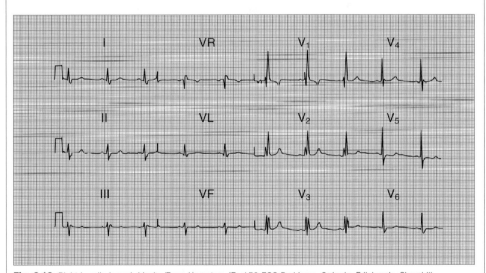

Fig. 6.13 Right bundle branch block. (From Hampton JR. 150 ECG Problems, 3rd edn. Edinburgh: Churchill Livingstone, 2008.)

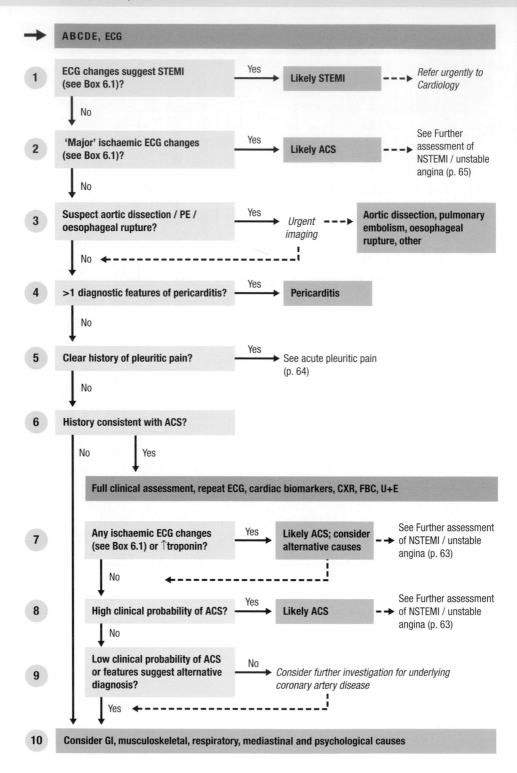

ABCDE, ECG

1 ECG changes suggest STEMI (see Box 6.1)? — Yes → **Likely STEMI** --→ *Refer urgently to Cardiology*

No

2 'Major' ischaemic ECG changes (see Box 6.1)? — Yes → **Likely ACS** --→ See Further assessment of NSTEMI / unstable angina (p. 65)

No

3 Suspect aortic dissection / PE / oesophageal rupture? — Yes → *Urgent imaging* --→ **Aortic dissection, pulmonary embolism, oesophageal rupture, other**

No

4 >1 diagnostic features of pericarditis? — Yes → **Pericarditis**

No

5 Clear history of pleuritic pain? — Yes → See acute pleuritic pain (p. 64)

No

6 History consistent with ACS?

No   Yes

Full clinical assessment, repeat ECG, cardiac biomarkers, CXR, FBC, U+E

7 Any ischaemic ECG changes (see Box 6.1) or ↑troponin? — Yes → **Likely ACS; consider alternative causes** --→ See Further assessment of NSTEMI / unstable angina (p. 63)

No

8 High clinical probability of ACS? — Yes → **Likely ACS** --→ See Further assessment of NSTEMI / unstable angina (p. 63)

No

9 Low clinical probability of ACS or features suggest alternative diagnosis? — No → *Consider further investigation for underlying coronary artery disease*

Yes

10 Consider GI, musculoskeletal, respiratory, mediastinal and psychological causes

1 ECG changes suggest STEMI (see Box 6.1)?

Patients with acute chest pain and ECG changes compatible with STEMI (see Box 6.1) are likely to benefit from immediate reperfusion therapy, e.g. primary angioplasty or thrombolysis.

Unless ECG changes are old, the history is incompatible with ACS (Box 6.4) or there is a strong clinical suspicion of aortic dissection (see below), make a diagnosis of STEMI.

- Attach cardiac monitoring and repeat ABCDE (p. 8) regularly.
- Establish the duration of the pain and whether it is ongoing.
- In younger patients with few or no risk factors for CAD, ask specifically about cocaine or amphetamine use.
- Seek urgent Cardiology input if there is diagnostic doubt, haemodynamic instability or if primary angioplasty services are available.
- If angioplasty is not available, confirm eligibility for thrombolysis (see Box 22.3, p. 207).

If ST elevation is present but does not meet the above criteria, repeat the ECG at frequent regular intervals and manage as per NSTEMI/unstable angina.

Seek urgent Cardiology input if there is any uncertainty regarding diagnosis or ECG interpretation.

2 'Major' ischaemic ECG changes (see Box 6.1)?

If the ECG shows 'major' ischaemic changes, clarify that the history is consistent with ACS (see Box 6.4) and proceed to further assessment of NSTEMI/unstable angina. Seek expert help if there is any doubt regarding ECG interpretation.

If the ECG is non-diagnostic, e.g. old left bundle branch block, paced ventricular rhythm:

- manage as per NSTEMI/unstable angina if clinical features strongly suggest ACS, e.g. pulmonary oedema or presenting symptoms very similar to previous MI
- consider a near-patient troponin assay, if available (these are specific, i.e. good to rule in, but not sensitive, i.e. not good enough to rule out, for MI)
- otherwise, await laboratory troponin results – check on admission; if negative, repeat up to 12 hours after maximal pain depending on your local protocol and local troponin assay. Some high sensitive troponin assays are more than 99% sensitive for MI at 6 hours after maximal pain, or even 3 hours at lower threshold values.

3 Suspect aortic dissection, PE or oesophageal rupture?

In the absence of clear ECG evidence of ischaemia/infarction, consider other life-threatening conditions such as aortic dissection, massive PE and oesophageal rupture. For all of these, a high index of suspicion is vital since delay in diagnosis may prove fatal and characteristic 'textbook' clinical features are often absent.

You must exclude aortic dissection in patients with severe acute chest pain and ANY of the features in Box 6.5. In the absence of these

---

Box 6.4 What symptoms are consistent with acute coronary syndrome?

Symptoms of myocardial ischaemia vary widely and often differ from textbook descriptions so, when confronted with compelling ECG evidence of ischaemia, you are likely to find that very few accounts of chest discomfort are inconsistent with ACS.

Any pain in the chest (or arms/jaw) that lasts >10 minutes, or that occurs repeatedly for minutes at a time with little or no exertion, is consistent with ACS. The task is to determine (using the ECG, cardiac biomarkers, the description of the pain and the underlying likelihood of CAD) whether the pain is likely to represent ACS.

Box 6.5 Features suggestive of acute aortic dissection

- Pain reaches maximal intensity within seconds of onset
- Main site of pain is interscapular
- Character of pain described as 'tearing' or 'ripping'
- Syncope or new focal neurological signs
- New early diastolic murmur (aortic regurgitation)
- Asymmetrical pulses (not previously documented)
- Inter-arm blood pressure differential greater than 20 mmHg
- Marfan's syndrome
- Widened mediastinum on CXR

features, consider the diagnosis in any patient with a first presentation of severe acute chest pain and no clear alternative diagnosis, especially if:

- there is a background of hypertension, previous aortic surgery, trauma or pregnancy, or
- the pain is described as 'sharp' or radiates to the back.

A normal CXR does not exclude the diagnosis. There are two characteristic age presentation peaks for dissection; by far the most common is in the 7th decade (majority male and associated with atherosclerosis) but there is also a small peak in the 3rd decade that mustn't be forgotten (mainly females and associated with connective tissue disease).

If you suspect dissection, arrange immediate contrast enhanced thoracic CT or transoesophageal echo; in unstable patients, consider bedside transthoracic echo, which will identify most type A dissections (but does not exclude the diagnosis).

Consider massive PE if there is sudden-onset, severe chest pain associated with any of the following features:

- marked dyspnoea or hypoxaemia in the absence of pulmonary oedema
- high risk of PE, e.g. malignancy, recent surgery, prolonged immobility or clinical evidence of DVT
- syncope or signs of shock (Box 30.1, p. 267) – especially with ↑JVP
- suggestive ECG changes (p. 58).

In hypotensive or peri-arrest patients, consider urgent transthoracic echo to look for evidence of acute right heart strain and exclude alternative diagnoses, e.g. cardiac tamponade and consider thrombolysis (after excluding contraindications; Box 22.3, p. 207). Otherwise, arrange prompt CT pulmonary angiography.

Suspect oesophageal perforation if acute severe chest pain arises after vomiting/retching or oesophageal instrumentation. Arrange immediate CXR if ≥1 hour after perforation (may show subcutaneous emphysema, pneumomediastinum or pleural effusion); otherwise, request water-soluble contrast barium swallow/CT and surgical review.

4 **More than one diagnostic features of pericarditis?**

Diagnose pericarditis if more than one of the following features is present:

- pain radiating to the trapezius ridge (highly specific for pericarditis) or has typical features (see p. 51)
- pericardial friction rub (85% of cases)
- typical ECG changes (p. 58; present in 80% of cases).

Request an echocardiogram to detect any associated effusion (urgently if any features of tamponade – p. 265) and assess LV function (may be impaired if associated myocarditis).

5 **Clear history of pleuritic pain?**

If the patient reports pain that clearly and consistently varies with respiratory movements, especially if described as 'sharp', 'knife-like', 'stabbing' or 'catching', then proceed to Acute pleuritic pain (p. 66). If there is any doubt, continue on the diagnostic pathway for non-pleuritic pain initially and reconsider if no clear diagnosis emerges or the patient's description becomes more suggestive of pleuritic pain.

6 **History consistent with ACS?**

Further assessment for ACS is generally not required in patients with:

- a single short-lived episode of pain, e.g. <10 minutes
- a typical episode of stable exertional angina
- a clear alternative cause for pain, e.g. herpes zoster; recent chest wall injury with tenderness on palpation
- an atypical history and very low risk of for CAD, e.g. <30 years with no risk factors.

Otherwise, consider admission for repeat ECG and cardiac biomarkers.

7 **Any ischaemic ECG changes (see Box 6.1) or ↑troponin?**

Repeat the ECG at least once and also during any further episodes of pain. Measure serum troponin concentration up to 12 hours from the onset of maximal pain, depending on the assay being used. If the ECG is non-diagnostic but you

---

Box 6.6 Conditions associated with elevation of serum troponin other than acute coronary syndrome

- Acute decompensated heart failure
- Tachy- or bradyarrhythmias
- Myocarditis/myopericarditis
- Aortic dissection
- Pulmonary embolism
- Prolonged severe hypotension/cardiac arrest
- Severe sepsis or burns
- Cardiac trauma/surgery/ablation
- Acute neurological disease, e.g. stroke, subarachnoid haemorrhage
- Congestive cardiac failure
- Infiltrative cardiac diseases, e.g. sarcoidosis, amyloidosis
- End-stage renal failure

Box 6.7 Angina symptom score

Retrosternal discomfort without atypical features[1]	1 point
Discomfort arises during physical exertion[2]	1 point
Discomfort is relieved by rest or GTN within 5–10 minutes	1 point

[1] Atypical pain features include a 'sharp' or 'stabbing' quality; significant variation with inspiration or position; or a high degree of localisation, e.g. point with tip of finger.
[2] Do not score point if discomfort is fleeting; occurs after but not during exertion; is induced only by specific movements/actions; or has inconsistent relationship, e.g. also occurs regularly without any provocation.

---

suspect ACS, check troponin early (laboratory or 'near-patient' testing) to expedite diagnosis, but always repeat at an appropriate interval after maximal pain if the initial test is negative (12 hours with conventional assays but often less with high sensitivity assays).

Diagnose ACS in patients with a convincing history of ischaemic chest pain accompanied by ↑troponin or any ECG evidence of ischaemia (see Box 6.1).

In patients with an atypical history or low underlying risk of CAD, first consider alternative causes of ↑troponin (Box 6.6) and ECG changes (see Box 6.1), e.g. PE, myopericarditis or aortic dissection, but proceed to further assessment of ACS if there is no clear alternative cause.

8 High clinical probability of ACS?

Now try to identify the subset of patients with unstable angina but no ECG evidence of ischaemia or significant myocyte necrosis. This presentation has become much less common since the advent of high sensitivity troponin assays. ACS is unlikely if biomarkers remain normal despite pain persisting at high intensity for a prolonged period, e.g. >1 hour since this degree of ischaemia would be expected to cause myocyte necrosis. However, consider unstable angina if the patient reports repeated shorter-lived episodes of chest discomfort occurring on minimal exertion or at rest, especially if:

- the symptoms mimic previous episodes of anginal chest discomfort, or
- the patient has established CAD or high likelihood of CAD (see Box 6.7) and the pain is characteristic of myocardial ischaemia (see above).

Refer patients with these features (or in whom the suspicion of ACS is otherwise high) to cardiology for further assessment.

9 Low clinical probability of ACS or features suggest alternative diagnosis?

In the absence of the features above, unstable angina is unlikely if any of the following is present:

- low likelihood of CAD (Box 6.3)
- the pain persisted at high intensity for >1 hour (would expect troponin rise if ischaemic pain) and an ECG during maximal pain was normal
- the symptoms mimic previous episodes of chest discomfort that are not suggestive of angina (Box 6.7).

Seek an alternative explanation for chest pain in these patients.

Further investigation (Box 6.8) may be helpful in patients who do not fall into either category, to look for evidence of underlying obstructive CAD.

Box 6.8 Investigations in suspected angina

- Investigations are used to seek evidence of myocardial ischaemia during cardiac stress or to confirm and/or refute underlying CAD.
- Exercise ECG and other 'stress tests' seek to establish whether increases in cardiac work induce myocardial ischaemia. During exercise, the development of typical symptoms with ST segment shift >1 mm suggests angina. Absence of symptoms and ECG changes at high workload argues against angina.
- Exercise ECG is often inconclusive and has a high 'false-positive' rate in low risk patients. Other forms of stress testing, e.g. myocardial perfusion scan or dobutamine stress echo, offer higher sensitivity/specificity and are particularly useful when the resting ECG is abnormal, e.g. left bundle branch block or the patient is unable to perform treadmill exercise.
- Stress tests are contraindicated in unstable angina, decompensated heart failure or severe hypertension.
- Coronary angiography is the definitive test for defining the presence, extent and severity of CAD. Severe stenosis in one or more vessels strongly suggests ischaemia as the cause of pain whilst the absence of significant coronary stenosis effectively excludes angina.
- In patients with a relatively low risk of CAD, CT coronary angiography is a useful, non-invasive method to rule out stable angina by excluding the presence of significant CAD.

10 Consider non-cardiac causes of chest pain

- Make a clinical diagnosis of GORD, musculoskeletal pain or herpes zoster if there are typical features (see p. 52).
- Consider paroxysmal tachyarrhythmia if the pain was accompanied by rapid palpitation and an ECG was not obtained during symptoms.
- Re-evaluate for aortic dissection or PE and consider echocardiogram/thoracic CT if ongoing pain, haemodynamic compromise or other clinical concern.
- Consider thoracic or respiratory review if there is an unexplained CXR abnormality, e.g. mediastinal/hilar mass.
- Reassess for pericarditis and arrange an echocardiogram to look for pericardial effusion, if there are any suggestive features (see step 4, above) or cardiomegaly on CXR.
- Consider hyperventilation or anxiety if there are suggestive clinical features (see p. 52) associated with $\downarrow PaCO_2$ (with normal PaO_2) and PE has been excluded.

Further assessment of NSTEMI/unstable angina

Step 1 Identify critically unwell patients

Attach cardiac monitoring to all patients with ongoing chest pain and review regularly with repeat ECG. Admit to a CCU/HDU and arrange urgent Cardiology review if you identify any of the following:

* shock (p. 267)
* pulmonary oedema
* ventricular arrhythmia, complete heart block (see Fig. 31.2, p. 279)
* ST elevation or refractory pain.

Step 2 Consider all potential factors contributing to myocardial ischaemia

In patients with ongoing pain:

* maintain SpO$_2$ ≥94%
* identify and treat tachyarrhythmias
* if any suspicion of anaemia or acute bleeding, e.g. pallor, haematemesis, melaena, check Hb urgently (prior to giving antiplatelet agents/anticoagulants)
* if tachycardic, assess and treat any ongoing pain, then consider beta-blockade (if no contraindications)
* evaluate the response to GTN spray; if pain improves, consider IV GTN infusion.

Consider paroxysmal tachyarrhythmia, e.g. atrial fibrillation, as the mechanism for NSTEMI in patients who did not have an ECG during pain, e.g. if pain associated with palpitation or previous history of arrhythmia.

Step 3 Identify high-risk patients

Risk-stratify patients using a validated scoring system such as the GRACE score (http://www.gracescore.org/website/WebVersion.aspx). The GRACE score predicts the risk of in-hospital and 6 month death in patients with ACS and can be used to aid the selection of patients for clinical and interventional procedures.

Step 4 Use cardiac biomarkers to differentiate unstable angina from NSTEMI

Measure serum troponin I or T up to 12 hours from the onset of maximal pain (can often be measured earlier with highly sensitive assays). If ↑, classify as NSTEMI; otherwise, classify as unstable angina.

6

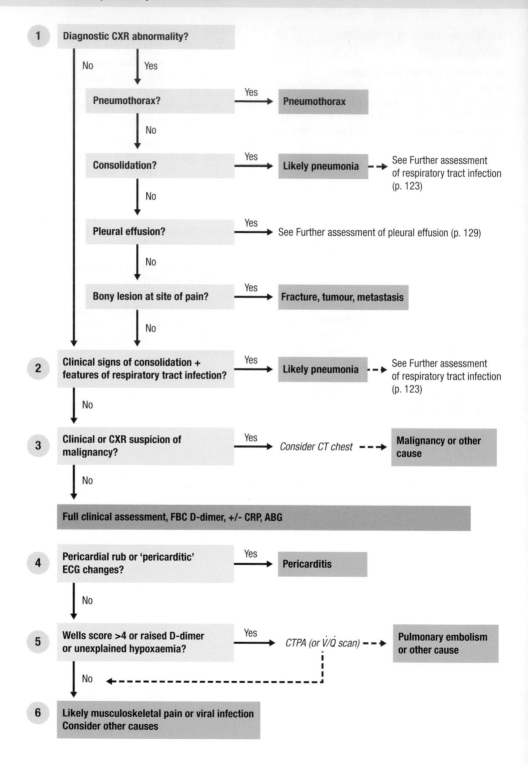

1   Diagnostic CXR abnormality?

Look carefully for:

- pneumothorax (see Fig. 12.5, p. 118) – small pneumothoraces are easily missed
- consolidation (see Figs 12.3 and 12.4, p. 118) – if present, go to further assessment of respiratory tract infection (RTI) (p. 123), especially if accompanied by cough, purulent sputum, dyspnoea or fever
- pleural effusion (see Fig. 12.6, p. 119) – if present, assess as on page 129
- rib fractures or metastatic deposits – if the latter are present, investigate for a primary lung, renal, thyroid, breast or prostate cancer or multiple myeloma.

2   Clinical signs of consolidation + features of respiratory tract infection?

Even in the absence of definitive CXR changes, pneumonia is the likely diagnosis if pleuritic pain is accompanied by:

- focal chest signs, e.g. crackles, bronchial breathing, and
- symptoms of RTI: productive cough, acute dyspnoea or fever.

If present, assess as per on page 123

3   Clinical or CXR suspicion of malignancy?

Consider further investigation with CT chest ± bronchoscopy in patients >40 years or with a history of smoking/asbestos exposure if pain is accompanied by:

- a history of weight loss
- recurrent or unexplained haemoptysis
- recent change in voice
- persistent cervical lymphadenopathy
- finger clubbing
- suspicious CXR changes (see Box 17.1, p. 163).

4   Pericardial rub or 'pericarditic' ECG changes?

Diagnose pericarditis if pleuritic pain is accompanied by typical ECG features of pericarditis (see Box 6.1) or a pericardial rub.

5   Wells score >4 or raised D-dimer or unexplained hypoxaemia?

You must exclude PE in any patient with acute pleuritic pain and no other obvious cause. A negative D-dimer test in patients with a Wells score ≤4 (see Fig. 12.7, p. 120) effectively rules out the diagnosis makes the diagnosis unlikely. Arrange further investigation with CTPA if the Wells score is >4 (irrespective of D-dimer), D-dimer is positive, or clinical suspicion is otherwise high, e.g. unexplained hypoxaemia, features of right heart strain on ECG (see Box 6.1).

CTPA may provide an alternative cause for the presentation in patients without PE.

6   Likely musculoskeletal pain or viral infection. Consider other causes

Seek a respiratory opinion and consider further imaging in patients with dyspnoea or a new CXR abnormality other than those described above. Consider drug-induced pleuritis, e.g. amiodarone, methotrexate, or pleurisy secondary to a connective tissue disorder, e.g. history or clinical features of systemic lupus erythematosus/ rheumatoid arthritis.

Otherwise, the most likely diagnoses are viral pleurisy or musculoskeletal pain. Suspect the former if there is fever, coryzal or 'flu-like' symptoms or a pleural rub; suspect the latter if there is any recent injury, prolonged severe coughing, unusually strenuous upper body activity, marked exacerbation of pain on movement or obvious tenderness on palpation.

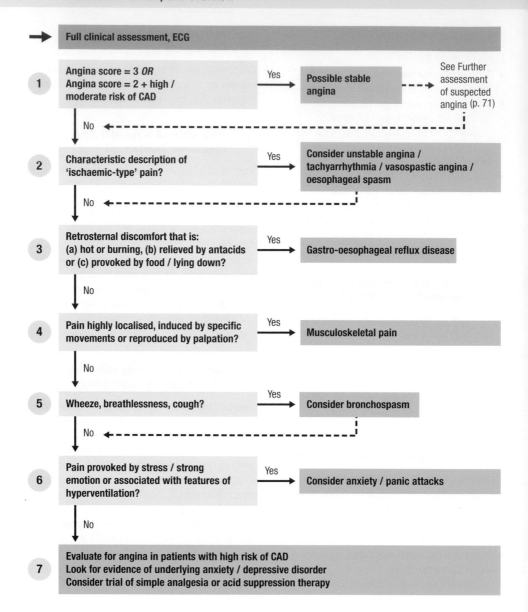

Full clinical assessment, ECG

1 Angina score = 3 *OR* Angina score = 2 + high / moderate risk of CAD — Yes → **Possible stable angina** ---▸ See Further assessment of suspected angina (p. 71)

No

2 Characteristic description of 'ischaemic-type' pain? — Yes → **Consider unstable angina / tachyarrhythmia / vasospastic angina / oesophageal spasm**

No

3 Retrosternal discomfort that is: (a) hot or burning, (b) relieved by antacids or (c) provoked by food / lying down? — Yes → **Gastro-oesophageal reflux disease**

No

4 Pain highly localised, induced by specific movements or reproduced by palpation? — Yes → **Musculoskeletal pain**

No

5 Wheeze, breathlessness, cough? — Yes → **Consider bronchospasm**

No

6 Pain provoked by stress / strong emotion or associated with features of hyperventilation? — Yes → **Consider anxiety / panic attacks**

No

7 Evaluate for angina in patients with high risk of CAD
Look for evidence of underlying anxiety / depressive disorder
Consider trial of simple analgesia or acid suppression therapy

1 Angina score = 3 *OR* Angina score = 2 + high/moderate risk of CAD?

The hallmark of stable angina is a correlation between symptoms and alterations in cardiac work. Retrosternal discomfort that consistently arises during exertion and is rapidly relieved (<5 minutes) by rest strongly suggests angina. The quality of the discomfort may vary widely and is frequently vague or non-specific. The likelihood of angina also depends on the risk of underlying CAD. With rare exceptions, coronary atherosclerosis is central to the pathogenesis of angina, so patients with a low risk of CAD have a correspondingly low risk of angina.

- Calculate the 'angina score' based on the three criteria in Box 6.7, then broadly stratify the a priori risk of CAD based on age, sex and risk factors (see Box 6.3).
- If angina score = 3, go to further assessment of possible angina, irrespective of risk factors.
- If angina score = 2, go to further assessment of possible angina unless 'low-risk' of CAD.
- Consider further assessment for possible angina in patients at high risk of CAD in whom the history is vague or unclear.

2 Characteristic description of 'ischaemic-type' pain?

The typical manifestation of myocardial ischaemia is a diffuse, poorly localized, retrosternal discomfort that radiates to the neck, jaw and left (or right) shoulder and/or arm, and has a tight, constricting, pressure-like, aching or heavy quality. It is frequently described as discomfort rather than pain. Patients often illustrate the sensation by placing a hand or fist over the centre of the chest.

Intermittent episodes of myocardial ischaemia unrelated to exertion may occur with critical coronary obstruction due to plaque rupture and thrombus formation (unstable angina), coronary artery spasm (vasospastic angina) or paroxysmal tachyarrhythmia (especially in the presence of an underlying coronary stenosis). Oesophageal spasm may closely mimic ischaemic-type discomfort and also lacks a consistent relationship to exertion.

Consider these diagnoses in patients with characteristic ischaemic-type discomfort that lacks a predictable relationship to exertion or (with the exception of unstable angina) in whom stress testing fails to demonstrate inducible myocardial ischaemia.

Suspect unstable angina and refer to cardiology if any of the following:

- new onset of symptoms within the preceding 2 weeks
- episodes of discomfort previously related to exertion but now occurring at rest
- new abnormality on resting ECG (see Box 6.1).

Suspect paroxysmal arrhythmia if any of the following:

- palpitation preceding or during symptoms
- previously documented tachyarrhythmia
- infrequent episodes of variable duration.

If suspected, attempt to document the rhythm during a typical episode of symptoms.

Suspect vasospastic angina if any of the following:

- no apparent triggers
- sudden onset of intense symptoms ± autonomic features
- short duration of episodes (2–5 minutes)
- episodes occurring in clusters.

If suspected, consider a trial of Holter ECG monitoring to look for evidence of ST elevation during symptomatic episodes.

Suspect oesophageal spasm if any of the following:

- intermittent dysphagia
- history or typical symptoms of GORD (see below)
- discomfort occurring predominantly at night or after eating.

If the history suggests GORD, consider reassessment after a trial of a proton pump inhibitor; otherwise, refer to the GI team for consideration of upper GI endoscopy/oesophageal manometry.

6

3 Retrosternal discomfort that is: (a) hot or burning, (b) relieved by antacids or (c) provoked by food/lying down?

If the pain is unlikely to be cardiac, seek typical features of other disorders. The above features suggest GORD; a symptomatic response to acid suppression therapy, e.g. proton pump inhibitor, effectively confirms the diagnosis. Upper GI endoscopy is usually not required but consider if symptoms are refractory.

4 Pain highly localized, induced by specific movements or reproduced by palpation?

Musculoskeletal pain may present in a multitude of ways. The above features are suggestive, as is a history of recent injury, strain or uncharacteristically vigorous activity. Further investigation is rarely necessary; a symptomatic response to simple analgesia helps to confirm the diagnosis.

5 Wheeze, breathlessness, cough?

Asthma and chronic obstructive pulmonary disease may be difficult to distinguish from angina on clinical grounds if symptoms are provoked by exertion and produce a sensation of chest 'tightness'. Helpful diagnostic features may include a history of cough or wheeze (especially nocturnal), diurnal variation in symptoms, the presence of wheeze on auscultation, a history of atopy and absence of risk factors for CAD. If asthma or chronic obstructive pulmonary disease is suspected, evaluate as described in Chapter 12.

6 Pain provoked by stress/strong emotion or associated with features of hyperventilation?

Attributing episodes of chest pain to anxiety can be challenging. Emotional distress increases cardiac work and may provoke angina, but symptoms that occur exclusively in this context are more likely to have a psychological origin. Associated features of panic or hyperventilation during episodes, e.g. breathlessness with 'inability to take in enough air' or a choking sensation, tingling in the extremities and light-headedness, support the diagnosis. Seek specialist input before attributing a new presentation of chest pain to anxiety in patients with a high risk of CAD.

7 Evaluate for angina in patients at high risk of CAD. Consider other causes.

In many patients it is not possible to reach a definite diagnosis. Reassess those with inconclusive investigations for angina or with a high likelihood of CAD (see Box 6.3) if symptoms persist. Where a cardiac cause has been ruled out and no other cause is apparent, patients often respond to simple reassurance. However, a minority experience severe, refractory symptoms and may merit specialist assessment for underlying psychological factors and/or management of chronic pain.

Further assessment of suspected angina

Step 1 Consider unstable angina and structural heart disease

An abrupt onset or sudden worsening of exertional chest pain indicates unstable angina - see p. 65.

Arrange echocardiography to exclude aortic stenosis and hypertrophic cardiomyopathy if the patient has an ejection systolic murmur, exertional syncope or ECG features of left ventricular hypertrophy (see Fig. 6.8).

Step 2 Confirm or refute the diagnosis

In patients >40 years with a typical history (angina score 3) and moderate/high likelihood of CAD (see Box 6.3), make a clinical diagnosis of stable angina and proceed to step 3.

If the risk of CAD is low (see Box 6.3), consider CT coronary angiography, if available, as a first-line investigation (Box 6.8). If negative, return to the algorithm for intermittent chest pain (re-enter at step 3). If positive, proceed to a stress test or invasive angiography.

Otherwise, consider a stress test (Box 6.8). If positive, diagnose stable angina and proceed to step 3. If negative, i.e. no evidence of inducible ischaemia at high stress, return to the algorithm for intermittent chest pain (re-enter at step 3). Seek input from cardiology if you have a high clinical suspicion and are unable to identify a clear alternative cause.

If results are equivocal, e.g. suboptimal test, minor abnormality, or typical symptoms without ECG changes), consider an alternative stress test or coronary angiography to clarify the diagnosis.

Step 3 Assess symptom severity and risk

The severity of angina is based not on the intensity of pain but the frequency of symptoms, impairment of exercise capacity and consequent functional limitation. As this information is used to guide treatment and monitor response, quantify symptoms accurately and determine their impact on work, hobbies and daily activities. Persistence of limiting symptoms despite anti-anginal therapy is an indication for angiography with a view to revascularisation.

Exercise ECG may identify high risk patients whose prognosis could be improved by revascularisation. Refer patients for angiography if there are any of the following abnormalities on exercise ECG:

- ST elevation
- severe or widespread ST depression
- ST depression at low workload or for a prolonged period in recovery
- fall or failure to rise in BP
- ventricular arrhythmia.

6

Consciousness is a poorly defined, ill-understood term. 'Normal' consciousness requires:

- an intact ascending reticular activating system (located in the brainstem and responsible for arousal) and
- normal function of the cerebral cortex, thalamus and their connections (responsible for cognition).

Altered consciousness results if either malfunctions. Minor defects, e.g. memory impairment, disorientation or slow cerebration, can be subtle and difficult to detect, especially if there are co-existent language, visual or speech problems. Consider multi-factorial causes contributing to altered consciousness, e.g. a patient who has taken alcohol falls in the street, sustaining a head injury, lying unnoticed for hours and becoming hypothermic.

The Glasgow Coma Scale (GCS; Table 7.1) was developed to assess/prognosticate head injury and is commonly used to record conscious level although it is less well validated in non-traumatic conditions. A GCS score <15/15 indicates altered consciousness. 'Coma' denotes a patient with no eye response and a GCS ≤8/15. Do not use terms such as semi-conscious, stuporous, obtunded, etc.

Minor disturbance of consciousness is a central feature of delirium, see Chapter 8. The assessment pathway in this chapter is appropriate for patients with a GCS <15 and:

- E <3, V <4 or M <5, i.e. >1 point drop in at least one domain
- known or suspected head injury
- a clinical picture not suggestive of delirium.

As the patient is unlikely to be able to give a clear history, it is essential to obtain a history from witnesses, relatives or ambulance crew. In particular, ask about:

- the circumstances in which the patient was found, e.g. exposure to temperature extremes or poisons
- the speed, nature and surrounding events, e.g. sudden onset – subarachnoid haemorrhage, seizure, trauma; gradual – expanding intracranial lesion, metabolic conditions; fluctuating – recurrent seizures; recent flu-like illness – meningitis, sepsis
- trauma, e.g. road traffic accident, falls, assault
- drug history (prescribed and over-the-counter), alcohol and recreational drug use
- past medical history. Important causes to consider are listed below.

Metabolic causes

- Hypo-/hyper-glycaemia.
- Hypo-/hyper-thermia.
- Hypo-/hyper-natraemia.
- Hypothyroidism.
- Metabolic acidosis.

Drugs/toxins

- Alcohol.
- Opioids, benzodiazepines, tricyclic antidepressants, barbiturates etc.
- 'Recreational' drugs, e.g. gamma-hydroxybutyrate (GHB), ketamine, mephedrone, etc.
- Carbon monoxide/other cellular toxins, e.g. cyanide.

Table 7.1 Glasgow Coma Scale

Criterion	Score
Eye opening	
Spontaneous	4
To speech	3
To pain	2
No response	1
Verbal response	
Orientated	5
Confused: talks in sentences but disorientated	4
Verbalizes: words not sentences	3
Vocalizes: sounds (groans or grunts) not words	2
No vocalization	1
Motor response	
Obeys commands	6
Localizes to pain, e.g. brings hand up beyond chin to supra-orbital pain	5
Flexion withdrawal to pain: no localisation to supra-orbital pain but flexes elbow to nail bed pressure	4
Abnormal flexion to pain	3
Extension to pain: extends elbow to nail bed pressure	2
No response	1
Record the GCS as a total and its three separate components e.g. GCS 9/15: E3, V2, M4	

CNS causes

- Trauma: intracranial bleeding (extradural, subdural, intracerebral, subarachnoid), diffuse axonal injury. Note that patients taking anticoagulants or with bleeding disorders may have intracranial bleeding following minor, unrecognized trauma.
- Infection: meningitis, encephalitis, cerebral abscess, cerebral malaria.
- Stroke: cortex or brainstem.
- Subarachnoid haemorrhage.
- Epilepsy.
- Intracranial space-occupying lesion, e.g. primary or secondary tumour.
- Hypertensive encephalopathy.
- Psychogenic.

Organ failure

- Shock.
- Respiratory failure (hypoxia and/or hypercapnia).
- Renal failure (uraemic encephalopathy).
- Liver failure (hepatic encephalopathy).

7

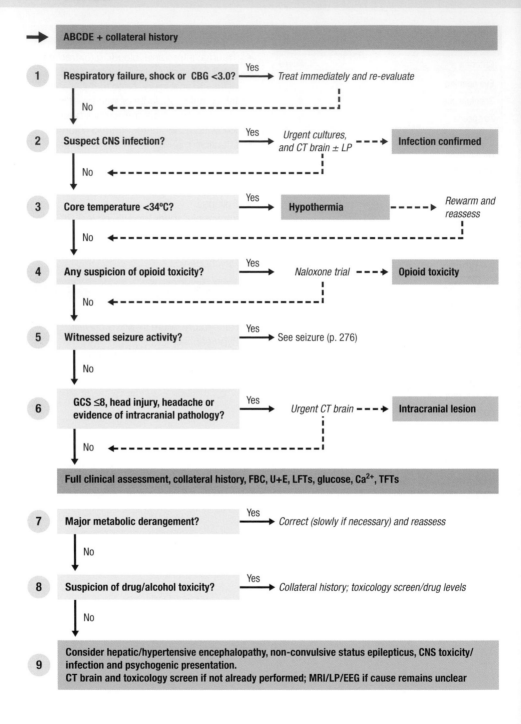

ABCDE + collateral history

1 Respiratory failure, shock or CBG <3.0? — Yes → *Treat immediately and re-evaluate*

No

2 Suspect CNS infection? — Yes → *Urgent cultures, and CT brain ± LP* - - - → **Infection confirmed**

No

3 Core temperature <34°C? — Yes → **Hypothermia** - - - → *Rewarm and reassess*

No

4 Any suspicion of opioid toxicity? — Yes → *Naloxone trial* - - - → **Opioid toxicity**

No

5 Witnessed seizure activity? — Yes → See seizure (p. 276)

No

6 GCS ≤8, head injury, headache or evidence of intracranial pathology? — Yes → *Urgent CT brain* - - - → **Intracranial lesion**

No

Full clinical assessment, collateral history, FBC, U+E, LFTs, glucose, Ca^{2+}, TFTs

7 Major metabolic derangement? — Yes → *Correct (slowly if necessary) and reassess*

No

8 Suspicion of drug/alcohol toxicity? — Yes → *Collateral history; toxicology screen/drug levels*

No

9 Consider hepatic/hypertensive encephalopathy, non-convulsive status epilepticus, CNS toxicity/infection and psychogenic presentation.
CT brain and toxicology screen if not already performed; MRI/LP/EEG if cause remains unclear

1 Respiratory failure, shock or CBG <3.0?

Ensure a patent airway and provide cervical spine control if you suspect trauma. As the GCS falls, particularly if GCS ≤8, definitive airway management, e.g. tracheal intubation, is likely to be required, so seek expert anaesthetic help early. Look for and treat rapidly reversible causes of ↓GCS as per the ABCDE assessment:

- assess oxygenation and ventilation by ABG analysis (p. 115). Treat hypoxia and hypercapnia urgently
- give a therapeutic/diagnostic trial of naloxone (see below) if $PaCO_2$ is ↑ or any evidence of respiratory depression
- look for shock (see Box 30.1, p. 267); if present, assess and treat as per Chapter 30
- check a capillary blood glucose reading ('CBG'); if <3.0 mmol/L, send blood for formal laboratory glucose measurement but treat immediately with IV dextrose or IV/IM glucagon *without waiting for the result*. In patients with malnutrition/chronic alcohol excess, consider slow IV thiamine to prevent the (theoretical) risk of precipitating Wernicke's encephalopathy.

Reassess if confusion persists despite effective correction of all of the above.

2 Suspect CNS infection?

Suspect CNS infection in any patient with ↓GCS accompanied by meningism (Box 18.2, p. 169), a new-onset maculopapular or purpuric rash, or fever. If malaria is a possibility, e.g. recent travel to endemic area, perform thick and thin blood films and seek immediate expert advice. Otherwise, take blood cultures and throat swabs, give empirical IV antibiotics/antivirals and arrange an urgent brain CT. If there is no clinical or CT contraindication, perform LP for CSF analysis (see Table 18.1, p. 171).

3 Core temperature <34°C?

Measure core temperature with a low-reading rectal thermometer in any patient with a tympanic reading <35°C or clinical suspicion of hypothermia, e.g. prolonged immobility or exposure to wet and cold conditions.

Suspect a contribution to altered consciousness from hypothermia if the core temperature is <34°C. Rewarm and reassess whilst searching for additional causes. Check TFTs and consider treatment with IV tri-iodothyronine (T3) or IV levothyroxine (T4) (preceded by IV corticosteroid) if there is any suspicion of myxoedema coma.

4 Any suspicion of opioid toxicity?

Give a therapeutic/diagnostic trial of naloxone if the patient has received any opioid medication, is a known or suspected 'recreational' user, has small pupils or has no obvious alternative cause for altered consciousness. Any rapid improvement in conscious level, increase in respiratory rate/depth or pupil dilation indicates that opioids are contributing, at least in part, to the clinical state. The half-life of naloxone is shorter than most opioid/opioid metabolites, so further doses or an infusion are likely to be needed.

5 Witnessed seizure activity?

A clear, detailed history from an eyewitness is crucial. ↓GCS is common post-ictal, but seizures can be precipitated by a wide spectrum of conditions including hypoglycaemia, head injury ± intracranial haematoma, alcohol withdrawal, drug overdose, e.g. tricyclic antidepressants, infection etc.

In status epilepticus, associated hypoxia/hypercapnia aggravates the cerebral injury and mortality is ~10%. Assess further as described in Chapter 31.

7

6 GCS ≤8, head injury, headache or evidence of intracranial pathology?

Once you have identified and treated major physiological derangement, life-threatening infection and rapidly reversible causes of ↓GCS, it is vital to identify an intracranial cause of altered consciousness. In general, immediate brain CT is required in patients with any of:

- GCS ≤8
- a history of headache, focal neurological symptoms, or lateralising neurological signs, e.g. unilateral pupillary abnormality, absence of limb movement or extensor plantar response, or signs of ↑ICP (Box 22.2, p. 199)
- known or suspected head injury
- CSF shunt in situ.

Patients must be accompanied throughout by an individual who can provide advanced airway/breathing support as intubation and controlled ventilation may be needed.

7 Major metabolic derangement?

Decreased GCS is common in hypo- and hypernatraemia. It tends to reflect the rate of sodium alteration rather than absolute values (see p. 88). If the disturbance is known to be acute, correct promptly then reassess; otherwise, correct cautiously, at a slow rate, with frequent remeasurement to avoid excessive neuronal fluid shifts and consequent cerebral oedema or central pontine myelinolysis. There may be a lag between correction of the metabolic derangement and return of normal conscious level.

Decreased GCS may be a feature of diabetic ketoacidosis (DKA). Always consider DKA if the patient has Type 1 diabetes mellitus; confirm the diagnosis by identifying metabolic acidosis on ABG, ketonuria on urinalysis or blood ketones.

Suspect Hyperosmolar Hyperglycaemic State (HHS), (formally HyperOsmolar Non-Ketotic coma - HONK) rather than DKA if there is marked hyperglycaemia (>30 mmol/L) and hyperosmolarity (>320 mOsm/kg) without significant hyperketonaemia (<3.0 mmol/L) or acidosis (pH >7.3, bicarbonate >15 mmol/L) – hypovolaemia and altered consciousness are common features.

Suspect a contribution to altered consciousness from uraemia or disturbances of plasma calcium, magnesium or phosphate, only if derangement is severe.

8 Suspicion of drug/alcohol toxicity?

Even in patients with a history or features of acute or chronic alcohol intake, never assume that altered consciousness is due to alcohol alone. The correlation between breath or blood alcohol levels and conscious level is poor, so beyond confirming that alcohol is present, these values are of limited help and can be potentially misleading. In particular, look for (and treat) alcohol-related hypoglycaemia, occult head injury, intracranial bleeding and recreational drug use or overdose.

Examine for characteristic clinical 'toxidromes' (Table 7.2) in any patient with suspected overdose but remember that mixed overdoses or cocktails of drugs (often with alcohol) are common and

Table 7.2 Common toxidromes associated with coma/altered consciousness

Symptom/signs	Drug
Respiratory depression, small pupils	Opioids
Dilated pupils, tachycardia, hyper-reflexia, ↑muscle tone, urinary retention. If severe: cardiac rhythm/ECG abnormalities, ↓BP, seizures	Tricyclic antidepressants
Hypotension, respiratory depression, bradycardia, ↓ muscle tone	Barbiturates, benzodiazepines
Tachycardia, ↑BP, arrhythmias, dilated pupils, tremor, agitation	Sympathomimetics, cocaine, ecstasy, amphetamines, SSRIs
Agitation, myoclonus, seizures, nausea, bradycardia, coma	Gamma-hydroxybutyrate (GHB)
Vivid hallucinations, agitation, dysphoria, nystagmus, autonomic disturbance, seizures, coma	Ketamine and phencyclidine (PCP)
Euphoria, drowsiness, arrhythmias, laryngospasm	Solvents

respiratory/cardiovascular depression (hypotension, arrhythmias etc.) may predominate in any severe poisoning. Measure paracetamol and salicylate levels (± lithium and iron, if indicated) and, if there is a strong suspicion of illicit drug use, perform a urine toxicology screen. See www.npis.org or http://www.toxbase.org for further information.

Consider carbon monoxide poisoning. The features of CO poisoning are non-specific; the 'classic' description of cherry-red mucous membranes/skin is very rare. Severe metabolic acidosis and ECG changes of ischaemia/infarction with arrhythmias and hypotension may be found. Some pulse oximeters can measure carboxyhaemoglobin (COHb), but confirm with measurement of COHb on arterial or venous blood sample. The COHb value at presentation is not a good guide to conscious level and the half-life of COHb (~4 hours breathing room air) will be significantly less if the patient has been given oxygen. Extrapolation back to the time of exposure will indicate the peak level more accurately.

9 Consider further investigation if no clear cause identified

If the cause remains unclear, arrange CT brain and send a toxicology screen if not already performed. Consider hepatic encephalopathy if the patient has known or suspected liver disease, or hypertensive encephalopathy if BP is consistently >180/120 mmHg with hypertensive retinopathy or evidence of renal involvement. Otherwise, seek neurological and/or critical care input and consider MRI (brainstem pathology), EEG (non-convulsive status, hepatic encephalopathy) and LP (CNS infection).

Psychogenic unresponsiveness is a diagnosis of exclusion, but consider it if comprehensive investigation fails to reveal an underlying cause and there are suggestive signs, e.g. response to tickling, resistance to passive eye opening and gaze deviating towards the floor in any position.

7

Confusion (impaired cognition) is global impairment of mental function.

Delirium is an abrupt decline in cognitive function that follows a fluctuating course and is accompanied by impaired attention, (e.g. easily distracted, unable to maintain focus) and disturbed consciousness ('hyperalert'/agitated or drowsy/↓awareness). Common associated features include reversal of the sleep–wake cycle, hallucinations, delusions and altered emotion/psychomotor behaviour.

Dementia is a chronic, progressive decline in cognitive function without disturbance of consciousness.

The initial challenge with confused patients is finding them (sometimes literally). Agitated, restless patients rapidly attract attention but those with 'hypoactive delirium' are quiet, withdrawn and easily missed. In patients with pre-existing dementia, delirium may be overlooked unless baseline cognitive function is established. It is also possible to mislabel dysphasic, deaf or depressed patients as confused.

Delirium

The differential diagnosis of delirium is wide and, in patients with a 'vulnerable brain' (Box 8.1), includes almost any acute physical, mental or environmental insult. Causes are listed below; those shown in bold are unlikely to be solely responsible for delirium, except in patients with a 'vulnerable brain'.

Drugs

- Alcohol*.
- Opioids*.
- Benzodiazepines*.
- Anticonvulsants.
- **Tricyclic antidepressants*.**
- **Anticholinergics.**
- **Antihistamines.**
- Antipsychotics*.
- Lithium.
- Corticosteroids (especially high-dose).
- Baclofen.
- Levodopa/dopamine agonists.
- Digoxin.

indicates that confusion may arise from either drug effects or withdrawal.

Metabolic/physiological disturbance

- Hypoxia.
- Hypercapnia.
- Shock.
- Hypo/hyperthermia.
- Hypo/hyperglycaemia.
- Hyponatraemia.
- **Hypo**/hypercalcaemia.
- **Dehydration.**
- Uraemia.
- Metabolic acidosis.
- Hepatic encephalopathy.
- Hypo/hyperthyroidism.

Infection

- CNS infection:
  - meningitis (bacterial, viral, fungal, tuberculosis)
  - encephalitis
  - cerebral abscess
  - cerebral malaria.
- Non-CNS infection:
  - sepsis
  - pneumonia
  - **urinary tract**
  - **biliary/intra-abdominal**
  - **endocarditis.**

Intracranial causes

- Seizures (post-ictal state).
- Haemorrhage.
- Space-occupying lesion.
- Head injury.
- ↑intracranial pressure.

Box 8.1 Delirium and the 'vulnerable brain'

When assessing delirium, consider predisposing factors, as well as acute precipitants. Elderly patients (especially >80 years) and those with pre-existing cognitive impairment (diagnosed or undiagnosed), frailty, multiple sensory deficits, chronic alcohol excess or any significant underlying brain disorder, e.g. cerebrovascular disease, Parkinson's disease, multiple sclerosis have a reduced threshold for developing delirium. These patients have a 'vulnerable brain' and delirium may result from relatively minor insults that would not normally impair cognitive function in healthy patients without such predisposing factors.

Other causes

- Pain.
- Postoperative.
- Constipation.
- Urinary retention.
- Acute abdominal pathology (pancreatitis, appendicitis).
- Myocardial infarction.
- Carbon monoxide.
- Acute thiamine deficiency (Wernicke's encephalopathy).
- Paraneoplastic syndromes.
- Cerebral vasculitis.
- Acute intermittent porphyria.
- Heavy metal poisoning, e.g. lead, arsenic.
- Unusual stimuli and sensory impairment.

Dementia/chronic cognitive impairment

Common causes

- Alzheimer's disease.
- Vascular disease.
- Lewy body dementia.

'Reversible' causes

- Vitamin B_{12}/folate deficiency.
- Subdural haemorrhage.
- Hypothyroidism.
- Normal pressure hydrocephalus.
- HIV.
- Neurosyphilis.
- Wilson's disease.

Other causes

- Frontotemporal dementias.
- Korsakoff's psychosis.
- Multiple sclerosis.
- Progressive multifocal leucoencephalopathy.
- Subacute sclerosing panencephalitis.
- (Variant) Creutzfeldt–Jakob disease.
- Huntington's disease.

Disorders that may mimic confusion

- Depression.
- Dysphasia.
- Deafness.
- Acute psychosis.
- Behavioural disturbance.
- Amnesic syndromes.

8

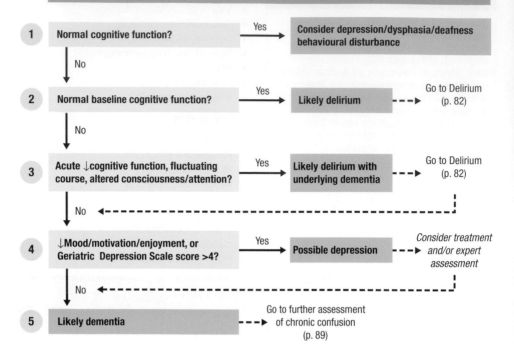

Full clinical assessment, collateral history, AMT (Box 2.4) & 4-AT test (Box 8.2)

1 Normal cognitive function? — Yes → Consider depression/dysphasia/deafness behavioural disturbance

No ↓

2 Normal baseline cognitive function? — Yes → Likely delirium - - -> Go to Delirium (p. 82)

No ↓

3 Acute ↓cognitive function, fluctuating course, altered consciousness/attention? — Yes → Likely delirium with underlying dementia - - -> Go to Delirium (p. 82)

No ←- - - - - - - - - - - - - - - - -

4 ↓Mood/motivation/enjoyment, or Geriatric Depression Scale score >4? — Yes → Possible depression - - -> *Consider treatment and/or expert assessment*

No ←- - - - - - - - - - - - - - - - -

5 Likely dementia - - -> Go to further assessment of chronic confusion (p. 89)

Clinical tool
The 4AT: rapid assessment test for delirium and cognitive impairment

The 4AT is a validated, sensitive tool for diagnosing delirium. It contains four elements. Scored as follows:
≥4: possible delirium +/– cognitive impairment
1–3: possible cognitive impairment
0: delirium or cognitive impairment unlikely (but delirium still possible if [4] information incomplete)

[1] Alertness
  Normal   0
  Mild sleepiness for <10 seconds after waking, then normal   0
  Clearly abnormal   4
  This includes patients who are drowsy, or agitated/hyperactive. Attempt to rouse with speech or gentle touch.

[2] AMT4
Age, date of birth, place (name of hospital or building), current year
  No mistakes   0
  1 mistake   1
  2 or more mistakes/untestable   2

[3] Attention
Ask the patient to recite the months of the year in backwards order, starting at December. One prompt is permitted to assist initial understanding.
  Achieves 7 months or more correctly   0
  Starts but scores <7 months/refuses to start   1
  Untestable (cannot start because unwell, drowsy, inattentive)   2

[4] Acute change or fluctuating course
Is there evidence of significant change or fluctuation in alertness/cognition/other mental function, e.g. paranoia/hallucinations arising over last 2 weeks and still evident in last 24 hours
  No   0
  Yes   4

1   Normal cognitive function?

Disorientation, forgetfulness and muddled thinking may be apparent from normal conversation but confirm with an objective assessment, e.g. the abbreviated mental test (AMT; Box 2.4, p. 14) or mini-mental state examination (MMSE). Use these tools to screen for confusion in all patients with a 'vulnerable brain' (Box 8.1). Ensure that apparent cognitive impairment is not due to communication problems (deafness, dysarthria, language barriers) or an isolated disorder of comprehension (receptive dysphasia), word-finding difficulty (expressive dysphasia), memory (amnesic syndrome), behaviour or mood. Patients with depression often score poorly in formal testing through refusal to volunteer answers rather than making mistakes – if these patients are encouraged (or treated), performance may improve.

2   Normal baseline cognitive function?

Establish baseline cognitive function and any recent change in mental status by speaking to relatives/friends/carers and checking previous cognitive assessments. Thorough questioning is important as relatives may have the impression that baseline cognition was normal – as the patient was in a familiar environment, seeing familiar people, talking about familiar topics and not being pressed on recent events – even if baseline cognition was, in fact, impaired.

3   Acute ↓cognitive function, fluctuating course, altered consciousness/attention?

Use the 4AT assessment test (Clinical tool, p. 80) to diagnose delirium. Having established baseline cognitive function, look for any evidence of an acute change. Spend time speaking with the patient and observing behaviour. In addition to direct observation, seek evidence of fluctuation through discussion with nursing staff or review of overnight reports. Delirium is frequently superimposed on dementia (acute on chronic confusion) – look for important clues such as sudden decline in cognitive abilities, alteration of consciousness, fluctuating course and difficulty concentrating.

4   ↓Mood/motivation/enjoyment, or Geriatric Depression Scale score >4?

8

Depression can mimic or exacerbate dementia. Ask patients if they feel low in mood but also enquire about things they take pleasure in (do they still enjoy them?), as well as biological symptoms (early morning waking, ↓appetite, ↓weight). During conversation, note expressions of guilt, worthlessness, pessimism and other negative thoughts (especially if exaggerated or incongruent with circumstances) and look for psychomotor retardation, lack of depth or variety in affect, and poor eye contact. Scoring systems, e.g. the geriatric depression scale (GDS), may assist diagnosis. If uncertain, refer for specialist evaluation or reassess after a trial of treatment.

5   Likely dementia

There is no absolute division between acute and chronic confusion in terms of timing or causes. Even if the cause has been removed, it can take many weeks for a delirium to resolve fully. Further, chronic confusion can fluctuate. However, if confusion has persisted for >12 weeks without an obvious acute cause or evidence of improvement, see 'Further assessment of chronic confusion' (p. 89).

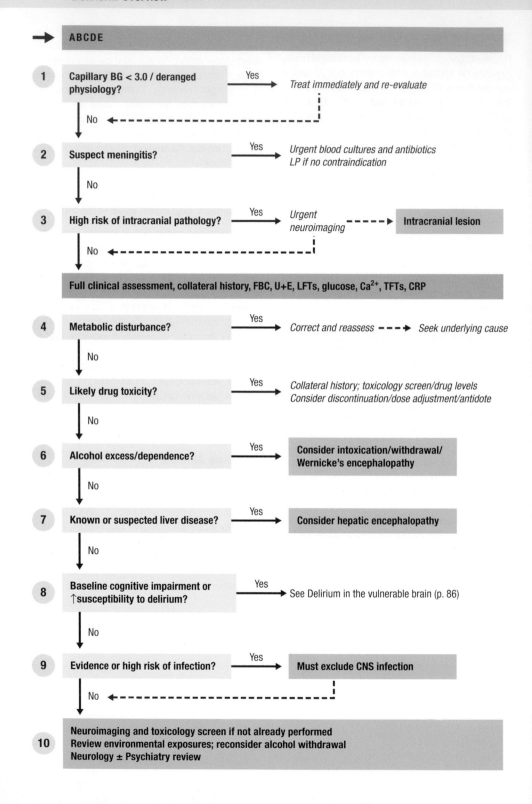

ABCDE

1 **Capillary BG < 3.0 / deranged physiology?** — Yes → *Treat immediately and re-evaluate*

No

2 **Suspect meningitis?** — Yes → *Urgent blood cultures and antibiotics*
LP if no contraindication

No

3 **High risk of intracranial pathology?** — Yes → *Urgent neuroimaging* ----→ **Intracranial lesion**

No

Full clinical assessment, collateral history, FBC, U+E, LFTs, glucose, Ca^{2+}, TFTs, CRP

4 **Metabolic disturbance?** — Yes → *Correct and reassess* ---→ *Seek underlying cause*

No

5 **Likely drug toxicity?** — Yes → *Collateral history; toxicology screen/drug levels*
Consider discontinuation/dose adjustment/antidote

No

6 **Alcohol excess/dependence?** — Yes → **Consider intoxication/withdrawal/ Wernicke's encephalopathy**

No

7 **Known or suspected liver disease?** — Yes → **Consider hepatic encephalopathy**

No

8 **Baseline cognitive impairment or ↑susceptibility to delirium?** — Yes → See Delirium in the vulnerable brain (p. 86)

No

9 **Evidence or high risk of infection?** — Yes → **Must exclude CNS infection**

No

10 **Neuroimaging and toxicology screen if not already performed**
Review environmental exposures; reconsider alcohol withdrawal
Neurology ± Psychiatry review

1 Capillary BG <3.0/deranged physiology?

Evaluate and treat respiratory failure (Ch. 12), shock (Ch. 30), depressed consciousness (Ch. 7), hypothermia and seizure (Ch. 31) before considering other causes of delirium. Exclude new or worsening hypercapnia in any patient with chronic type 2 respiratory failure or significant chronic lung disease. If the capillary BG is <3.0 mmol/L, send blood for laboratory glucose measurement but treat immediately, without waiting for the result. Reassess if confusion persists despite effective correction.

2 Suspect meningitis?

Assume meningitis/encephalitis if the patient has meningism (Box 18.2, p. 169), a purpuric rash or a febrile illness with headache, seizures, focal neurological signs or no obvious alternative source. Take blood cultures and throat swabs and give empirical IV antibiotics immediately. If there are no contraindications, perform an LP (p. 170). Request CT prior to LP if seizure, focal neurological signs, GCS <15 or papilloedema.

3 High risk of intracranial pathology?

Consider urgent CT brain to exclude a structural CNS cause if any of the following are present:

- new focal neurological signs or ataxia
- first seizure
- drowsiness (if you suspect opioid toxicity, give a trial of naloxone before CT)
- recent head injury
- sudden severe headache
- any fall/trauma in a patient on anticoagulation.

In patients with active malignancy, immunosuppression or recent falls, look for other causes of delirium, but have a low threshold for early neuroimaging to exclude intracranial metastases/abscess/haemorrhage.

4 Metabolic disturbance?

Review blood chemistry for metabolic disturbance; check laboratory glucose, even if capillary BG is within the normal range. The healthy brain is relatively resistant to metabolic insult so do not attribute confusion solely to modest biochemical derangement. However, delirium is likely to be explained by hypoglycaemia, hypothyroidism or, if severe: dehydration, acidosis, $\downarrow Na^+$ (especially <120 mmol/L), $\uparrow Ca^{2+}$ (>3.0 mmol/L) or hyperglycaemia, e.g. hyperosmolar hyperglycaemic state (p. 297 [Ch. 34]). Uraemia is an unusual cause of acute confusion in the non-vulnerable brain but may result in toxic accumulation of medication.

The vulnerable brain is more sensitive to metabolic derangement – even mild dehydration, renal impairment or glycaemic/electrolyte/thyroid disturbance may impair cognition. Correct any disturbances but continue to search for additional contributing factors.

See 'Further assessment of hyponatraemia' (p. 88) in any patient with unexplained $\downarrow Na^+$.

5 Likely drug toxicity?

Illicit drug use or poisoning

Substance abuse is a common cause of acute confusion/psychosis in younger patients. If it is suspected, use all available sources of information to establish what has been taken and when. Look for characteristic clinical features of toxicity (see Table 7.2, p. 76) and consider a urine toxicology screen. See www.npis.org for further information. Give naloxone in patients with features of acute opioid toxicity – a response should occur within seconds to minutes; observe closely for symptoms of acute opioid withdrawal (sweating, tremor, agitation, seizures).

Prescribed medication

Anticonvulsants, lithium, sedatives and opioids can cause confusion, even in healthy brains. Many other drugs may precipitate delirium in the vulnerable brain (see Box 8.1), especially tricyclic antidepressants, anticholinergics, e.g. oxybutynin, antipsychotics and antihistamines. Even if they are normally well tolerated, these agents may contribute to delirium in the context of other acute insults. Benzodiazepines can have a paradoxical effect, worsening confusion and agitation. Abrupt withdrawal of benzodiazepines and opioids can also precipitate delirium, often several days after stopping.

Verify all drugs and dosages with the patient/relatives/carers. Check how frequently PRN medications, especially benzodiazepines and opioids, are used at home and ensure they have not been inadvertently omitted, reduced or reinstated in hospital. Consider a trial cessation or ↓dose of any drug with potential CNS side-effects (see Table 7.2, p. 76), especially if recently introduced or increased. Weigh the likelihood of toxicity against ongoing treatment benefit and predictable problems on discontinuation. Where necessary, taper the dose gradually to avoid withdrawal symptoms.

6   Alcohol excess/dependence?

Acute alcohol intoxication

Acute alcohol intoxication is the most common cause of altered mental status in the emergency department but may coexist with other pathology, e.g. head injury, liver injury, nutritional deficiency. Confirm the presence of alcohol with breath or blood tests but always search for additional causes of confusion.

Alcohol withdrawal

This may present early, e.g. 6–12 hours after cessation of drinking, or late, e.g. 2–3 days after hospital admission. Typical symptoms include confusion, agitation, hallucinations and adrenergic over-stimulation (tremor, sweating, tachycardia). The diagnosis is obvious in patients with a florid presentation and clear history of alcohol excess/dependence but consider it in all cases of unexplained delirium. Screen all patients for alcohol problems (Box 2.1, p. 11), identify elderly patients with subtle alcohol dependence, e.g. 'large' daily sherry. If in doubt, obtain a collateral history and look for an isolated increase in GGT/mean cell volume. Seizures may complicate severe withdrawal but consider neuroimaging

if first fit, focal neurological signs or evidence of head injury.

Wernicke's encephalopathy

Consider thiamine deficiency and the need for supplementation in all patients with acute confusion on a background of chronic alcohol excess. Give immediate IV thiamine if there is short-term memory loss, diplopia, gaze palsy, nystagmus, ataxia or severe malnutrition.

7   Known or suspected liver disease?

Suspect hepatic encephalopathy in any patient with an existing diagnosis or clinical features of cirrhosis. Constructional apraxia (inability to draw a star) and/or asterixis (Fig. 19.1, p. 180), together with the absence of florid hallucinations/adrenergic features may differentiate hepatic encephalopathy from alcohol withdrawal in patients with alcoholic liver disease. If you suspect encephalopathy, seek and treat potential precipitants, including spontaneous bacterial peritonitis (an ascitic tap is mandatory if ascites is present), other infections, dehydration, constipation, subclinical GI bleeding and drugs with CNS toxicity.

Consider acute liver failure and seek urgent expert advice in patients without cirrhosis who have jaundice and very high ALT or ↑PT. Perform an ABG to exclude hypercapnia if there is asterixis without features of liver disease.

8   Baseline cognitive impairment or ↑susceptibility to delirium?

The diagnostic approach now depends on the underlying threshold for developing delirium. If any feature in Box 8.1 is present, proceed to 'Delirium in the vulnerable brain: overview of further assessment'.

9 Evidence or high risk of infection?

Suspect CNS infection in patients with ↑temperature/WBC/CRP or ↑susceptibility (foreign travel, immunosuppression, animal bite). Do not attribute confusion to minor non-CNS infections.

Seek urgent input from an ID unit if the patient has recently travelled to the developing world, has received an animal or tick bite, is HIV-positive or is taking immunosuppressive therapy, e.g. long-term steroids, chemotherapy. Send blood for thick and thin films if travel to a malaria-endemic region has been undertaken within the last 3 months. Otherwise, undertake LP to exclude CNS infection.

If CNS infection has been excluded, treat any other apparent source of infection but continue to search for additional causes of confusion.

10 Neuroimaging and toxicology screen. Consider other causes. Neurology ± Psychiatry review

If not already carried out, perform neuroimaging and LP to exclude CNS infection and structural disease. If CT is non-diagnostic, consider MRI brain. Check carboxyhaemoglobin levels for carbon monoxide toxicity if there is associated headache or if the patient has been exposed to smoke/exhaust fumes (though levels may correlate poorly with symptoms). Measure urinary porphyrins (liaising with the biochemistry laboratory in advance), especially if there is associated abdominal pain. Test for HIV.

If the cause is still not apparent, seek expert neurological ± psychiatric input. EEG may assist in the diagnosis of atypical seizures, toxic encephalopathies or unusual neurodegenerative diseases. Other tests to consider include autoimmune/vasculitis antibodies (cerebral vasculitis?), syphilis/Lyme disease serology, antineuronal antibodies (paraneoplastic syndrome?) and heavy metal levels in blood and urine.

8

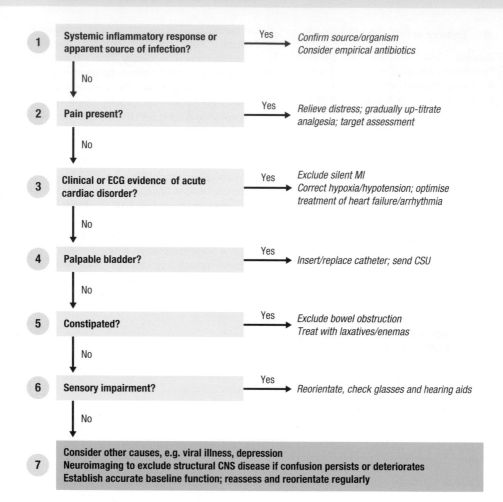

1 Systemic inflammatory response or apparent source of infection? — Yes → *Confirm source/organism*
Consider empirical antibiotics

No

2 Pain present? — Yes → *Relieve distress; gradually up-titrate analgesia; target assessment*

No

3 Clinical or ECG evidence of acute cardiac disorder? — Yes → *Exclude silent MI*
Correct hypoxia/hypotension; optimise treatment of heart failure/arrhythmia

No

4 Palpable bladder? — Yes → *Insert/replace catheter; send CSU*

No

5 Constipated? — Yes → *Exclude bowel obstruction*
Treat with laxatives/enemas

No

6 Sensory impairment? — Yes → *Reorientate, check glasses and hearing aids*

No

7 Consider other causes, e.g. viral illness, depression
Neuroimaging to exclude structural CNS disease if confusion persists or deteriorates
Establish accurate baseline function; reassess and reorientate regularly

1 Likely source of infection or systemic inflammatory response?

In the vulnerable brain, even minor infections can trigger delirium. Infections may present 'atypically' lacking characteristic symptoms and signs.

In patients with ↑temperature/WBC/CRP, take blood cultures and look for a septic focus (p. 142). Also consider atypical presentations of acute abdominal pathologies, e.g. perforation, pancreatitis, appendicitis, cholecystitis or diverticulitis. Re-examine regularly, check amylase and have a low threshold for abdominal imaging – especially if there is any pain/tenderness or deranged LFTs. Consider LP if the source remains elusive.

Even in the absence of ↑temperature/WBC/ CRP, consider empirical antibiotic treatment if there is a convincing focus of infection, e.g. positive MSU or new purulent sputum, but weigh the likelihood of bacterial infection against complications such as GI upset or *Clostridium difficile* diarrhoea.

2 Pain present?

Pain can cause or contribute to delirium in the vulnerable brain and may be difficult to assess if the patient is agitated or muddled. Wherever possible, identify and treat the underlying cause using simple analgesia/non-pharmacological measures as first-line treatment but do not leave patients in distress. Where opioids are required, carefully up-titrate and monitor.

3 Clinical or ECG evidence of acute cardiac disorder?

Occasionally, myocardial infarction (MI) presents as delirium. Seek urgent cardiology input if the ECG meets the criteria for ST elevation MI. Check troponin and assess further for acute coronary syndrome if there are other indicative ECG changes (p. 51). Cardiac failure may contribute to delirium through hypoxia or cerebral hypoperfusion. Avoid hypotension where possible (review medication) and correct hypoxia and anaemia. Treat any brady- or tachyarrhythmias and consider diuretic if there is fluid overload.

4-6 Palpable bladder/Constipated/Sensory impairment?

Actively look for and treat urinary retention, constipation and nutritional deficiency (including B_{12}/folate). If a urinary catheter is required, it may be possible to withhold anticholinergic drugs for detrusor instability. Patients with moderate to severe dementia are at high risk of becoming acutely confused when presented with unusual surroundings, people and stimuli. Provide frequent reassurance and reorientation, encourage visits from family members, check that patients have their normal glasses and hearing aids, and ensure adequate lighting.

7 Consider other causes. Neuroimaging. Establish baseline function

In the absence of another indication for brain imaging, it may be reasonable to persevere with the above measures for several days. However, arrange CT brain to exclude subdural haemorrhage and other structural pathology if the patient fails to improve or deteriorates. Review medications daily and reassess regularly for pain, metabolic disturbance or infection. Make a detailed assessment of baseline cognitive ability and level of function. Finally, consider rarer causes, as described for the non-vulnerable brain.

8

Further assessment of hyponatraemia

Step 1 Confirm true hyponatraemia

Apparent hyponatraemia may result from drip arm contamination, laboratory/labelling error, or 'pseudohyponatraemia' due to hyperlipidaemia, hyperproteinaemia, hyperglycaemia or high plasma ethanol. Check plasma osmolality (usually normal in pseudohyponatraemia) and recheck Na^+ if the result appears spurious.

Step 2 Estimate the rate of Na⁺ decline

A rapid $\downarrow$ in plasma Na^+ may lead to life-threatening cerebral oedema, and requires prompt correction. In contrast a gradual $\downarrow$ in Na^+ allows osmotic adaptation by cerebral neurons and rapid correction may lead to irreversible and brainstem damage (central pontine myelinolysis).

It is therefore critical to distinguish acute (<72 hours) from chronic (>72 hours) hyponatraemia. Suspect chronic if any of the following features is present:

- recent U+E results demonstrating a progressive decline in plasma Na^+
- slowly progressive onset of symptoms, e.g. anorexia, lethargy, confusion
- asymptomatic or only mild symptoms with a plasma Na^+ ≤125 mmol/L
- no clear cause for a sudden decrease in plasma Na^+ (see below).

In these patients, correct Na^+ with extreme care. Recheck U+E every 2–4 hours, and aim for a rise in plasma Na^+ of ≤8 mmol/day.

Suspect acute hyponatraemia if:

- abrupt onset of symptoms within the last 48 hours OR
- major symptoms (severe confusion, $\downarrow$ GCS, seizures) with Na^+ ≥ 120 mmol/L,

especially with a history of sudden increase in free water intake, e.g., excessive IV dextrose administration (especially postoperatively) or polydipsia.

If you suspect acute hyponatraemia, seek urgent expert advice but, in an emergency, aim to increase plasma Na^+ by 4–6 mmol/L over 1–2 hours then reassess.

Step 3 Assess volume status

Clear evidence of either $\uparrow$ or $\downarrow$ECF volume is very helpful in determining the underlying cause. Categorize the patient as:

- 'hypervolaemic' if there is evidence of fluid overload, e.g. oedema, $\uparrow$JVP, ascites

- 'hypovolaemic' if there is evidence of fluid depletion, e.g. dry mucous membranes, $\downarrow$skin turgor, thirst, $\downarrow$JVP
- 'euvolaemic' if neither of the above are present.

The most common causes of hypervolaemic hyponatraemia are cardiac failure, cirrhosis, oliguric renal failure and nephrotic syndrome. If the cause is not obvious, check for proteinuria, perform an echocardiogram and assess for evidence of cirrhosis (p. 176).

In hypovolaemic hyponatraemia there is Na^+ and water depletion, with relatively greater Na^+ loss. The most common causes are excessive diuretic therapy and acute diarrhoea/vomiting.

If the source of Na^+ and water loss is not obvious, measure urine sodium. The normal response of the kidneys to salt and water depletion is to minimize Na^+ excretion. If urine Na^+ is appropriately low (<20 mmol/L), suspect GI tract losses, e.g. diarrhoea, vomiting or 'third space' losses, e.g. pancreatitis, burns. If urine Na^+ is (>20 mmol/L), then there is a contribution to salt and water depletion from renal losses, e.g. adrenal insufficiency, renal tubular acidosis or 'salt-wasting' renal disease.

Step 4 If euvolaemic, or if cause unclear, measure urine sodium and osmolality

If feasible, discontinue any diuretics for 10 days and recheck U+E alongside plasma and urine osmolality and urine Na^+.

Low urine Na^+ (<20 mmol/L) implies that $\downarrow$plasma Na^+ is not due to excessive renal Na^+ losses. The cause may be hypovolaemic hyponatraemia due to extra-renal losses (see above) but without obvious clinical manifestations of hypovolaemia. In this case, urine osmolality will be $\uparrow$ (>150 mmol/kg) due to the presence of other solutes. If urine osmolality is <150 mmol/kg, the likely cause is excessive water intake. In hospitalized patients check for recent administration of hypotonic IV fluids, e.g. 5% dextrose. In non-hospitalized patients consider psychogenic polydipsia.

If hyponatraemia is accompanied by $\uparrow$urine Na^+ (>20 mmol/L) and osmolality (>150 mmol/kg), consider diuretic use, adrenal insufficiency, hypothyroidism, salt-wasting renal disease and the syndrome of inappropriate ADH secretion (SIADH).

Check TFTs and a 9 a.m. cortisol. High or high–normal plasma urea/uric acid may indicate subtle ↓ECF volume; if present, consider salt-wasting diseases or occult diuretic use. Otherwise, the likely diagnosis is SIADH.

If you suspect SIADH, look for an underlying cause (Box 8.2). Consider trial cessation of any suspected causative agent. If the cause remains unclear, request a CXR and CT brain and assess the response to fluid restriction (<1 L/day).

Further assessment of chronic confusion

The approach to progressive cognitive decline over a period of months to years differs from the approach to acute confusion. Exclude the reversible causes from p. 79 with a CT brain and blood tests; if no reversible cause is identified, refer for specialist evaluation and care.

Box 8.2 Causes of SIADH

- Tumours, especially small-cell lung cancer
- CNS disorders: stroke, trauma, infection
- Pulmonary disorders, e.g. pneumonia, tuberculosis
- Drugs
  - Anticonvulsants, e.g. carbamazepine
  - Psychotropics, e.g. haloperidol
  - Antidepressants, e.g. fluoxetine
  - Cytotoxics, e.g. cyclophosphamide
  - Hypoglycaemics, e.g. chlorpropamide
  - Opioids, e.g. morphine
  - Proton-pump inhibitors, e.g. omeprazole
- Sustained pain, stress, nausea, e.g. postoperative state
- Acute porphyria
- Idiopathic

Consider psychiatric illness

Perform an objective measure of cognition (at least MMSE) to ensure the presentation fits with a chronic decline in cognition dementia. Depression can mimic or exacerbate dementia and may be difficult to diagnose. Consider using tools such as the Cornell scale to assist diagnosis and, if you suspect depression, reassess cognitive function after a trial of anti-depressant therapy.

Assess for reversible causes

Perform a CT brain in every patient with chronic confusion. This may identify reversible causes, e.g. subdural haemorrhage or normal pressure hydrocephalus (ataxia and incontinence should raise the index of suspicion), or suggest possible aetiological factors, e.g. vascular disease. Measure TFTs in all patients, as hypothyroidism can present as dementia and responds to treatment. Take a careful alcohol history and consider Wernicke–Korsakoff syndrome in any patient with chronic alcohol misuse. Look for and correct nutritional deficiencies, e.g. B_{12}, folate.

Consider rare causes

Perform a more intensive work-up if the patient has an unusual pattern of cognitive impairment, e.g. preserved recent memory or personality/speech change, unexplained neurological findings on examination, a rapid course of cognitive decline or onset at a young age. This should usually include an HIV test, copper studies, Lyme/syphilis serology, MRI brain and LP ± further specialist assessment, e.g. EEG.

8

Diarrhoea may be defined as the passage of ≥3 loose or liquid stools/day. Patients often have difficulty describing their stools. The Bristol Stool Form Scale https://www.niddk.nih.gov/health-information/health-communication-programs/bowel-control-awareness-campaign/Documents/Bristol_Stool_Form_Scale_508.pdf can be helpful. The differential diagnosis depends on symptom duration. Acute diarrhoea (<2 weeks) is usually infectious but occasionally is due to drugs or a first presentation of inflammatory bowel disease. Chronic/relapsing diarrhoea may reflect colorectal cancer or inflammatory bowel disease, but the most frequent cause is irritable bowel syndrome.

Infectious diarrhoea

Infectious diarrhoea is due to faecal–oral transmission of viruses, bacteria, bacterial toxins or parasites. Most cases are self-limiting and a pathogen is rarely identified. Viruses and toxins predominantly affect the stomach and small bowel, causing large-volume, watery diarrhoea and pronounced vomiting; in toxin-mediated diarrhoea, e.g. *Staphylococcus aureus*, the incubation period is typically <12 hours. Invasive intestinal pathogens, including certain strains of *Escherichia coli*, and *Shigella*, may cause bloody diarrhoea, often with severe abdominal cramps and systemic upset (dysentery). *Clostridium difficile* infection (CDI) is an important cause of hospital-acquired diarrhoea, especially following broad-spectrum antibiotic therapy; CDI ranges from mild diarrhoeal illness to life-threatening pseudomembranous colitis. Diarrhoea that persists for >10 days is unlikely to be infective, but consider protozoal infections, e.g. giardiasis, amoebiasis or *Cryptosporidium* infection, in patients who are immunocompromised or have recently travelled to the tropics.

Irritable bowel syndrome

Irritable bowel syndrome is the most common cause of chronic diarrhoea. The predominant bowel habit may alternate between diarrhoea and constipation, and diagnosis is based on typical clinical features (Box 9.1) in the absence of apparent organic disease. Symptoms tend to follow a relapsing and remitting course, often exacerbated by psychosocial stress.

Drugs

Many drugs, including numerous over-the-counter preparations, cause diarrhoea (Box 9.2).

Colorectal cancer

Colorectal cancer may present with diarrhoea, especially if left-sided/distal. Suggestive features include weight loss, rectal bleeding, a palpable mass or iron-deficiency anaemia, but the absence of these features DOES NOT exclude malignancy.

Box 9.1 Rome III criteria for diagnosis of irritable bowel syndrome

Recurrent abdominal pain or discomfort on at least 3 days per month during the previous 3 months that is associated with two or more of the following:
- relieved by defecation
- onset associated with a change in stool frequency
- onset associated with a change in stool form or appearance.

Supporting symptoms include:
- altered stool frequency
- altered stool form
- altered stool passage (straining and/or urgency)
- mucorrhoea
- abdominal bloating or subjective distension.

Box 9.2 Drugs that frequently cause diarrhoea

- Laxatives (including occult laxative abuse)
- Antibiotics (especially macrolides)
- Alcohol (especially chronic alcohol excess)
- NSAIDs
- Metformin
- Colchicine
- Orlistat (steatorrhoea)
- Proton pump inhibitors
- SSRIs
- Nicorandil
- Cytotoxic agents

Box 9.3 Extra-intestinal features of inflammatory bowel disease

- General: fever, malaise, weight loss
- Eyes: conjunctivitis, episcleritis, iritis
- Joints: arthralgia of large joints, sacroiliitis/ankylosing spondylitis
- Skin: mouth ulcers, erythema nodosum, pyoderma gangrenosum
- Liver: fatty liver, gallstones, sclerosing cholangitis, cholangiocarcinoma (ulcerative colitis)

The diagnosis must be considered in any patient >45 years with new-onset, persistent diarrhoea and is usually confirmed by colonoscopy with biopsy.

Inflammatory bowel disease

Ulcerative colitis (UC) is confined to the large bowel and typically presents with bloody diarrhoea and cramping lower abdominal pain ± tenesmus, mucous discharge, fever and constitutional upset. Crohn's disease can affect any part of the alimentary tract and may present with large bowel symptoms similar to those of UC, or with small bowel symptoms, e.g. watery, non-bloody diarrhoea accompanied by abdominal pain and weight loss. Both disorders are associated with a range of extra-intestinal features (Box 9.3).

Disorders causing malabsorption

Fat malabsorption causes pale, greasy, offensive stools that float and are difficult to flush (steatorrhoea). Other features of malabsorption include undigested foodstuffs in stool, weight loss, bloating and nutritional deficiencies. The usual underlying cause is small bowel disease, e.g. coeliac disease, Crohn's disease, tropical sprue, lymphoma, small bowel resection or pancreatic insufficiency.

Other causes

- Diverticulitis, ischaemic colitis.
- Hyperthyroidism, autonomic neuropathy.
- Carcinoid tumour, gastrinoma, VIPoma.
- Severe constipation with overflow.

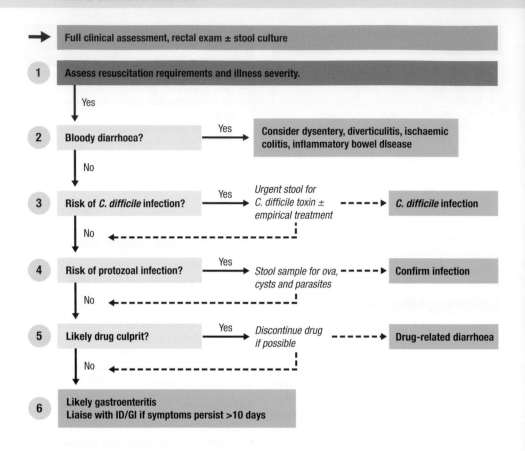

➡️ Full clinical assessment, rectal exam ± stool culture

1 Assess resuscitation requirements and illness severity.

Yes

2 Bloody diarrhoea? → Yes → Consider dysentery, diverticulitis, ischaemic colitis, inflammatory bowel disease

No

3 Risk of *C. difficile* infection? → Yes → Urgent stool for *C. difficile* toxin ± empirical treatment ⟶ *C. difficile* infection

No

4 Risk of protozoal infection? → Yes → Stool sample for ova, cysts and parasites ⟶ Confirm infection

No

5 Likely drug culprit? → Yes → Discontinue drug if possible ⟶ Drug-related diarrhoea

No

6 Likely gastroenteritis
Liaise with ID/GI if symptoms persist >10 days

---

1 Assess resuscitation requirements and illness severity

Step 1 Are there features of shock?
Look for ↑HR, ↓BP (a late sign) or evidence of tissue hypoperfusion (see Box 30.1, p. 267). If present, provide aggressive IV fluid resuscitation and reassess. Although hypovolaemia from GI losses is the likeliest cause of shock, also consider intra-abdominal SIRS/sepsis, medication and adrenal insufficiency (diarrhoea is a common feature of acute adrenal crisis).

Step 2 Is there acute renal impairment?
Hypovolaemia may result in severe 'pre-renal' acute kidney injury (AKI), especially if compounded by antihypertensive or nephrotoxic medication, e.g. diuretics, ACE inhibitors, NSAIDs. Patients with AKI require IV rehydration with close monitoring of fluid balance, urine output and U+E. If

AKI occurs in the context of bloody diarrhoea, look for features of haemolytic uraemic syndrome, e.g. ↓Hb, ↓platelets, ↑bilirubin/LDH/reticulocytes.

Step 3 Does the patient otherwise require IV fluids/hospital admission?
Patients with clinical evidence of dehydration (thirst, dry mucous membranes, ↓skin turgor) and concomitant vomiting, or those who are unable to match oral intake to ongoing losses require IV fluids.

Other features that may indicate a need for hospital admission include
- fever
- ↑WBC
- bloody diarrhoea
- abdominal tenderness/guarding/rigidity
- frail, elderly or immunocompromised patient
- significant comorbidity, e.g. heart/renal/hepatic failure.

2 Bloody diarrhoea?

The frequent passage of bloody stools suggests either

- infection with invasive organisms, e.g. *Campylobacter*, *Shigella* or *Amoeba*, or cytotoxin-producing organisms, e.g. *C. difficile*, *E. coli* O157 OR
- non-infectious colitis, e.g. ischaemic colitis inflammatory bowel disease.

It is often difficult to differentiate dysentery from a first attack of inflammatory bowel disease in the early stages: both may be accompanied by abdominal pain, tenesmus, mucus, constitutional upset and a systemic inflammatory response (see Box 14.1, p. 141).

- Send FBC, CRP and three stool samples in all patients, plus blood cultures if fever is present.
- Test stool for *C. difficile* toxin (CDT) if the patient has risk factors (see below), severe systemic upset or ↑↑WBC.
- Liaise with the ID team and request analysis of stool for ova, cysts and parasites if recent foreign travel.
- Request an abdominal X-ray to look for colonic dilatation (see Fig. 4.5B, p. 32) if there is abdominal tenderness/distention or a pronounced systemic inflammatory response.

If the duration of symptoms is ≤7 days, suspect an infectious cause unless there are specific pointers to an alternative diagnosis. Consider ischaemic colitis if bloody diarrhoea was preceded by sudden onset of left-sided lower abdominal pain or in any patient >50 years with known atherosclerotic disease or a source of systemic embolism, e.g. atrial fibrillation.

Refer any patient with known inflammatory bowel disease, extra-intestinal manifestations (see Box 9.3), previous similar episodes or symptoms >7 days for specialist GI evaluation.

Seek an urgent surgical review if there is evidence of peritonism or toxic megacolon, or you suspect ischaemic colitis or diverticulitis.

3 Risk of *C. difficile* infection?

Send stool for CDT in any patient who lives in an institution, e.g. nursing home, has recently been hospitalized, received antibiotics within the last 3 months or is >65 years. In high-risk patients send ≥3 samples before ruling out the diagnosis. If *C. difficile* confirmed, assess severity at least daily (Box 9.4).

Box 9.4 Assessing the severity of *Clostridium difficile* infection	
Mild	WBC not elevated <3 episodes of loose stools/day
Moderate	↑WBC (but <15 × 10⁹/L) 3–5 loose stools/day
Severe	WBC >15 × 10⁹/L or Serum creatinine >50% above baseline or Temp >38.5°C or Evidence of severe colitis (abdominal or radiological signs)
Life-threatening	Signs of shock (p. 267) Partial or complete ileus Toxic megacolon or CT evidence of severe disease

Adapted from Public Health England 2013. Updated guidance on the management and treatment of Clostridium difficile *infection. Public Health England. http://www.hpa.org.uk*

4 Risk of protozoal infection?

Send three stool samples on consecutive days for ova, cysts and parasites in patients with a history of recent foreign travel, when there is known or suspected immunocompromised, e.g. chemotherapy, HIV or in men who have sex with men.

5 Likely drug culprit?

Suspect drug-related diarrhoea if the onset of symptoms corresponds with initiation or ↑dose of drug, especially those listed in Box 9.2. Seek an alternative explanation if diarrhoea does not resolve on drug discontinuation.

6 Likely gastroenteritis. Liaise with ID/GI if symptoms persist >10 days

Most cases are self-limiting viral or toxin-mediated infections and do not require further investigation or antimicrobial treatment. If symptoms persist >10 days, seek specialist advice and consider further assessment as for chronic/relapsing diarrhoea (see below).

9

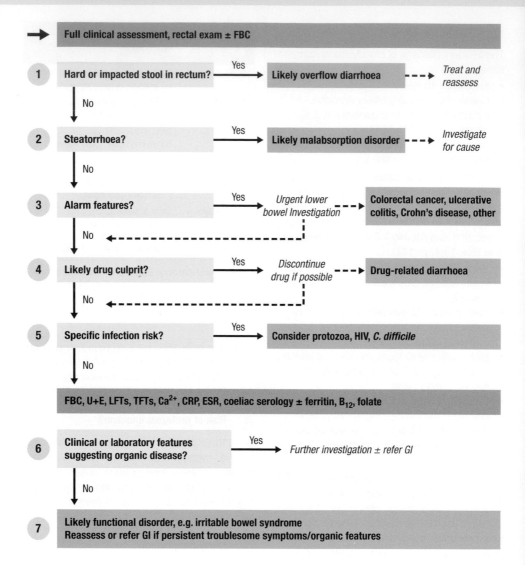

Full clinical assessment, rectal exam ± FBC

1 Hard or impacted stool in rectum? —Yes→ Likely overflow diarrhoea - - -> *Treat and reassess*

No

2 Steatorrhoea? —Yes→ Likely malabsorption disorder - - -> *Investigate for cause*

No

3 Alarm features? —Yes→ *Urgent lower bowel Investigation* - - - Colorectal cancer, ulcerative colitis, Crohn's disease, other

No

4 Likely drug culprit? —Yes→ *Discontinue drug if possible* - - -> Drug-related diarrhoea

No

5 Specific infection risk? —Yes→ Consider protozoa, HIV, *C. difficile*

No

FBC, U+E, LFTs, TFTs, Ca^{2+}, CRP, ESR, coeliac serology ± ferritin, B$_{12}$, folate

6 Clinical or laboratory features suggesting organic disease? —Yes→ *Further investigation ± refer GI*

No

7 Likely functional disorder, e.g. irritable bowel syndrome
Reassess or refer GI if persistent troublesome symptoms/organic features

1 Hard or impacted stool in rectum?

Have a high index of suspicion for overflow diarrhoea in frail, immobile or confused elderly patients. Always do a rectal examination. If the stool is hard or impacted, treat with faecal softeners and laxatives, then reassess. If the rectal examination is normal, overflow diarrhoea is unlikely (90% of impactions are rectal), but consider an abdominal X-ray if there is strong clinical suspicion.

2 Steatorrhoea?

Steatorrhoea signifies fat malabsorption but its absence does not exclude a malabsorptive disorder. If steatorrhoea is present, ensure that the patient is not taking orlistat (available over the counter in the UK) and check coeliac serology and faecal elastase ($\downarrow$in pancreatic insufficiency). If $\downarrow$faecal elastase or a strong suspicion of pancreatic disease, e.g. suggestive symptoms or cystic fibrosis, consider pancreatic imaging (CT/MRCP); otherwise, consider small bowel investigation, e.g. duodenal biopsy, MRI. Screen for nutritional deficiencies, e.g. iron, B_{12}, folate, Ca^{2+}, Mg^{2+}, PO_4^{3-}, albumin, in any patient with suspected malabsorption.

3 Alarm features?

Expedite lower bowel investigation to exclude colorectal cancer/inflammatory bowel disease if the patient has persistent diarrhoea associated with any of the following:

- rectal bleeding
- palpable rectal/abdominal mass
- weight loss
- iron deficiency anaemia
- new presentation in a patient >45 years.

Consider flexible sigmoidoscopy as a first-line investigation in patients <45 years or colonoscopy if >45 years.

4 Likely drug culprit?

Look for a temporal relationship between potential drug culprits (see Box 9.2) and the onset of diarrhoea. Consider trial discontinuation where feasible but change only one agent at any time and restart the drug if symptoms continue unaltered. Always ask about alcohol excess.

5 Specific infection risk?

Exclude protozoal infection in patients with a history of travel to the tropics, e.g. giardiasis, amoebiasis, or with known HIV infection/other immunocompromised, e.g. cryptosporidiosis – send three fresh stool samples for examination for ova cysts and parasites. Liaise with the ID team if stool samples are negative but there is ongoing clinical suspicion of infection. Test for HIV in any patient with chronic diarrhoea and risk factors.

C. difficile diarrhoea may be chronic or relapsing – send stool to test for CDT in any patient with risk factors (see above).

6 Clinical or laboratory features suggesting organic disease?

Screen for hyperthyroidism, hypercalcaemia and coeliac disease. Refer to GI for further small bowel investigation if large-volume, non-bloody stool, previous gastric/small bowel surgery or evidence of nutritional deficiencies: albumin, B_{12}, folate, Ca^{2+}, Mg^{2+}, PO_4^{3-}.

Exclude inflammatory bowel disease if there is a positive family history, mouth ulcers, fever, $\uparrow$CRP/ESR or extra-intestinal manifestations (see Box 9.3). Refer to GI for further evaluation if any of the above features is present or there are other findings that suggest organic disease, e.g. weight loss, anorexia, painless diarrhoea, prominent nocturnal symptoms or recent onset of symptoms in a patient >45 years. Faecal calprotectin levels can assist in the differentiation between inflammatory and non-inflammatory bowel disease.

7 Likely functional disorder

If none of the above is present, a functional cause, e.g. irritable bowel syndrome, is likely – particularly when typical symptoms are present (Box 9.1). Provide reassurance and explanation but refer to GI if symptoms are progressive, distressing or disabling.

9

10 Dizziness

The key to assessing dizziness lies in establishing the exact nature of the patient's symptoms. Occasionally, transient alteration of consciousness or focal neurological deficit will be described as a dizzy turn. However, most patients with dizziness have vertigo, light-headedness/presyncope or a sensation of unsteadiness.

Disorders causing vertigo

Vestibular neuronitis

This is inflammation of the vestibular nerve, possibly due to viral infection. There is abrupt onset of severe vertigo, associated with nausea and vomiting. Labyrinthine involvement (labyrinthitis) causes tinnitus and/or hearing impairment.

Benign paroxysmal positional vertigo (BPPV)

BPPV is caused by particles in the semicircular canals which alter endolymph flow. Brief episodes of vertigo, typically lasting 10–60 seconds, are provoked by changes in head position.

Ménière's disease

Recurrent attacks of vertigo, fluctuating low-frequency hearing loss, tinnitus and a sense of aural fullness are caused by increased volume of endolymph in the semicircular canals.

Acoustic neuroma

This cerebellopontine angle tumour usually presents with unilateral sensorineural hearing loss. Vertigo may occur but is rarely the predominant problem.

Brainstem pathology

Vertigo may be due to infarction, haemorrhage, demyelination or a space-occupying lesion. There will usually be associated features of brainstem dysfunction, e.g. diplopia, dysarthria or cranial nerve palsies. Vertigo, nausea, vomiting and nystagmus tend to be constant and protracted. Vertebrobasilar transient ischaemic attacks (TIAs) may cause recurrent, transient episodes of vertigo.

Other causes

These include migraine-associated vertigo, ototoxicity, e.g. gentamicin, furosemide, cisplatin, herpes zoster oticus (Ramsay Hunt syndrome) and perilymphatic fistula.

Disorders causing presyncope/light-headedness

Reflex presyncope (vasovagal episode)

Reflex vasodilatation and/or bradycardia occur in response to a 'trigger' such as intense emotion or noxious stimuli, e.g. venesection. There is a prodrome of nausea, sweating and 'greying-out' of vision/loss of peripheral vision. Syncope often ensues but may be averted by lying down.

Orthostatic hypotension

Orthostatic hypotension may result from anti-hypertensive medication, hypovolaemia (dehydration, blood loss) or autonomic dysfunction, especially in elderly or diabetic patients.

Arrhythmia

Brady- and tachyarrhythmia can reduce cardiac output and thereby compromise cerebral perfusion. There may be associated palpitation, ECG abnormalities or a cardiac history.

Structural cardiac disease

Severe left ventricular outflow tract obstruction, e.g. aortic stenosis or hypertrophic obstructive cardiomyopathy, can result in light-headedness by reducing cardiac output. Episodes may be provoked by exertion. There will usually be abnormalities on examination, e.g. systolic murmur, and ECG, e.g. left ventricular hypertrophy.

Disorders causing unsteadiness

Ataxia

Lack of coordination of muscle movements may cause profound unsteadiness and difficulty walking; it is most commonly due to cerebellar pathology.

Multisensory impairment

Balance requires input from multiple sensory modalities (visual, vestibular, touch, proprioceptive); reduced function in more than one of these modalities, even if relatively minor, may cause unsteadiness. This is most often seen in the elderly.

Weakness

Lesions anywhere in the motor tract (cerebral cortex, upper motor neuron, lower motor neuron, motor endplate or muscle) can result in unsteadiness due to weakness.

Other causes

Loss of confidence, joint problems, Parkinson's disease and gait dyspraxia may all cause unsteadiness.

Other disorders causing dizziness

Many other conditions can cause dizziness, including hypoglycaemia, partial (temporal lobe) seizure, migraine variants, normal pressure hydrocephalus, hyperventilation and anxiety.

10

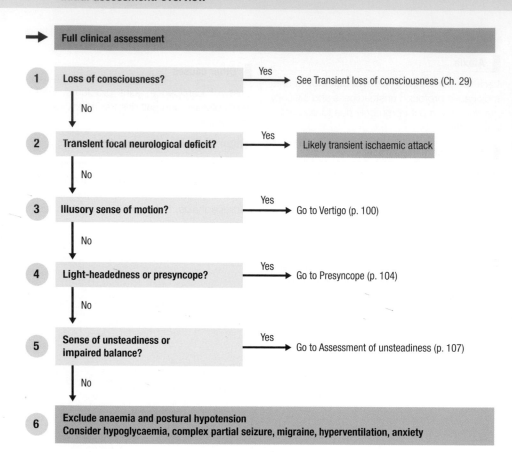

Full clinical assessment

1 Loss of consciousness? — Yes → See Transient loss of consciousness (Ch. 29)

No

2 Transient focal neurological deficit? — Yes → Likely transient ischaemic attack

No

3 Illusory sense of motion? — Yes → Go to Vertigo (p. 100)

No

4 Light-headedness or presyncope? — Yes → Go to Presyncope (p. 104)

No

5 Sense of unsteadiness or impaired balance? — Yes → Go to Assessment of unsteadiness (p. 107)

No

6 Exclude anaemia and postural hypotension
Consider hypoglycaemia, complex partial seizure, migraine, hyperventilation, anxiety

1 Loss of consciousness?

Establish this first, as loss of consciousness requires a different diagnostic approach (see Ch. 31). If at all possible, obtain an eyewitness account of the episode; otherwise, suspect transient loss of consciousness if there is a history of 'coming to' on the ground or if facial injuries were sustained.

2 Transient focal neurological deficit?

A TIA is often described by the patient as a 'funny turn' and careful questioning may be required to elicit a history of transient focal neurological disturbance (usually <3 hours). The most common presentations include hemiparesis, hemisensory disturbance, facial droop, speech disturbance, diplopia and monocular visual loss (amaurosis fugax). Vertigo may occur with a vertebrobasilar TIA, usually accompanied by other brainstem features.

3 Illusory sense of motion?

Vertigo is an illusory sensation of motion (usually spinning or rotatory). When present, it is invariably aggravated by movement. If the nature of the dizziness is not apparent from the patient's own account, then ask: 'When you have dizzy spells, do you simply feel light-headed or do you see the world spin around you as if you had just got off a playground roundabout?' The latter indicates vertigo.

4 Light-headedness or presyncope?

Consider presyncope in patients who describe a feeling of light-headedness, 'as if I might faint or pass out', or one that is akin to the familiar transient sensation experienced after standing up quickly. If any of the episodes has been associated with blackout, assess as described for transient loss of consciousness (Ch. 31).

5 Sense of unsteadiness or impaired balance?

In some patients with dizziness, the principal problem is impaired sense of balance associated with falls or the feeling that one might fall. This usually occurs while standing and is aggravated by walking. The patient may need to hold on to furniture or other people. Examination of the gait (p. 215) may be revealing. The underlying problem is often impaired central processing of the body's position in space, e.g. cerebellar disorders, impaired proprioception, peripheral neuropathy, visual loss, poorly compensated vestibular disorders, which may be exacerbated by reduced muscle strength or confidence, particularly in the elderly.

10

6 Consider other causes

If the description of dizziness is unclear, ask for more details: 'Imagine you are having one of your dizzy turns now. Talk me through exactly what happens and what you feel.' If the account is not consistent with any of the above categories, consider alternative causes.

- Suspect hypoglycaemic attacks if the patient is taking insulin or sulphonylurea drugs or reports relief of symptoms with sugar intake; a CBG and lab glucose measurement taken during an episode will confirm or exclude the diagnosis.
- Seek neurological advice if there are repeated episodes of amnesia, altered consciousness or unusual behaviour.
- In all patients with orthostatic symptoms, perform an FBC to exclude anaemia and measure erect and supine BP.
- Anxiety is the most common cause of 'dizzy turns' in patients under 65 years but is a diagnosis of exclusion.

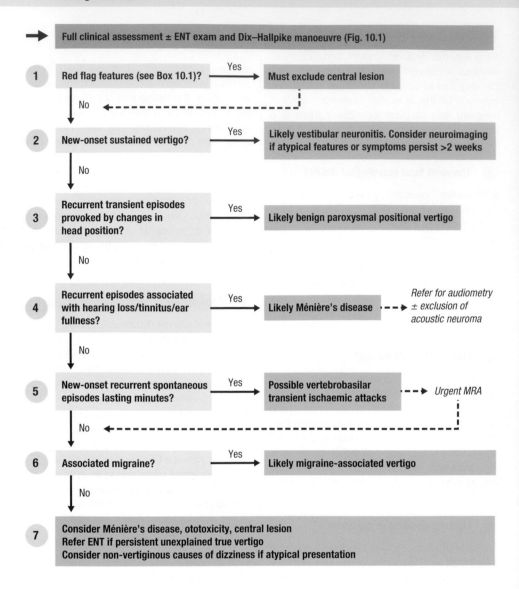

Full clinical assessment ± ENT exam and Dix–Hallpike manoeuvre (Fig. 10.1)

1 Red flag features (see Box 10.1)? — Yes → Must exclude central lesion

No

2 New-onset sustained vertigo? — Yes → Likely vestibular neuronitis. Consider neuroimaging if atypical features or symptoms persist >2 weeks

No

3 Recurrent transient episodes provoked by changes in head position? — Yes → Likely benign paroxysmal positional vertigo

No

4 Recurrent episodes associated with hearing loss/tinnitus/ear fullness? — Yes → Likely Ménière's disease ⤏ *Refer for audiometry ± exclusion of acoustic neuroma*

No

5 New-onset recurrent spontaneous episodes lasting minutes? — Yes → Possible vertebrobasilar transient ischaemic attacks ⤏ *Urgent MRA*

No

6 Associated migraine? — Yes → Likely migraine-associated vertigo

No

7 Consider Ménière's disease, ototoxicity, central lesion
Refer ENT if persistent unexplained true vertigo
Consider non-vertiginous causes of dizziness if atypical presentation

1   Red flag features (Box 10.1)?

The presence of any of the features in Box 10.1 raises the possibility of serious intracranial pathology.

If the presentation is sudden, consider acute haemorrhagic or ischaemic stroke and arrange urgent neuroimaging. Where less acute, the main concern is to exclude intracranial mass lesion.

CT is usually the initial imaging modality but MRI offers superior visualization of the posterior fossa. All patients with progressive sensorineural hearing loss require MRI to exclude acoustic neuroma.

2   New-onset sustained vertigo?

In the absence of red flag features, new-onset sustained vertigo is most likely due to vestibular neuronitis. The usual story is of abrupt-onset severe vertigo with nausea and vomiting but without hearing loss or tinnitus. The patient has difficulty walking but can usually stand unsupported. There is unilateral nystagmus enhanced by asking the patient to look to the side or by blocking visual fixation (place a blank piece of paper a few inches in front of the eyes and inspect from the side). A positive head thrust test (Box 10.2) confirms the diagnosis.

Consider neuroimaging (preferably MRI) if the patient has a negative head thrust test, is unable to stand without support or has a history of vascular disease – primarily to exclude acute cerebellar stroke.

In vestibular neuronitis, severe vertigo typically persists for several days and full recovery occurs within 3–4 weeks; reassess if symptoms persist beyond this period.

3   Recurrent transient episodes provoked by changes in head position?

A history of repeated, brief episodes of vertigo provoked by changes in head position, e.g. turning over in bed or looking up, strongly suggests BPPV. Episodes may occur in bouts lasting several weeks interspersed with periods of remission. A positive Dix–Hallpike test (Fig. 10.1) confirms the diagnosis but, even if negative, BPPV remains the likely diagnosis.

10

Box 10.1   Red flag features in vertigo

- Focal neurological symptoms or signs: dysarthria, diplopia, facial weakness, swallowing difficulties, dysdiadochokinesis or focal limb weakness
- Papilloedema, drowsiness or ↓GCS
- Inability to stand or walk
- Atypical nystagmus (down-beating, bi-directional gaze evoked, pure torsional, not suppressed with fixation on object)
- New-onset headache: sudden onset and severe or worse in morning/lying down
- Progressive unilateral hearing loss

Box 10.2   The head thrust test

With intact vestibular function, changes in head position trigger reflex eye movements in the opposite direction to maintain visual fixation via the vestibulo-ocular reflex (VOR). The head thrust test assesses the VOR on both sides. Stand in front of the patient, grasp his/her head in your hands and instruct him/her to focus on your nose. Turn the head as rapidly as possible to one side by 15° (do not perform in patients with known or suspected neck pathology) and observe eye movements. Failure to maintain fixation on the target is evidenced by the need for a voluntary, corrective eye movement back towards the target. This indicates peripheral vestibular dysfunction on the side to which the head was turned. Perform the test in both directions. Unilateral impairment of VOR is seen in vestibular neuronitis and excludes a central cause for vertigo. See the video at the website of the *Journal of Neurology, Neurosurgery, and Psychiatry:* http://jnnp.bmj.com/content/suppl/2007/09/13/ jnnp.2006.109512.DC1/78101113webonlymedia.mpg

Recurrent episodes associated with hearing loss/tinnitus/ear fullness?

Diagnosis of Ménière's disease requires the following criteria:

- recurrent attacks of vertigo lasting minutes to hours (± nausea and vomiting)
- fluctuating sensorineural hearing loss, especially for low frequencies (audiometry is usually required to detect this)
- tinnitus or a sense of pressure/fullness in the ear.

To exclude acoustic neuroma, consider ENT referral for any patient with unilateral hearing loss and vertigo, especially if the presentation is recent in onset or atypical for Ménière's disease.

 New-onset recurrent spontaneous episodes lasting minutes?

Vertebrobasilar TIAs are normally associated with other neurological features, e.g. diplopia, dysarthria, facial numbness, but occasionally present with episodes of vertigo as the only symptom. Patients with a crescendo pattern of symptoms may have impending thrombosis and require prompt referral for imaging of the posterior circulation, e.g. MR angiography.

6 **Associated migraine?**

Enquire about possible migrainous symptoms in all patients with episodic vertigo. Those who fulfil the diagnostic criteria for migraine (see Table 18.2, p. 173) and have episodic vertigo with no other obvious cause have probable migraine-associated vertigo; definitive diagnosis requires a temporal association between vertigo and migraine headache or aura.

 Consider other causes/ENT referral

In Ménière's disease, the patient is often unaware of low-frequency hearing loss or tinnitus during attacks, and hearing may have returned to normal by the time of audiometry. In these circumstances, recurrent attacks of spontaneous vertigo may be the only presenting feature.

Suspect ototoxicity in any patient with new-onset vertigo or other balance/hearing disturbance if gentamicin, furosemide or cisplatin has recently been prescribed. Persistent symptoms despite drug cessation may indicate irreversible vestibulocochlear dysfunction.

Reassess all patients for red flag features and arrange an MRI of the brain if there is any suspicion of a central lesion.

Patients with dizziness present constantly over weeks or whose dizziness is not improved by remaining still are unlikely to have true vertigo. Otherwise, refer to ENT for further evaluation.

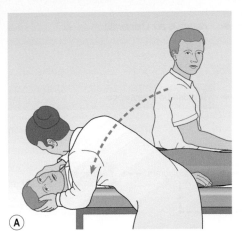 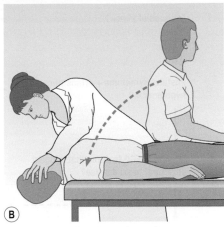

(A)   (B)

10

Fig. 10.1 The Dix–Hallpike test. Start with the patient sitting upright on the couch. Explain what you are going to do. [A] Rapidly lie the patient supine with the head (supported by your hands) extended over the end of the couch and turned to the right. Maintain this position for at least 30 seconds, asking the patient to report any symptoms whilst observing for nystagmus. [B] Repeat with the head turned to the left. The test is positive if the patient develops symptoms of vertigo and nystagmus. (From Boon NA, Colledge NR, Walker BR. Davidson's Principles & Practice of Medicine, 20th edn. Edinburgh: Churchill Livingstone, 2006.)

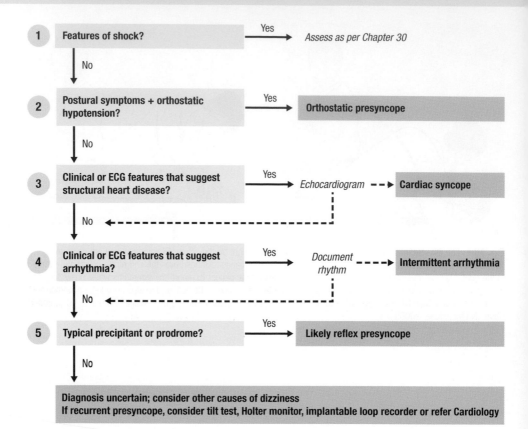

1 Features of shock? — Yes → *Assess as per Chapter 30*

No ↓

2 Postural symptoms + orthostatic hypotension? — Yes → **Orthostatic presyncope**

No ↓

3 Clinical or ECG features that suggest structural heart disease? — Yes → *Echocardiogram* ---▶ **Cardiac syncope**

No ◀------

4 Clinical or ECG features that suggest arrhythmia? — Yes → *Document rhythm* ---▶ **Intermittent arrhythmia**

No ◀------

5 Typical precipitant or prodrome? — Yes → **Likely reflex presyncope**

No ↓

Diagnosis uncertain; consider other causes of dizziness
If recurrent presyncope, consider tilt test, Holter monitor, implantable loop recorder or refer Cardiology

1 Features of shock?

Acute light-headedness may signify haemodynamic instability. Look for shock (Box 30.1, p. 267), including early features, e.g. ↑HR, narrow pulse pressure, pallor or postural ↓BP. If present, assess as described in Chapter 30.

2 Postural symptoms + orthostatic hypotension?

A secure diagnosis of orthostatic presyncope requires:
- a clear temporal relationship between light-headedness and standing up
- demonstration of a significant postural BP drop (≥20 mmHg in systolic BP or ≥10 mmHg in diastolic BP within 3 minutes of changing from a lying to a standing position).

If orthostatic presyncope is detected, search for underlying causes, e.g. antihypertensives, dehydration, autonomic neuropathy.

3 Clinical or ECG features that suggest structural heart disease?

Consider echocardiography to exclude structural heart disease in patients with:
- exertional presyncope
- a family history of sudden unexplained death

- a history or clinical signs of aortic stenosis/ hypertrophic cardiomyopathy
- clinical features of cardiac failure
- relevant ECG abnormalities, e.g. severe left ventricular hypertrophy, right heart strain, deep anterior T-wave inversion.

4 Clinical or ECG features that suggest arrhythmia?

Suspect an arrhythmic aetiology if episodes of light-headedness are associated with palpitation or occur whilst supine, if there are significant ECG abnormalities (see Box 31.3, p. 273), or if the patient has a history of myocardial infarction.

The key to clinching the diagnosis is to document the rhythm during a typical episode. If episodes are relatively frequent, arrange Holter monitoring, e.g. 24-hour tape; if less frequent, a patient-activated external recorder or implantable loop recorder may be more helpful.

5 Typical precipitant or prodrome?

Consider whether episodes of light-headedness occurred while the patient was standing and had a clear precipitating trigger, e.g. intense emotion, venepuncture or prolonged standing and/or were accompanied by other 'prodromal' features such as nausea, sweating and disturbance of vision. A tilt test may help to clinch the diagnosis.

10

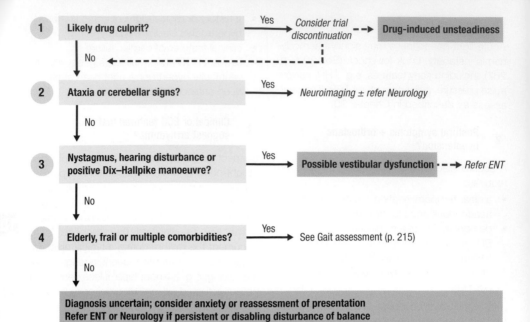

1 Likely drug culprit? → Yes → *Consider trial discontinuation* - -> **Drug-induced unsteadiness**

↓ No ← -

2 Ataxia or cerebellar signs? → Yes → *Neuroimaging ± refer Neurology*

↓ No

3 Nystagmus, hearing disturbance or positive Dix–Hallpike manoeuvre? → Yes → **Possible vestibular dysfunction** - - -> *Refer ENT*

↓ No

4 Elderly, frail or multiple comorbidities? → Yes → *See Gait assessment (p. 215)*

↓ No

Diagnosis uncertain; consider anxiety or reassessment of presentation
Refer ENT or Neurology if persistent or disabling disturbance of balance

1 Likely drug culprit?

Drug causes of unsteadiness are numerous and common but close attention should be paid to the following agents:

- alcohol
- antihypertensives
- sedatives, e.g. benzodiazepines
- antipsychotics, e.g. haloperidol
- antidepressants, e.g. amitriptyline
- anticonvulsants, e.g. carbamazepine.

If safe to do so, discontinue potential drug culprits and reassess.

2 Ataxia or cerebellar signs?

Suspect cerebellar dysfunction if there is ataxia (broad-based, unsteady gait; inability to heel–toe walk) or other typical clinical features, e.g. intention tremor, dysdiadochokinesis, past-pointing, dysarthria or nystagmus. If any of these is present, enquire about current and previous alcohol intake and consider an MRI of the brain and/or neurology referral.

3 Nystagmus, hearing disturbance or positive Dix–Hallpike manoeuvre?

Even if the patient's account of dizziness is not suggestive of vertigo, the presence of nystagmus, hearing disturbance or a positive Dix–Hallpike manoeuvre suggests vestibular dysfunction. Refer to ENT.

4 Elderly, frail or multiple comorbidities?

Multiple factors may contribute to unsteadiness, particularly in the elderly, including limb weakness, sensory neuropathy, impaired proprioception, joint disease, impaired visual acuity and loss of confidence. Several factors commonly coexist. If the patient has evidence of more than one of these, is frail/elderly or exhibits unsteadiness during walking, assess as described for mobility problems (Ch. 24).

10

Patients with dysphagia require prompt assessment to exclude serious pathology. Unless the history clearly points to a functional oropharyngeal cause, oesophageal investigation is necessary to rule out mechanical obstruction – in particular, malignancy.

Oropharyngeal dysphagia

Bulbar palsy

Lower motor neuron palsies of cranial nerves IX–XII result in weakness of the tongue and muscles of chewing/swallowing. The tongue is flaccid with fasciculation, often with a change in voice (Table 11.1). Causes include motor neuron disease (MND) and brainstem tumour or infarction.

Pseudobulbar palsy

Bilateral upper motor neuron lesions of cranial nerves IX–XII produce a small, contracted and slowly moving tongue and pharyngeal muscles with a brisk jaw jerk (Fig. 11.1). There may be associated speech disturbance and emotional lability (Table 11.1). Causes include cerebrovascular disease, demyelination and MND.

Myasthenia gravis

Fatigability of oropharyngeal muscles causes increasing swallowing difficulty after the first few mouthfuls. Dysphagia may occur before other features of myasthenia are readily apparent.

Pharyngeal pouch

The pouch is formed by posterior herniation of the pharyngeal mucosa between the thyropharyngeus and cricopharyngeus muscle, and is usually found in elderly patients. In addition to dysphagia, there is classically regurgitation of undigested food, halitosis, the feeling of a lump in the neck and gurgling after swallowing liquids.

Parkinson's disease and stroke

These frequently cause swallowing difficulty but other features are usually more prominent.

Inadequate saliva

Inadequate saliva, e.g. anticholinergics, connective tissue disease, such as Sjögren's syndrome, may lead to problems with forming a manageable bolus.

Other causes

These include myopathies, myotonic dystrophy and tumours of the pharynx or larynx.

Oesophageal dysphagia (structural)

Both structural disease and dysmotility may cause dysphagia. Structural causes usually cause dysphagia for solids; motility disorders may cause dysphagia for solids and liquids.

Food bolus obstruction

There is sudden onset of complete dysphagia, often with an inability to swallow even saliva. The diagnosis is usually obvious from the history but it may be the first manifestation of an underlying stricture.

Malignant stricture

Patients with oesophageal cancer typically present with progressive, painless dysphagia to solid foods. Weight loss may be marked, especially if presentation is delayed. Cachexia and lymphadenopathy are suggestive but physical signs are typically absent.

Benign stricture

Most commonly, benign stricture is due to *gastro-oesophageal reflux*, especially in the elderly. Rarer causes include *oesophageal webs* (seen in iron deficiency, typically posterior to

Table 11.1 Comparison of signs in bulbar and pseudobulbar palsy		
	Bulbar	**Pseudobulbar**
Speech	Nasal tone; difficulty forming consonants (especially 'R'); may become slurred	'Donald duck' voice
Tongue	Weak, wasted with fasciculation	Small, stiff
Jaw jerk	Normal or absent	Brisk
Gag reflex	Absent	Present
Emotions	Normal	Labile (e.g. uncontrollable laughing/crying)

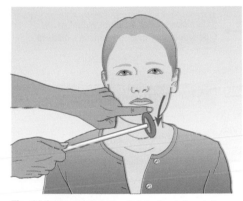

Fig. 11.1 The jaw jerk. To elicit the jaw jerk, ask the patient to let his/her mouth hang open, place your index finger on the patient's chin and strike your finger with a tendon hammer. (From Ford MJ, Hennessey I, Japp A. Introduction to Clinical Examination, 8th edn. Edinburgh: Churchill Livingstone, 2005.)

the cricoid), *Schatzki rings* (benign idiopathic strictures of the lower oesophagus), ingestion of caustic substances, eosinophilic oesophagitis or, rarely, benign oesophageal tumours and radiotherapy.

Hiatus hernia

Hiatus hernia with an associated intrathoracic stomach can present with dysphagia and vomiting. Urgent treatment is required to prevent strangulation of the stomach.

Extrinsic compression

Lung cancer, thyroid goitre, mediastinal nodes, an enlarged left atrium or a thoracic aortic aneurysm may, rarely, produce dysphagia by compressing the oesophagus.

Oesophageal dysphagia (dysmotility)

Achalasia

This is an uncommon disorder characterized by loss of peristalsis in the distal oesophagus and impaired relaxation of the lower oesophageal sphincter. Dysphagia is of slow onset (often years), occurs for liquids and solids and may initially be intermittent. Dysphagia for liquids is the most prominent symptom. Retrosternal discomfort and regurgitation are common.

Chagas disease

Chagas disease can present with achalasia; consider it in patients originating from endemic areas in Central and South America and confirm with serological testing.

Scleroderma

Oesophageal involvement is seen in ~90% of cases; impaired peristalsis results from replacement of muscle with fibrous tissues and severe gastro-oesophageal reflux occurs due to incompetence of the lower oesophageal sphincter. Other features of scleroderma, e.g. calcinosis, Raynaud's disease, telangiectasia, may be apparent.

Diffuse oesophageal spasm

This may cause transient episodes of dysphagia, although episodic chest pain that mimics angina is usually the predominant symptom.

11

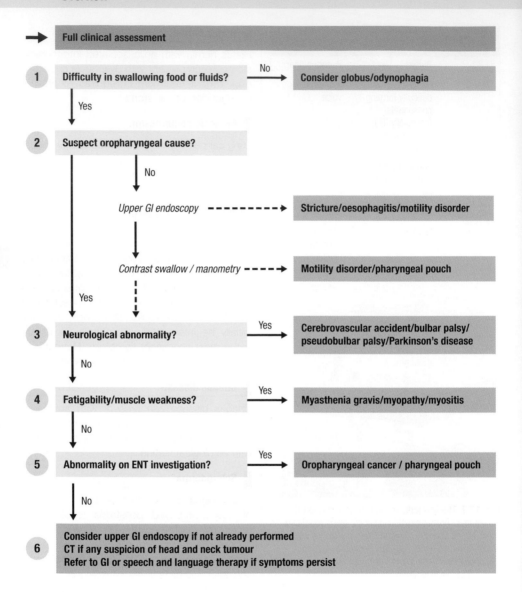

➡ **Full clinical assessment**

1 **Difficulty in swallowing food or fluids?** —— No ——▶ **Consider globus/odynophagia**

Yes

2 **Suspect oropharyngeal cause?**

No

Upper GI endoscopy ---------▶ **Stricture/oesophagitis/motility disorder**

Contrast swallow / manometry -----▶ **Motility disorder/pharyngeal pouch**

Yes

3 **Neurological abnormality?** —— Yes ——▶ **Cerebrovascular accident/bulbar palsy/ pseudobulbar palsy/Parkinson's disease**

No

4 **Fatigability/muscle weakness?** —— Yes ——▶ **Myasthenia gravis/myopathy/myositis**

No

5 **Abnormality on ENT investigation?** —— Yes ——▶ **Oropharyngeal cancer / pharyngeal pouch**

No

6 **Consider upper GI endoscopy if not already performed**
CT if any suspicion of head and neck tumour
Refer to GI or speech and language therapy if symptoms persist

---

1 **Difficulty in swallowing foods or fluids?**

Features of true dysphagia include difficulty initiating swallowing or the sensation of food 'sticking' after swallowing. Globus is the sensation of a lump in the throat; it is unrelated to swallowing and often associated with anxiety or strong emotion. Odynophagia is pain on swallowing and suggests oesophageal inflammation or ulceration.

2 **Suspect oropharyngeal cause?**

Suspect oropharyngeal dysphagia if the patient does NOT report food sticking in the lower throat or retrosternum and one or more of the following features is present:
- drooling/spillage of food from the mouth
- immediate sensation of a bolus 'catching' in the neck

- difficulty initiating swallow – repeated attempts are required to clear the bolus
- choking/coughing on swallowing.

If none of these features are present, investigate for an oesophageal cause. Arrange a UGIE to look for a structural cause, especially oesophageal cancer. UGIE may also reveal features of certain motility disorders, e.g. achalasia, but can be normal, especially in scleroderma or diffuse oesophageal spasm.

If no cause is identified on UGIE, consult a GI specialist, as further investigation for a motility disorder, e.g. contrast swallow or oesophageal manometry, may be required. If all GI investigations are reassuring, re-evaluate for a possible oropharyngeal cause.

3 Neurological abnormality?

If the history suggests an oropharyngeal aetiology for dysphagia, neurological evaluation is essential. Although swallowing difficulty is common in stroke, Parkinson's disease and multiple sclerosis, it is very rarely the primary presenting problem. However, dysphagia may be the principal complaint in bulbar palsy and pseudobulbar palsy so look carefully for the relevant clinical features (Table 11.1); if they are present, look for other features of MND and perform neuroimaging to exclude vascular or structural brainstem disease.

4 Fatigability/muscle weakness?

Myasthenia gravis is rare and easily missed. The dysphagia typically presents with increasing difficulty in swallowing after the first few mouthfuls and difficulty in chewing. Ask specifically about/ examine for:

- fatigable weakness of muscles: initial strength is normal but there is a rapid decline with activity
- weak voice with prolonged speaking
- diplopia
- ptosis

- muscle fatigability (ask the patient to count to 50 or hold the arms above the head). Refer to a Neurologist if you suspect the diagnosis.

5 Abnormality on ENT investigation?

Exclude oropharyngeal cancer if the patient has an oropharyngeal pattern of dysphagia (see step 2) without evidence of underlying neurological/ neuromuscular disorder – especially if risk factors (smoking, alcohol, human papillomavirus infection) or other suggestive clinical features, e.g. palpable neck lump, halitosis, cough, hoarseness, sore throat, ear pain (referred pain), weight loss. Refer to an ENT specialist for investigation, e.g. nasendoscopy and CT/MRI scanning.

Investigate for a pharyngeal pouch, e.g. contrast swallow or nasoendoscopy, if there is associated regurgitation or a lump in the neck that appears after eating (occasionally may be compressed by hand, expunging the food contents of the pouch), +/– halitosis (from food lodged in the pouch), weight loss, aspiration or chronic cough.

6 Consider further investigation/referral to GI or speech and language therapy

If not already done, arrange urgent UGIE unless there is clear evidence of neurological or neuromuscular dysfunction. Request a CT if you suspect cancer of the head and neck, e.g. local mass or lymphadenopathy. Once significant pathology of the oropharynx and oesophagus is actively excluded, refer patients with suspected oropharyngeal dysphagia of uncertain cause to the speech and language therapy team for a detailed swallow evaluation with formal speech and ± videofluoroscopy. This will confirm the presence of oropharyngeal dysfunction and help to clarify the mechanism. If you still suspect oesophageal dysphagia, refer to a GI specialist for further assessment.

The sensation of breathlessness occurs when there is a mismatch between instructions for ventilation sent by the brainstem, and sensory feedback from the thorax. When evaluating a patient with breathlessness, remember that severity is highly subjective. Some individuals may not experience dyspnoea despite severe impairment of gas exchange.

Acute dyspnoea

Acute dyspnoea is defined here as new-onset or abruptly worsening breathlessness within the preceding 2 weeks. When accompanied by severe hypoxaemia, hypercapnia, exhaustion or ↓GCS, it may herald life-threatening pathology. The diagnosis can usually be made by combining clinical evaluation and monitoring with key investigations including CXR, ECG and ABG. In the initial phase of assessment, diagnosis and treatment should be concurrent, and the cycle of intervention and reassessment should continue until the patient is stable. Important causes of acute dyspnoea are listed below.

Upper airway obstruction

- Inhaled foreign body.
- Anaphylaxis.
- Epiglottitis.
- Extrinsic compression, e.g. rapidly expanding haematoma.

Lower airway disease

- Acute bronchitis.
- Asthma.
- Acute exacerbation of chronic obstructive pulmonary disease (COPD).
- Acute exacerbation of bronchiectasis.
- Anaphylaxis.

Parenchymal lung disease

- Pneumonia.
- Lobar collapse.
- Acute respiratory distress syndrome (ARDS).

Other respiratory causes

- Pneumothorax.
- Pleural effusion.
- Pulmonary embolism (PE).
- Acute chest wall injury.

Cardiovascular causes

- Acute cardiogenic pulmonary oedema.
- Acute coronary syndrome.
- Cardiac tamponade.
- Arrhythmia.
- Acute valvular heart disease.

Other causes

- Metabolic acidosis.
- Psychogenic breathlessness (acute hyperventilation).

Chronic dyspnoea

Chronic dyspnoea is defined here as breathlessness of >2 weeks' duration. Use the Medical Research Council (MRC) dyspnoea scale (Box 12.1) to assess the severity of breathlessness.

Important causes of chronic dyspnoea are listed below.

For many causes, the diagnosis can be made by combining clinical evaluation with PFTs, ECG, CXR, FBC and pulse oximetry. However, early presentations of common problems, such as COPD and congestive cardiac failure, may have no clinical signs and a normal CXR. In 1 in 3

Box 12.1 **MRC dyspnoea scale**

Grade 1 Not troubled by breathlessness except on strenuous exercise

Grade 2 Short of breath when hurrying or walking up a slight hill

Grade 3 Walks slower than contemporaries on level ground because of breathlessness, or has to stop for breath when walking at own pace

Grade 4 Stops for breath after walking about 100 m or after a few minutes on level ground

Grade 5 Too breathless to leave the house, or breathless when dressing or undressing

Source: Adapted from Fletcher CM, Elmes PC, Fairbairn MB et al. 1959. The significance of respiratory symptoms and the diagnosis of chronic bronchitis in a working population. Br Med J. 2:257–266.

patients, there is more than one underlying diagnosis to explain dyspnoea, so assess dyspnoeic patients thoroughly, even after a possible explanation has been found, particularly if the severity of pathology found is not commensurate with the severity of symptoms.

Respiratory causes

- Asthma.
- COPD.
- Pleural effusion.
- Lung cancer: bronchial carcinoma, mesothelioma, lymphangitis carcinomatosis.
- Interstitial lung disease (ILD), e.g. sarcoidosis, idiopathic pulmonary fibrosis, extrinsic allergic alveolitis.
- Chronic pulmonary thromboembolism.
- Bronchiectasis.
- Cystic fibrosis.
- Pulmonary hypertension (primary or secondary).
- Pulmonary vasculitis.
- Tuberculosis (TB).
- Laryngeal/tracheal stenosis, e.g. extrinsic compression, malignancy.

Cardiovascular causes

- Chronic heart failure.
- Coronary artery disease ('angina equivalent').
- Valvular heart disease.
- Paroxysmal arrhythmia.
- Constrictive pericarditis.
- Pericardial effusion.
- Cyanotic congenital heart disease.

Other causes

- Severe anaemia.
- Obesity.
- Chest wall disease, e.g. kyphoscoliosis.
- Physical deconditioning.
- Diaphragmatic paralysis.
- Psychogenic hyperventilation.
- Neuromuscular disorder, e.g. myasthenia gravis, muscular dystrophies.
- Cirrhosis (hepatopulmonary syndrome).
- Tense ascites.

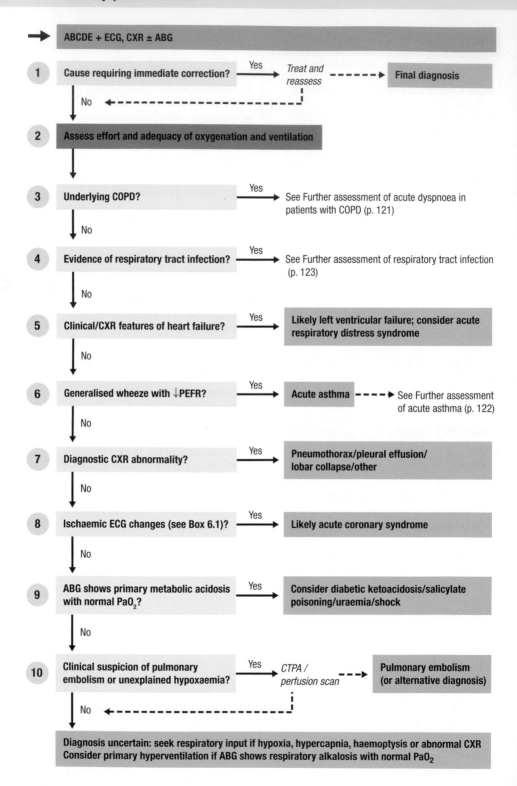

ABCDE + ECG, CXR ± ABG

1 Cause requiring immediate correction? — Yes → *Treat and reassess* ---→ **Final diagnosis**

No

2 Assess effort and adequacy of oxygenation and ventilation

3 Underlying COPD? — Yes → See Further assessment of acute dyspnoea in patients with COPD (p. 121)

No

4 Evidence of respiratory tract infection? — Yes → See Further assessment of respiratory tract infection (p. 123)

No

5 Clinical/CXR features of heart failure? — Yes → **Likely left ventricular failure; consider acute respiratory distress syndrome**

No

6 Generalised wheeze with ↓PEFR? — Yes → **Acute asthma** ---→ See Further assessment of acute asthma (p. 122)

No

7 Diagnostic CXR abnormality? — Yes → **Pneumothorax/pleural effusion/lobar collapse/other**

No

8 Ischaemic ECG changes (see Box 6.1)? — Yes → **Likely acute coronary syndrome**

No

9 ABG shows primary metabolic acidosis with normal PaO_2? — Yes → **Consider diabetic ketoacidosis/salicylate poisoning/uraemia/shock**

No

10 Clinical suspicion of pulmonary embolism or unexplained hypoxaemia? — Yes → *CTPA / perfusion scan* ---→ **Pulmonary embolism (or alternative diagnosis)**

No

**Diagnosis uncertain: seek respiratory input if hypoxia, hypercapnia, haemoptysis or abnormal CXR
Consider primary hyperventilation if ABG shows respiratory alkalosis with normal PaO_2**

1 **Cause requiring immediate correction?**

As part of the ABCDE assessment process (p. 8), identify and provide immediate corrective treatment for:

- airway obstruction
- tension pneumothorax
- anaphylaxis
- arrhythmia with cardiac compromise.

Seek specialist input if necessary and repeat the assessment following intervention.

2 **Assess effort and adequacy of oxygenation and ventilation**

This is fundamental to the assessment of acute respiratory compromise and should be reassessed frequently to monitor progress and evaluate the effects of interventions.

Assess the effort of breathing by repeated clinical observation of rate, depth and pattern of respiration; look for use of accessory muscles and features of exhaustion. Monitor the SpO_2 by pulse oximetry in all patients and perform ABG analysis if any of the following features is present:

- a need for airway or ventilatory support
- SpO_2 <92% (or unreliable), central cyanosis or high O_2 requirements
- features of hypercapnia: drowsiness, confusion, asterixis
- severe, prolonged or worsening respiratory distress
- background of COPD and/or chronic type 2 respiratory failure
- smoke inhalation (carboxyhaemoglobin)
- suspected metabolic acidosis or primary hyperventilation.

Use the $SpO_2 \pm PaO_2$ to assess adequacy of oxygenation.

Correct hypoxia by administration of supplemental O_2. Titrate the inspired O_2 concentration (FiO_2) to the minimum required to achieve a target SpO_2:

- 94–98% for previously well patients.
- normal baseline SpO_2 for patients with chronic hypoxia.

Monitor FiO_2 requirements carefully to maintain the target SpO_2.

Use the $PaCO_2$ to assess adequacy of ventilation (see Clinical tool, p. 116).

Distinguish acute and acute-on-chronic ventilatory failure from chronic compensated hypercapnia.

Look for reversible factors contributing to ventilatory impairment, e.g. bronchospasm, sedation, respiratory depressants. Be vigilant for loss of hypoxic drive in patients with chronic type 2 respiratory failure receiving supplemental O_2 but suspect an alternative cause, e.g. exhaustion, airways obstruction, if the patient exhibits marked breathlessness or increased effort of breathing.

Seek input from the critical care team and consider the need for respiratory support, e.g. non-invasive ventilation or tracheal intubation and mechanical ventilation if any of the following features is present:

- impending exhaustion
- acute/acute-on-chronic ventilatory failure not resolving with the measures described above
- progressively rising $PaCO_2$
- SpO_2 <90% or PaO_2 <8 kPa despite maximal respiratory assistance
- progressively rising FiO_2 requirements to maintain target SpO_2.

12

3 **Underlying COPD?**

See 'Further assessment of acute dyspnoea in COPD' if the patient has known or suspected COPD.

In the absence of a pre-existing diagnosis, suspect COPD in any patient with a smoking history and either:

- clinical (Fig. 12.1) or CXR features of hyperinflation, or
- chronic exertional dyspnoea with wheeze and/or a chronic productive cough.

4 **Evidence of respiratory tract infection (RTI)?**

Having considered the above conditions, go to 'Further assessment of respiratory tract infection' if any of the following features is present:

- new cough with purulent sputum or significant increase in purulent sputum
- temperature ≥38°C or <35°C
- acute illness with sweating, shivers and myalgia
- clinical/CXR signs of consolidation (Figs 12.2 and 12.3) with ↑WBC/CRP.

Clinical tool
Interpretation of arterial blood gases

Assessment of ventilation

$PaCO_2$ is directly determined by alveolar ventilation – the volume of air transported between the alveoli and the outside world in any given time. Therefore, $\uparrow PaCO_2$ (hypercapnia) implies ventilatory failure – type 2 respiratory failure.

A slow, gradual rise in $PaCO_2$ (chronic type 2 respiratory failure) is usually accompanied by an increase in HCO_3^- that serves to maintain overall acid–base balance (H^+ within normal range). However, this metabolic compensation occurs over days/weeks so any acute rise in $PaCO_2$ (acute or acute-on-chronic type 2 respiratory failure) will lead to an increase in H^+ (Table 12.1).

In type 2 respiratory failure, the rate of rise in $PaCO_2$ and the associated increase in H^+ provide a better guide to severity than the absolute value of $PaCO_2$.

A $\downarrow PaCO_2$ implies hyperventilation. If PaO_2 is also lowered (or just within normal limits), the hyperventilation is probably an appropriate response to hypoxia. Alternatively, if HCO_3^- is decreased, it may reflect respiratory compensation for a primary metabolic acidosis, e.g. diabetic ketoacidosis. A $\downarrow PaCO_2$ with normal PaO_2 and HCO_3^- (on room air) suggests primary (psychogenic) hyperventilation but this is a diagnosis of exclusion (see below).

Assessment of oxygenation

A $\downarrow PaO_2$ implies impairment of oxygenation. A corresponding normal $PaCO_2$ indicates that this is due to ventilation/perfusion mismatch – type 1 respiratory failure. In contrast, $\uparrow PaCO_2$ indicates that it is due, at least in part, to failure of ventilation – type 2 respiratory failure.

The administration of supplemental O_2 makes ABG analysis more complex as it can be difficult to judge whether the PaO_2 is appropriate for the FiO_2 and, hence, whether oxygenation is impaired. A useful rule of thumb is that the difference between FiO_2 (%) and PaO_2 (in kPa) should be ≤10. A patient breathing room air (FiO_2 of 21%) should have a PaO_2 of at least 11 kPa. If subtle impairment is suspected, repeat the ABG on room air.

It is important to note the distinction between impaired oxygenation ($\downarrow PaO_2$) and inadequate oxygenation (insufficient PaO_2 to support normal aerobic metabolism). Consider a patient with a PaO_2 of 8.5 kPa: oxygenation

is clearly impaired, suggesting the presence of important lung disease. However, this PaO_2 would usually result in an SaO_2 (arterial oxygen saturation) >90%, a level which will allow adequate delivery of O_2 to tissues (provided that haemoglobin and cardiac output are normal).

Assessment of acid–base status

An acidosis is any process that acts to lower blood pH ($\uparrow H^+$); an alkalosis is one that acts to raise blood pH ($\downarrow H^+$). An $\uparrow PaCO_2$ indicates a respiratory acidosis; a $\downarrow PaCO_2$ indicates a respiratory alkalosis.

A $\downarrow HCO_3^-$ indicates a metabolic acidosis; an $\uparrow HCO_3^-$ indicates a metabolic alkalosis.

A respiratory or metabolic acid–base disturbance usually triggers an adjustment by the other system to limit the change in blood pH (compensation). Respiratory compensation happens over minutes; metabolic compensation takes days to weeks.

Having identified the presence of any metabolic or respiratory disturbances, look next at H^+ (or pH) to assess the overall impact on acid–base status. If the metabolic and respiratory processes oppose each other, the H^+ helps to differentiate the primary disturbance from the compensatory response: an $\uparrow H^+$ (or upper limit of normal) suggests that the acidosis is the primary disturbance and vice versa.

Primary respiratory acidosis (ventilatory failure) and alkalosis (hyperventilation) are dealt with above.

Causes of metabolic acidosis and alkalosis are shown in Box 12.2. If there is a primary metabolic acidosis, calculate the anion gap:

$$\text{Anion gap} = (Na^+ + K^+) - (Cl^- + HCO_3^-)$$
$$[\text{Normal} = 10{-}18 \, mmol/L]$$

Table 12.1 Arterial blood gases in different patterns of type 2 respiratory failure

	$PaCO_2$	HCO_3^-	pH
Acute	↑	→	↓
Chronic	↑	↑	→
Acute-on-chronic	↑	↑	↓

---

5   Clinical/CXR features of heart failure?

Acute decompensated heart failure is the likely cause of breathlessness if any of the following are present:

- CXR evidence of pulmonary oedema or congestion (Fig. 12.4)

- a recent history of orthopnoea, nocturnal dyspnoea or progressively worsening exertional dyspnoea
- signs of fluid overload: peripheral oedema, $\uparrow JVP$

Always suspect the diagnosis in patients with a background of chronic heart failure or

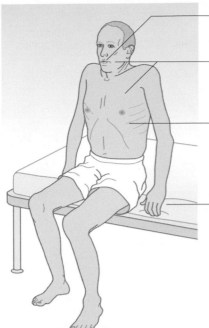

- Pursed lips

- Increased rate and depth of breathing

- Intercostal indrawing

- Sitting forward and gripping bed (increases action of accessory muscles)

Signs of hyperinflation
↑Antero-posterior diameter
Intercostal indrawing
Decreased cricosternal distance
Poor chest expansion (<5 cm)

12

Fig. 12.1 Clinical features of COPD.

Box 12.2 Causes of metabolic acidosis and alkalosis

Metabolic acidosis (low HCO_3^-)

With raised anion gap
- Lactic acidosis, e.g. hypoxaemia, shock, sepsis, infarction
- Ketoacidosis (diabetes, starvation, alcohol excess)
- Renal failure
- Poisoning (aspirin, methanol, ethylene glycol)

With normal anion gap
- Renal tubular acidosis
- Diarrhoea
- Ammonium chloride ingestion
- Adrenal insufficiency

Metabolic alkalosis (high HCO_3^-)

- Vomiting
- Potassium depletion, e.g. diuretics
- Cushing's syndrome
- Conn's syndrome (primary hyperaldosteronism)

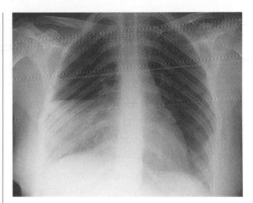

Fig. 12.2 Pneumonia of the right middle lobe.

other predisposing cardiac condition, e.g. previous MI, LV systolic dysfunction or valvular disease but assess carefully for alternative causes of acute decompensation (especially if the above features are absent) and remember that acute heart failure can also present *de novo*.

Difficulty may arise when the CXR is not diagnostic, e.g. in early or mild cases, and when auscultatory findings resemble those heard in other disorders, e.g. pulmonary fibrosis, bilateral pneumonia. A therapeutic trial may assist diagnosis: rapid improvement of symptoms with vasodilators/diuretics is strongly suggestive of heart failure as the aetiology of dyspnoea.

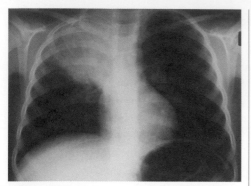

Fig. 12.3 Right upper lobe pneumonia containing air bronchograms.

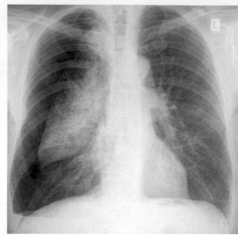

Fig. 12.5 Right pneumothorax.

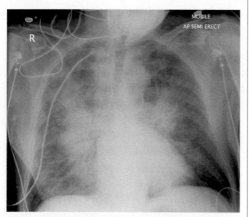

Fig. 12.4 Left ventricular failure. Note the hazy perihilar shadowing ('bat's wings'), the prominent, dilated upper lobe veins and the basal Kerley B lines, all characteristic of pulmonary oedema. There is also cardiomegaly.

Consider non-cardiogenic pulmonary oedema in acutely dyspnoeic patients with bilateral pulmonary infiltrates but no other evidence of heart failure – especially in the setting of severe acute pathology such as trauma, burns, pancreatitis or sepsis.

Echocardiography, to assess ventricular and valvular function, is a key diagnostic test and is particularly useful in patients without a pre-existing diagnosis of heart failure or in those with possible non-cardiogenic pulmonary oedema.

If available, brain-type natriuretic peptide (BNP) testing can help to rule out acute heart failure. Low plasma BNP (<100 pg/mL) or N-terminal-pro BNP (<300 pg/mL) make the diagnosis unlikely.

However, BNP is also raised in a wide variety of other cardiac and non-cardiac conditions so elevated levels do not automatically confirm a diagnosis of acute heart failure.

6 Generalized wheeze with ↓PEFR?

See 'Further assessment of acute asthma exacerbation' in patients with known asthma and either:

• generalized wheeze, or
• ↓PEFR.

Consider other causes of acute dyspnoea, e.g. pneumothorax or PE, if neither of these features is present.

Suspect a first presentation of asthma (and proceed to 'Further assessment of acute asthma exacerbation') if there is widespread wheeze with no evidence of COPD, anaphylaxis or pulmonary oedema (see above). Assess with pulmonary function tests (PFTs) ± PEFR diary following resolution of the acute episode.

7 Diagnostic CXR abnormality?

CXR may be more sensitive than clinical examination for detecting some lung abnormalities, e.g. pneumothorax (Fig. 12.5), pleural effusion (Fig. 12.6) or lobar collapse (see Figs 17.3 and 17.4, p. 163).

See below (p. 129) for 'Further assessment of pleural effusion'.

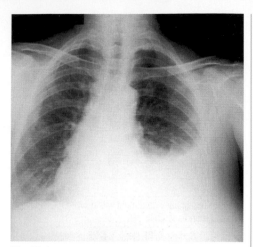

Fig. 12.6 Left pleural effusion.

If the patient has lobar collapse, consider further investigation, e.g. bronchoscopy to exclude a proximal obstructing lesion.

If CXR appearances are non-specific or uncertain, continue through the diagnostic process and attempt to correlate with clinical findings. Consider further imaging, e.g. CT thorax, or specialist respiratory input if no firm diagnosis emerges.

8 Ischaemic ECG changes (see Box 6.1, p. 51)?

Dyspnoea may be the predominant manifestation of myocardial ischaemia/infarction. If there is ECG evidence of ischaemia (Box 6.1) and no obvious alternative cause for breathlessness, assess as described in Chapter 6.

9 ABG shows primary metabolic acidosis with normal PaO$_2$?

Identify the presence of metabolic acidosis by ABG analysis (see Clinical tool, p. 116). If present, look for an underlying cause (see Box 12.2)

- examine for evidence of shock or mesenteric infarction
- test urine for glucose and ketones
- check U & E
- measure plasma glucose, lactate, salicylate levels
- calculate the anion gap.

Do not attribute dyspnoea solely to metabolic acidosis if there is evidence of hypoxaemia.

Table 12.2 Clinical and chest X-ray findings in patients with suspected PE in the emergency department (with and without confirmed PE on further investigation)

Feature	Confirmed PE (n = 1,880)	No PE identified (n = 528)
Clinical findings		
Dyspnoea at rest	50%	51%
Pleuritic chest pain	39%	28%
Cough	23%	23%
Haemoptysis	8%	5%
Syncope	6%	6%
Signs of DVT (unilateral limb swelling)	24%	18%
CXR findings		
Normal	40%	41%
Atelectasis	17%	15%
Infiltrate	14%	14%
Pleural effusion	16%	14%

Adapted from Pollack CV et al. 2011. Clinical characteristics, management, and outcomes of patients diagnosed with acute pulmonary embolism in the emergency department: initial report of EMPEROR (Multicenter Emergency Medicine Pulmonary Embolism in the Real World Registry). J Am Coll Cardiol. 57(6):700–706.

10 Clinical suspicion of PE?

PE is under-diagnosed. Clinical and CXR findings, in isolation, lack diagnostic sensitivity and specificity (Table 12.2). Use a clinical decision tool such as that shown in Fig. 12.7 and Table 12.3 to evaluate for PE in patients with acute dyspnoea and any of the following:

- relevant risk factors, e.g. active malignancy, recent surgery or prolonged immobility
- haemoptysis, pleuritic chest pain or evidence of deep vein thrombosis (DVT)
- unexplained hypoxaemia
- ECG features of right heart strain (see p. 58)
- no clear alternative diagnosis

D-dimer is less useful in hospitalized patients so in this setting consider further investigation if the Wells score is ≥2. Have a low threshold for performing ABG as subtle oxygenation abnormalities may not be detected by SpO$_2$. Where imaging is performed to exclude PE, CT pulmonary angiography offers greater sensitivity than a ventilation/perfusion scan and may demonstrate an alternative diagnosis.

12

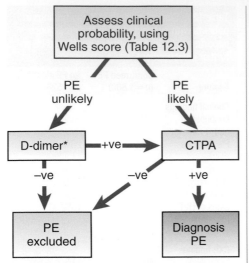

Fig. 12.7 Algorithm for the assessment of suspected pulmonary embolism using the Wells score. *Highly sensitive assay.

Table 12.3 Wells score (pulmonary embolism)	
Clinical variable	Points
Clinical signs and symptoms of DVT[1]	3
No alternative diagnosis is more likely than PE	3
Heart rate >100 bpm	1.5
Immobilisation or surgery in the previous 4 weeks	1.5
Previous DVT/PE	1.5
Haemoptysis	1
Active malignancy (treatment within last 6 months or palliative)	1
Score >4: PE likely; ≤4: PE unlikely	

[1]Minimum of leg swelling and pain elicited upon palpation of the deep veins.

Further assessment of acute dyspnoea in patients with COPD

Step 1 Clarify cause for acute deterioration

- Ensure that there is no new CXR abnormality: look carefully for evidence of collapse, consolidation, pneumothorax or pleural effusion. If there are features of consolidation, treat as pneumonia rather than 'infective exacerbation of COPD'.
- Ask about cough and sputum: treat as an infective exacerbation of COPD if there is an increase in sputum volume or purulence with no evidence of consolidation.
- If wheeze is predominant and there are no features of infection, the likely diagnosis is non-infective exacerbation of COPD. Look for precipitants, e.g. beta-blocker, non-compliance with inhalers, environmental trigger.
- Evaluate for PE (see Fig. 12.7) if there is a sudden increase in breathlessness or hypoxia without wheeze, change in sputum or new CXR abnormality.

Step 2 Establish pre-exacerbation status and details of previous exacerbations

This provides a comprehensive picture of underlying disease severity, helping to guide the goals and limits of therapy.

- Baseline performance: quantify normal exercise tolerance, ask about activities that provoke dyspnoea and ascertain ability to perform activities of daily living (ADLs).
- Baseline lung function: refer to previous ABG/ SpO_2 measurements and PFTs to provide an objective estimate of disease severity and look for evidence of chronic hypercapnia (see above).
- Trajectory of disease: consider changes in the above severity measures over time, the frequency of admissions and previous requirement for respiratory support, e.g. non-invasive and invasive ventilation.
- Previous sputum cultures: antibiotic prescribing should be guided by local protocols but knowledge of previous pathogens may permit more effective tailored therapy; discuss with the microbiology team if unusual or resistant organisms have been grown on previous cultures.

Step 3 Compare current status to baseline and monitor response to treatment

- Oxygenation and ventilation: compare current ABG values and SpO_2 to previous records. Give supplemental O_2 to return SpO_2/PaO_2 to baseline. If the patient has chronic type 2 respiratory failure, monitor for loss of ventilatory drive and repeat an ABG after any increase in FiO_2.
- Airways obstruction: assess PEFR and the presence/extent of wheeze; monitor changes to gauge response to bronchodilator therapy.
- Functional reserve: assess overall work of breathing (rate, depth, use of accessory muscles). Very high respiratory work cannot be maintained for long; refer to critical care if there is impending exhaustion.
- Following recovery, record pre-discharge PEFR, SpO_2 and ABG on air.

12

Further assessment of acute asthma exacerbation

Step 1 Assess severity and need for hospital admission

Assess severity in any patient with suspected acute asthma according to Table 12.4; perform an ABG if there are life-threatening features or SpO_2 <92%. Admit patients to hospital if they have:

- any life-threatening features
- features of a severe attack persisting after initial treatment
- PEFR <75% or significant ongoing symptoms after 1 hour of treatment
- other features causing concern, e.g. previous near-fatal asthma, poor compliance.

If there are ongoing features of a severe attack, monitor in a critical care environment with repeated assessment of SpO_2, PEFR, RR, HR and work of breathing ± ABG. Refer urgently to the intensive care unit if $PaCO_2$ is >6 kPa or rising, or there is worsening hypoxia, exhaustion or ↓GCS.

Step 2 Look for treatable precipitants

Seek evidence of infection, e.g. pyrexia, purulent sputum, ↑WBC, physical/CXR signs of consolidation (see Figs 12.2 and 12.3) and flitting upper lobe infiltrates, suggesting allergic bronchopulmonary aspergillosis. Culture sputum if this is purulent and blood if temperature is ≥38°C. Carefully review the CXR to exclude pneumothorax (see Fig. 12.5).

Step 3 Assess baseline control

Establish:

- frequency and severity of exacerbations
- baseline symptoms between exacerbations
- best PEFR
- current inhaler regimen, technique and compliance
- frequency of PRN inhaler use
- frequency of oral steroids (need for bone protection?)
- current smoking status.

Look for avoidable precipitants, e.g. pollen, pets, cold air, exercise, smoking, occupational triggers, beta-blockers, NSAIDs.

Table 12.4 Clinical features of severe asthma		
Severity	PEFR	or Other features
Moderate	50–75% best or predicted	Increased symptoms
Severe	33–50% best or predicted	Any of: RR >25 HR >110 Inability to complete sentences in one breath
Life-threatening	<33% best or predicted	Any of: PaO_2 <8 kPa 'Normal' $PaCO_2$ (>4.6–6.0 kPa) SpO_2 <92% Silent chest Cyanosis Exhaustion/altered conscious level Poor respiratory effort Arrhythmia Hypotension
Near-fatal		$PaCO_2$ >6 kPa

Modified from British Thoracic Society, Scottish Intercollegiate Guidelines Network 2014. British guideline on the management of asthma. Thorax. 69(Suppl 1):1–192.

Further assessment of respiratory tract infection

Step 1 Classify the type of RTI

In patients with features of RTI, distinguish pneumonia from non-pneumonic infection by the presence of focal chest signs, e.g. crackles, bronchial breathing and/or new CXR shadowing (see Figs 12.2 and 12.3). Classify as community-acquired pneumonia (CAP) if infection has been acquired out of hospital, and hospital-acquired pneumonia (HAP) if the onset of illness occurred ≥2 days after hospital admission or within 90 days of discharge from hospital after an admission of 2 or more days. In previously well patients without focal chest signs or CXR abnormality, the likely diagnosis is non-pneumonic RTI, e.g. acute bronchitis. In patients with known bronchiectasis, consider an infective exacerbation if the sputum becomes more purulent or offensive; assessment of patients with underlying COPD is described above.

Step 2 Assess severity

The CURB-65 score (Table 12.5) can help to risk-stratify patients with CAP. Consider referral to critical care for monitoring/intervention in patients with a CURB-65 score >2. Patients with a low CURB-65 may still require admission to hospital if they require supplementary oxygen.

Step 3 Look for predisposing factors

Assess for factors associated with immunocompromise, e.g. chronic disease (AIDS, diabetes, cirrhosis, malnutrition), acute disease (any critical illness), drugs (steroids, cancer chemotherapy) or previous splenectomy. Suspect aspiration in patients with a history of swallowing difficulty, stroke, alcoholism or recent unconsciousness. Pneumonia may occur distal to a bronchial carcinoma – repeat the CXR to ensure resolution of changes in patients with risk factors and consider further investigation, e.g. bronchoscopy, if there are persistent symptoms/CXR features or recurrent pneumonia at the same site. Preceding viral infection, especially influenza, may predispose to severe secondary bacterial infection. Consider endocarditis in patients with multiple discrete or flitting shadows on CXR, especially IV drug users.

Step 4 Gather information to inform antimicrobial choice

In any patient requiring hospitalisation for RTI, culture blood and sputum, perform serological assessment for atypical pathogens and (during influenza outbreaks) take a viral throat swab. In patients with severe pneumonia (CURB-65 >2), send urine (*Legionella*) and blood/sputum (*Pneumococcus*) for rapid antigen detection by PCR. Aspirate pleural fluid for microscopy and culture if there is an associated parapneumonic effusion. Send multiple sputum samples (induced with nebulized hypertonic saline if necessary) for Ziehl–Neelsen staining and TB culture if there is a suspicion of TB:

- significant immunocompromise or debility
- previous residence in an endemic TB area
- recent close contact with a smear-positive TB patient
- CXR evidence of previous TB
- a background of persistent productive cough with weight loss, night sweats or other constitutional symptoms.

Table 12.5 CURB-65 score

Feature	Score
Confusion	Abbreviated Mental Test <8/10
Urea	>7 mmol/L
RR	≥30/min
BP	Systolic <90 or diastolic <60 mmHg
Age	≥65 years

Total score	30-day mortality risk
0	0.6%
1	3.2%
2	13.0%
3	17.0%
4	41.5%
5	57.0%

Lim W, et al. 2003. Defining community acquired pneumonia severity on presentation to hospital: an international derivation and validation study. Thorax. 58(5):377–382.

12

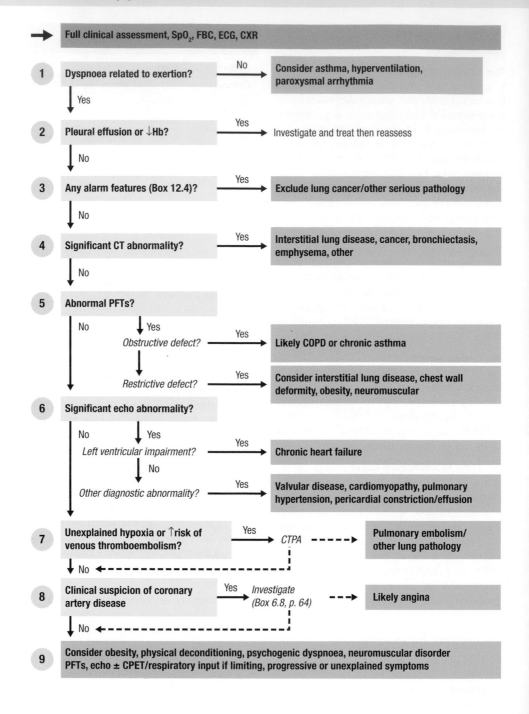

→ Full clinical assessment, SpO$_2$, FBC, ECG, CXR

1 Dyspnoea related to exertion? — No → Consider asthma, hyperventilation, paroxysmal arrhythmia

↓ Yes

2 Pleural effusion or ↓Hb? — Yes → Investigate and treat then reassess

↓ No

3 Any alarm features (Box 12.4)? — Yes → Exclude lung cancer/other serious pathology

↓ No

4 Significant CT abnormality? — Yes → Interstitial lung disease, cancer, bronchiectasis, emphysema, other

↓ No

5 Abnormal PFTs?

No ↓ ↓ Yes

Obstructive defect? — Yes → Likely COPD or chronic asthma

↓

Restrictive defect? — Yes → Consider interstitial lung disease, chest wall deformity, obesity, neuromuscular

6 Significant echo abnormality?

No ↓ ↓ Yes

Left ventricular impairment? — Yes → Chronic heart failure

↓ No

Other diagnostic abnormality? — Yes → Valvular disease, cardiomyopathy, pulmonary hypertension, pericardial constriction/effusion

7 Unexplained hypoxia or ↑risk of venous thromboembolism? — Yes → *CTPA* - - - - → Pulmonary embolism/ other lung pathology

↓ No

8 Clinical suspicion of coronary artery disease — Yes → *Investigate (Box 6.8, p. 64)* - - - → Likely angina

↓ No

9 Consider obesity, physical deconditioning, psychogenic dyspnoea, neuromuscular disorder PFTs, echo ± CPET/respiratory input if limiting, progressive or unexplained symptoms

1 Dyspnoea related to exertion?

Chronic dyspnoea arising from organic disease is almost always provoked or exacerbated by exertion, so episodic dyspnoea unrelated to exertion has a limited range of diagnoses.

Suspect asthma if there is:

- associated cough or wheeze
- a reproducible precipitant for episodes, e.g. cold air, pollen, house dust, pets
- diurnal variation in symptoms with prominent nocturnal or early morning symptoms (especially if sleep is disturbed), or
- a history of atopy.

Seek objective evidence of airflow reversibility or variability to confirm the diagnosis: the former by spirometry (≥15% improvement in FEV_1 following inhaled bronchodilators), the latter by asking the patient to keep a diary of peak-flow recordings (look for >20% diurnal variation on ≥3 days/week for 2 weeks). Consider specialist assessment if the diagnosis is uncertain, especially if occupational asthma is suspected.

Paroxysmal tachyarrhythmia may present with discrete episodes of breathlessness without any clear precipitant (although dyspnoea, when present, is usually aggravated by exertion). Consider this if:

- dyspnoea is accompanied by palpitation
- episodes arise 'out of the blue' with an abrupt onset, or
- the ECG shows evidence of pre-excitation (see Fig. 26.2, p. 233).

If paroxysmal tachyarrhythmia is suspected, attempt to document the rhythm during symptoms (see p. 237) if necessary using an ambulatory recorder or smart phone ECG monitor.

Dyspnoea that occurs predominantly at rest with no consistent relationship to exertion may be functional. Suspect this if the patient exhibits typical features (Box 12.3) in the absence of objective evidence of cardiorespiratory disease (normal examination, SpO_2, CXR ± PFTs/serial PEFR). Refer for specialist assessment if there is diagnostic doubt or symptoms are troublesome or disabling despite explanation and reassurance.

2 Pleural effusion or ↓Hb?

Consider these conditions early as they can be easily confirmed or excluded. Go to 'Further evaluation of pleural effusion' if there is CXR ± clinical evidence of unilateral effusion (see Fig. 12.6). Always check Hb in patients with exertional dyspnoea, as pallor is an insensitive sign. If Hb is decreased, evaluate as described on page 136 but consider other causes – especially if Hb is only slightly decreased or symptoms persist despite correction.

3 Any alarm features (Box 12.4)?

Change in voice or stridor may indicate laryngeal/tracheal obstruction secondary to intrinsic cancer or extrinsic compression (lymphoma, thyroid tumour or retrosternal goitre); if present, refer the patient urgently for endoscopic evaluation, e.g. fibre optic bronchoscopy/nasoendoscopy.

Refer for urgent specialist evaluation with bronchoscopy ± CT to exclude lung cancer if the patient has risk factors (>40 years or smoking history) accompanied by any suspicious clinical or CXR features (see Box 12.4); these include

---

Box 12.3 Features suggestive of psychogenic dyspnoea

- Provoked by stressful situations
- Inability to take a deep breath or 'get enough air'
- Frequent deep sighs
- Digital/perioral tingling
- ↓$PaCO_2$ with normal PaO_2 on ABG
- Short breath-holding time

Box 12.4 Alarm features in chronic dyspnoea

Clinical features

- Stridor
- Haemoptysis
- Weight loss
- Change in voice
- Persistent or non-tender cervical lymphadenopathy
- Finger clubbing

CXR features (see also Box 17.1, p. 163)

- Lung mass
- Cavitation
- Hilar enlargement
- Lobar collapse (persistent)

N.B. These features are especially worrying if the patient is a smoker, is >40 years or has had asbestos exposure.

12

lobar collapse, which may indicate a proximal obstructing tumour.

In younger non-smokers consider initial further evaluation with CT thorax; refer for specialist assessment if CT suggests malignant disease, fails to reveal a clear alternative cause or is not readily available. Evaluate patients with haemoptysis as described in Chapter 17.

4 Significant CT abnormality?

Arrange high-resolution CT to look for evidence of ILD if the patient has any of the relevant features listed in Box 12.5.

Box 12.5 Criteria for investigations in chronic dyspnoea

PFTs if there is:

- wheeze
- prominent nocturnal or early morning symptoms
- symptoms precipitated by cold weather or common allergens
- history of atopy
- clinical or CXR features of hyperinflation (see Fig. 12.2)
- smoker aged >40 years
- chronic productive cough (≥3 consecutive months for ≥2 successive years)
- occupational dust exposure, treatment with methotrexate/amiodarone or previous radiotherapy
- ↓SpO_2 (at rest or on exertion) with no apparent alternative cause
- major or progressive decrease in effort tolerance without other obvious cause.

Echocardiogram if there is:

- significant ECG abnormality, e.g. left bundle branch block, evidence of LVH, pathological Q waves, frequent ventricular ectopics, atrial fibrillation
- previous MI or chronic hypertension (especially if target organ damage)
- ↑JVP or peripheral oedema
- murmur (not previously investigated)
- clinical/CXR evidence of pulmonary congestion, cardiomegaly or pulmonary hypertension
- elevated BNP (BNP ≥35 pg/mL; N-terminal-pro BNP ≥125 pg/mL).

High-resolution CT thorax if there is:

- interstitial shadowing on CXR (Fig. 12.8)
- unexplained restrictive lung defect or ↓gas transfer
- strong clinical suspicion of interstitial lung disease, e.g. hypoxia or end-inspiratory crackles in a patient with previous exposure to birds, dust or hay.

Refer for specialist evaluation if CT shows evidence of ILD or other serious pathology, e.g. cancer, bronchiectasis. Arrange further investigation with PFTs, if these have not been performed already, if the CT shows features of emphysema.

5 Abnormal PFTs?

Have a low threshold for requesting PFTs (Box 12.5 and Tables 12.6 and 12.7).

Diagnose COPD if FEV_1/FVC is <70% (indicating airways obstruction) with a post-bronchodilator FEV_1 <80% predicted (indicating incomplete reversibility). Look for other characteristic abnormalities, including ↑TLC and RV (which helps to differentiate from ILD in borderline cases) and ↓gas transfer (indicative of significant emphysema). Exclude alpha$_1$-antitrypsin deficiency in younger patients. If SpO_2 is ≤92%, perform an ABG to identify patients with type 2 respiratory failure or those who might qualify for home oxygen therapy.

Diagnose asthma if there is an obstructive ventilatory defect with ≥15% improvement in FEV_1 following inhaled bronchodilators. If not, consider further assessment with repeat spirometry, PEFR

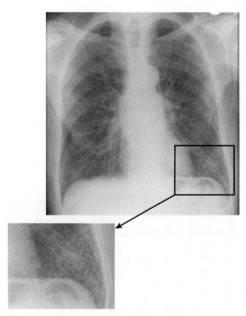

Fig. 12.8 CXR in interstitial lung disease.

Table 12.6 Pulmonary function tests

Test	Description	Measures	Examples of relevant diagnoses
Spirometry	Airflow at the mouth is measured during a forced exhalation	FEV_1, FVC	Obstructive lung disease: disproportionate reduction in FEV_1 (FEV_1:FVC ratio <0.8) Restrictive lung disease: proportionate reduction in FEV_1 and FVC
Reversibility	Spirometry is repeated after giving bronchodilators	FEV_1, FVC	Complete reversibility of obstruction is common in asthma, incomplete reversibility common in COPD
Lung volumes	Gas dilution or whole-body plethysmography	TLC, RV	COPD (normal or increased TLC), restrictive lung disease (reduced TLC and RV)
Diffusion capacity	Carbon monoxide uptake from alveoli is measured	DLCO, Dm	Interstitial pneumonitis (low DLCO, low Dm), pulmonary haemorrhage (high DLCO, normal Dm)

DLCO – lung diffusion of carbon monoxide; Dm – membrane component of diffusion; FEV_1 – forced expired volume in 1 second; FVC – forced vital capacity; RV – residual volume; TLC – total lung capacity.

12

Table 12.7 Severity of airflow obstruction

Severity	FEV_1
Mild	50–80% predicted
Moderate	30–49% predicted
Severe	<30% predicted

Source: Modified from Boon NA, Colledge NR, Walker BR, Hunter JAA. Davidson's Principles and Practice of Medicine, 20th edn. Edinburgh: Churchill Livingstone, 2006 (Box 19.30, p. 680).

diary or specialist evaluation if there is high clinical suspicion or borderline spirometry results.

In patients with a restrictive lung defect (see Table 12.6), evaluate for an underlying cause:

- arrange echocardiography and reassess following treatment if there is evidence of pulmonary congestion
- look for major chest wall deformity, e.g. severe kyphoscoliosis
- exclude ILD with high-resolution CT if there are suggestive clinical/CXR features (Fig. 12.8) or there is no clear alternative cause
- measure BMI to identify massive obesity, e.g. BMI >40.

Suspect extrapulmonary compression (e.g. neuromuscular disorder, chest wall deformity) if there is a decrease in TLC with normal RV, and an intrapulmonary cause, e.g. ILD, if there is a proportionate decrease in TLC and RV.

6 Significant echocardiographic abnormality?

Refer for cardiology evaluation if the echo shows major valvular abnormality, e.g. severe mitral regurgitation or aortic stenosis or pericardial effusion.

In chronic heart failure, exertional dyspnoea may be the sole presenting feature, but significant cardiac dysfunction is unlikely in the absence of the features in Box 12.5. The presence and severity of left ventricular systolic dysfunction can be determined by echocardiography. Consider cardiology referral if left ventricular systolic function is normal but the patient has clinical features suggestive of heart failure, e.g. elevated JVP, oedema or CXR evidence of pulmonary congestion – especially if there is left ventricular hypertrophy/left atrial dilatation (heart failure with preserved ejection fraction) or a history of previous cardiac surgery/radiotherapy (constrictive pericarditis).

If the echo suggests pulmonary hypertension without significant LV impairment or valvular disease, evaluate fully for underlying chronic lung disease, e.g. PFTs, high-resolution CT chest, sleep studies, CTPA. In the absence of hypoxaemia or significant lung disease, refer for specialist assessment.

7 **Unexplained hypoxia or ↑risk of venous thromboembolism?**

Exclude chronic thromboembolic disease in any patient with unexplained hypoxia or risk factors for DVT. Ventilation/perfusion lung scanning may have higher sensitivity for detection of chronic PE but CT pulmonary angiography is more likely to identify alternative lung pathology, e.g. ILD, emphysema.

8 **Clinical suspicion of coronary artery disease?**

Angina occasionally manifests as a sensation of breathlessness without chest discomfort. Evaluate for angina with an exercise ECG or other stress test (see Box 6.8, p. 63) if the patient has risk factors for coronary artery disease (see Box 6.3, p. 52) and symptoms are consistently provoked by exertion and relieved within 5 minutes by rest. Relief of symptoms with anti-anginal therapy or coronary revascularisation confirms the diagnosis.

9 **Consider other causes. Further investigation if limiting, progressive or unexplained symptoms**

Obesity rarely causes significant cardiorespiratory impairment unless BMI is >40. However, lesser degrees of obesity and/or physical deconditioning are frequently responsible for exertional breathlessness and ↓exercise capacity; suspect this in patients with ↑BMI (especially >30), recent weight gain or a sedentary lifestyle.

If there are features of hyperventilation (see Box 12.3) or symptoms are disproportionate to objective findings, perform an ABG on room air (ideally during symptoms) and consider referral for formal evaluation of psychogenic dyspnoea.

At this stage, review any abnormalities detected and determine whether they are sufficient to account for the presentation. In patients with multiple possible causes for dyspnoea, e.g. obesity, left ventricular impairment and airways disease, cardiopulmonary exercise testing (in which ECG, respiratory gas exchange and minute ventilation are recorded during exercise) may help to establish the predominant mechanism. Patients with a major change or progressive decline in exercise capacity without adequate explanation require further evaluation; arrange an echocardiogram and PFTs if these have not yet been performed, and consider referral for specialist evaluation, e.g. cardiac catheterisation or cardiopulmonary exercise testing.

Box 12.6 Causes of abnormal pleural fluid collections

Serous effusions

Transudate
- Cardiac failure
- Hepatic failure
- Renal failure
- Nephrotic syndrome
- Hypoalbuminaemia
- Peritoneal dialysis
- Constrictive pericarditis
- Hypothyroidism
- Meigs' syndrome (pleural effusion, benign ovarian fibroma and ascites)

Exudate
- Parapneumonic (usually bacterial)
- Bronchial carcinoma
- TB
- Connective tissue disease
- Pancreatitis
- Mesothelioma
- Post-MI syndrome
- Sarcoidosis

Other fluids

Pus
- Empyema; most commonly caused by acute bacterial infection of the pleura

Chyle
- Chylothorax; caused by lymphatic obstruction, most commonly by metastatic cancer

Blood
- Haemothorax; causes acute dyspnoea, usually following trauma

Box 12.7 Light's criteria for differentiation of pleural exudate and transudate

The pleural fluid is likely to be an exudate if ≥1 of the following criteria is present:
- pleural fluid protein : serum protein ratio >0.5
- pleural fluid LDH : serum LDH ratio >0.6
- pleural fluid LDH >two-thirds of the upper limit of normal serum LDH.

Further assessment of pleural effusion

Box 12.6 lists the causes of abnormal collections of fluid in the pleura. Initial assessment depends on laboratory analysis of the fluid.

- Use Light's criteria to distinguish exudative from transudative effusions (Box 12.7).
- Review pleural fluid biochemistry. The presence of amylase indicates pancreatitis; pH <7.3 suggests bacterial infection or cancer; rheumatoid factor suggests connective tissue disease.
- Identify evidence of infection: Gram stain, culture, microscopy for acid-fast bacilli. TB culture may take months.
- Look for evidence of malignancy: cytology may identify malignant cells; CT thorax ± needle biopsy may reveal malignancy; pleural biopsy of regions identified as abnormal may provide a diagnostic specimen.

12

Fatigue is physical and/or mental exhaustion. It is very common and non-specific, so identifying significant underlying disease is difficult. Acute fatigue is usually caused by self-limiting infections or transient life circumstances. This guide pertains to fatigue of at least 2 weeks' duration.

A careful history may reveal that the problem is actually something other than fatigue, e.g. breathlessness, in which case this should be pursued. If a localizing or more specific feature, e.g. haemoptysis, fever, jaundice, comes to light, make it the primary focus of assessment.

Causes of fatigue are shown below, with an emphasis on conditions that frequently present with fatigue as the chief complaint. Important problems to differentiate from fatigue are described in Box 13.1.

Non-organic causes

- Psychological stress/overwork.
- Depression.
- Fibromyalgia.
- Chronic fatigue syndrome.

Medications

- Beta-blockers.
- Chronic alcohol excess.
- Benzodiazepines and other sedatives.
- Corticosteroids.
- Chemotherapeutic agents.

Malignancy

- Haematological.
- Solid organ.
- Disseminated.

Respiratory causes

- Obstructive sleep apnoea.
- Chronic obstructive pulmonary disease.

Cardiac causes

- Congestive cardiac failure.
- Bradyarrhythmias.

Haematological causes

- Anaemia.
- Haematological malignancy, e.g. lymphoma.

Endocrine causes

- Hypothyroidism.
- Hypercalcaemia.
- Diabetes mellitus.
- Adrenal insufficiency.
- Hypopituitarism.

Infection

- Infectious mononucleosis.
- Tuberculosis.
- HIV.
- Infective endocarditis.
- Lyme disease.

Chronic inflammatory conditions

- Rheumatoid arthritis.
- Inflammatory bowel disease.
- Connective tissue disorders, e.g. systemic lupus erythematosus.

Box 13.1 Presentations that must be distinguished from fatigue

Exertional dyspnoea

Establish if the true complaint is reduced exercise tolerance. Quantify how far the patient can walk in meters/other tangible distance. Assess as described in Chapter 12.

Muscle weakness

Ask specifically about muscle weakness and formally assess muscle group power (see Table 22.1). If detected, evaluate muscle weakness as per Chapter 22.

Excessive sleepiness

This may result from depression, insomnia or sleep disordered breathing, e.g. obstructive sleep apnoea (OSA). Assess with the Epworth sleep score. Ask the patient's partner about snoring and episodes of apnoea/hypoapnoea during sleep. If OSA is suspected, refer the patient for formal sleep studies.

Loss of motivation

This may result from depression, chronic stress or other psychosocial problems – consider it whenever a patient no longer participates in hobbies, interests and other activities. 'Tiredness' or 'lack of energy' is often cited as the reason for giving up these activities and careful questioning may be required to distinguish true physical limitation from a lack of inclination or will.

General debility

Ask about a change in weight, appearance or clothes size. Measure weight and compare with previous records if available. Look for evidence of malnutrition and reduced muscle bulk. If present, evaluate thoroughly for an underlying malignant, inflammatory, GI or endocrine cause.

Concealed concerns

Fatigue may act as a 'proxy' complaint for an issue that the patient is reluctant to raise directly, e.g. problems with finances, employment, alcohol or personal/sexual relationships. Enquire with tact, allow time and opportunity for the patient to voice concerns and ask specifically about alcohol intake (see Box 2.1, p. 11).

13

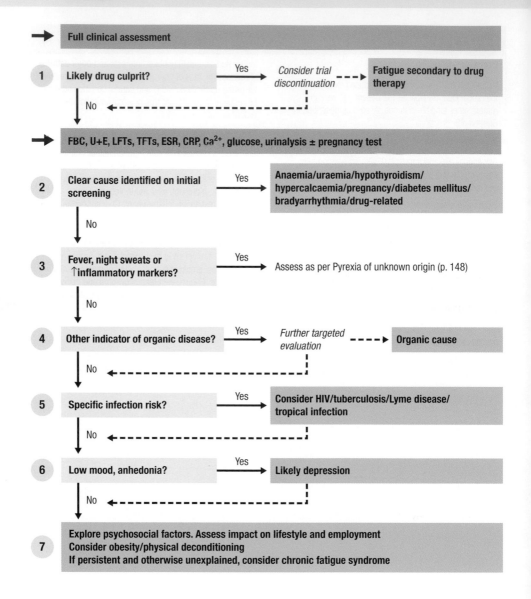

→ **Full clinical assessment**

1   **Likely drug culprit?**   Yes → *Consider trial discontinuation* ----▶ **Fatigue secondary to drug therapy**

No

→ **FBC, U+E, LFTs, TFTs, ESR, CRP, Ca²⁺, glucose, urinalysis ± pregnancy test**

2   **Clear cause identified on initial screening**   Yes → **Anaemia/uraemia/hypothyroidism/ hypercalcaemia/pregnancy/diabetes mellitus/ bradyarrhythmia/drug-related**

No

3   **Fever, night sweats or ↑inflammatory markers?**   Yes → Assess as per Pyrexia of unknown origin (p. 148)

No

4   **Other indicator of organic disease?**   Yes → *Further targeted evaluation* ----▶ **Organic cause**

No

5   **Specific infection risk?**   Yes → **Consider HIV/tuberculosis/Lyme disease/ tropical infection**

No

6   **Low mood, anhedonia?**   Yes → **Likely depression**

No

7   **Explore psychosocial factors. Assess impact on lifestyle and employment Consider obesity/physical deconditioning If persistent and otherwise unexplained, consider chronic fatigue syndrome**

1   Likely drug culprit?

Review all medications – prescribed and over-the-counter. Suspect a drug cause if there is a temporal relationship between a likely culprit (see above) and the onset of symptoms. If possible, stop or replace suspect medications and review symptoms after an appropriate interval. Alcohol in excess or used chronically can cause fatigue. Toxic environmental exposures, e.g. carbon monoxide, lead, mercury, arsenic, are less common, but potentially reversible causes.

2   Definite cause identified on examination or screening investigations?

If any of the abnormalities listed below are detected, reassess fatigue after appropriate evaluation and treatment.

Anaemia

This may cause fatigue but is also a common feature of chronic disease. See 'Further assessment of anaemia' (p. 136) in any patient with ↓Hb.

Renal failure

Uraemia is a cause of fatigue. If there is new or worsening renal impairment, see 'Further assessment of renal failure' (p. 230).

Hypercalcaemia

Fatigue and other symptoms, e.g. abdominal pain, vomiting, constipation, polyuria, confusion and anorexia, may occur if corrected serum calcium is >3.0 mmol/L. Hypercalcaemia may reflect serious underlying disease, e.g. bony metastases, squamous cell lung cancer and multiple myeloma.

Firstly, check a parathyroid hormone (PTH) level:

- an ↑ or →PTH suggests primary hyperparathyroidism. Refer to Endocrinology
- if ↓PTH, examine the breasts (p. 48) and prostate, perform a CXR, a radioisotope bone scan and myeloma 'screen', review drugs (especially calcium or vitamin D supplements). If no cause is identified, consider a CT scan of the chest, abdomen and pelvis to look for underlying malignancy.

Diabetes mellitus

Formally evaluate for diabetes if the patient has other suggestive symptoms or an elevated fasting or random blood glucose (see Clinical tool: Diagnosing diabetes and glycaemic complications, p. 299).

Poor glycaemic control in known diabetes cases may cause fatigue. Review the blood glucose diary and HbA_{1c} to determine whether control is adequate and, if not, reassess the fatigue after correction. Repeated episodes of hypoglycaemia may also cause fatigue, and should be addressed.

Hypothyroidism

Ask about symptoms of cold intolerance, constipation and weight gain, and look for hypothyroid facies, dry skin, brittle hair and nails, myxoedema and goitre. In patients with known hypothyroidism, consider whether thyroxine replacement is adequate and ask about compliance. ↑TSH and ↓T_4 confirms primary hypothyroidism. Beware the low TSH with low T_4 – this may indicate secondary hypothyroidism so perform a full pituitary hormone profile.

Bradycardia

If HR is <60 bpm, perform an ECG and consider a 24-hour tape. Refer to a cardiologist if there is evidence of complete heart block, a resting HR <50 bpm or a blunted HR response to exercise.

Pregnancy

Consider in any woman of child-bearing age and, if necessary, perform a pregnancy test.

3   Fever, night sweats or ↑inflammatory markers?

Fatigue is a common, and often predominant, symptom in patients with systemic inflammatory or malignant disease, e.g. lymphoma, endocarditis, myeloma, tuberculosis. If there is a history of fever or night sweats or an ↑ESR/CRP, review as described for fever and pyrexia of unknown origin (Chapter 14).

4   Other indicator of organic disease?

Look for the following indicators of organic disease during your assessment.

13

Abnormalities on FBC or blood film

High or low cell counts, abnormal cells, e.g. blasts, or morphological abnormalities, e.g. target cells, may indicate important haematological or systemic disease. Seek haematological advice for any unusual or unsuspected abnormality.

Lymphadenopathy

Enlarged lymph nodes may occur with malignancy (lymphoma, leukaemia or secondary deposits) or in reaction to infection/inflammation. The most important conditions to consider are HIV, tuberculosis (TB), infectious mononucleosis and malignancy.

- Search for a local source of infection/ inflammation if swelling is localized to one lymph node group.
- Suspect haematological malignancy if there is generalized painless lymphadenopathy.
- Consider lymph node biopsy if the cause is not apparent or you suspect malignancy.

Evidence of cardiorespiratory dysfunction

- Look for features of cardiac failure (↑JVP, peripheral oedema, pulmonary congestion) or a new murmur; if present, arrange an ECG and echocardiogram.
- Check SpO_2 at rest ± on exertion; if low, perform an ABG on room air and look for an underlying cause.
- Ask about smoking history and consider CXR/pulmonary function tests (see Table 12.5, p. 126).

Some patients find it difficult to differentiate between fatigue and dyspnoea; if there is a clear history or objective evidence of reduced effort tolerance, consider a similar approach to that of chronic exertional dyspnoea (see Ch. 12).

Features of chronic liver disease or deranged LFTs

Look for stigmata of chronic liver disease (Box 19.5, p. 176). If jaundiced, assess as per Ch. 19. If LFTs are abnormal, enquire about alcohol intake and discontinue hepatotoxic drugs; if the abnormality persists, consider a 'liver screen' (Box 19.7, p. 181).

Features of adrenal insufficiency

Look for pigmentation of sun-exposed areas, recent scars, palmar creases and mucosal membranes; vitiligo/other autoimmune conditions; postural hypotension and $\downarrow Na^+/\uparrow K^+$. Confirm with a short ACTH (Synacthen) stimulation test.

5 Specific infection risk?

Consider HIV if the patient:
- has had unprotected sex, a blood transfusion, done health-care work or has been resident in an HIV endemic area
- has engaged in high-risk sexual activity
- is an IV drug user, past or present.

Consider a CXR ± Mantoux test if the patient has:
- had previous TB or been resident in a TB endemic area
- had recent exposure to a patient with active TB
- immunosuppression.

Consider Lyme serology if the patient has:
- a history of a recent tick bite
- a history of an erythema chronicum migrans
- recently travelled to an endemic area.

Discuss with an ID unit if the patient has:
- recently undertaken foreign travel beyond Europe and North America
- a history of a recent animal bite.

6 Low mood, anhedonia?

Suspect depression if the patient has lost enjoyment or interest in life (ask about previous interests, hobbies and so on), reports low mood or expresses negative thoughts (guilt, pessimism, low self-esteem) out of proportion to the circumstances. Look for blunted affect, psychomotor retardation and biological symptoms, e.g. loss of libido, early morning waking. Consider psychiatric referral or a trial of antidepressants.

7 Explore psychosocial factors and impact on lifestyle. Consider obesity, physical deconditioning, chronic fatigue syndrome

If the patient has a BMI >30 or lacks physical fitness, encourage appropriate lifestyle changes and reassess. If not already excluded consider coeliac disease, infectious mononucleosis and Lyme borreliosis. Chronic fatigue syndrome is a diagnosis of exclusion with specific criteria (Box 13.2).

Box 13.2 Diagnostic criteria for chronic fatigue syndrome

Fatigue for ≥4 months with all of the following:
- a clear starting point
- persistent and/or recurrent symptoms
- unexplained by other conditions
- a substantial reduction in activity level
- characterized by post-exertional malaise and/or fatigue (feeling worse after physical activity)

and one or more of the following:
- difficulty sleeping or insomnia
- muscle and/or joint pain without inflammation
- headaches
- painful lymph nodes that are not enlarged
- sore throat or general malaise or flu-like symptoms
- cognitive dysfunction, such as difficulty with thinking
- physical or mental exertion that makes symptoms worse
- dizziness and/or nausea
- palpitation, without heart disease

13

Further assessment of anaemia

Step 1 Use the mean cell volume (MCV) to narrow the differential diagnosis

In the UK, *microcytic anaemia* (MCV <76 fL) is usually due to iron deficiency.

First, confirm iron deficiency. Serum ferritin is more indicative of total body iron than serum iron but may be increased by liver disease or systemic inflammation.

- ↓ferritin confirms iron deficiency.
- If ferritin is normal, transferrin saturation <20% suggests iron deficiency.

If iron deficiency is confirmed, identify the underlying cause.

- Review the diet and consider inadequate iron intake, especially in vegetarians.
- Ask about blood loss: haematemesis, melaena, haemoptysis, epistaxis, haematuria, menorrhagia, trauma.
- Arrange UGIE and colonoscopy unless there is a clear non-GI source of bleeding, e.g. menorrhagia, haematuria.

Where the cause remains unclear

- exclude coeliac disease: serology ± duodenal biopsy at the time of UGIE
- refer to GI for further investigation, e.g. small bowel pathology.

Reassess symptoms and FBC after iron supplementation and treatment of any underlying cause.

Refer patients with a ↓MCV and normal iron stores to a haematologist for investigation of alternative diagnoses, e.g. thalassaemia, sideroblastic anaemia.

In patients with a *macrocytic anaemia* (MCV >98 fL), measure vitamin B_{12} and fasting serum folate.

In the absence of pregnancy, causative drugs, e.g. methotrexate, phenytoin, or haemolysis (see below), ↓folate is likely to be due to poor dietary intake (fruit, leafy vegetables) but always check coeliac serology.

↓B_{12} is unlikely to be due to dietary deficiency unless the patient is a strict vegan. Check for previous gastrectomy or small bowel surgery, then investigate for pernicious anaemia. Intrinsic factor antibodies are diagnostic but only present in 60% of cases; anti-parietal cell antibodies are non-specific but their absence makes pernicious anaemia less likely (present in 90% of cases). Seek Haematology advice in difficult cases.

If B_{12} and folate are normal, exclude hypothyroidism, pregnancy and alcoholic liver disease, and then evaluate for haemolysis (Step 2) and myelodysplasia (Step 3), as described below.

Measure iron studies and vitamin B_{12}/folate in patients with *normocytic anaemia*, as combined iron and B_{12} or folate deficiencies, e.g. nutritional deficiency, small bowel disease, may result in a normocytic picture.

Step 2 Investigate for haemolysis

Consider haemolysis in patients with normal or ↑MCV.

Seek evidence of ↑red cell destruction:

- ↑bilirubin/LDH
- ↑urinary urobilinogen
- red cell fragments on blood film

and a compensatory increase in red cell production:

- ↑reticulocytes
- polychromasia
- nucleated red cell precursors on blood film.

If present, distinguish intravascular from extravascular haemolysis to narrow the differential diagnosis.

Intravascular haemolysis, e.g. in microangiopathic haemolytic anaemia (MAHA), defective mechanical heart valve, malaria – releases free Hb into the plasma, leading to

- ↓plasma haptoglobins (mop up free Hb then cleared by the liver)
- methaemalbuminaemia (once haptoglobin binding is saturated)
- haemosiderinuria (once albumin binding capacity exceeded)
- haemoglobinuria (black urine if fulminant, e.g. in malaria).

With extravascular haemolysis, e.g. hereditary spherocytosis, autoimmune haemolysis or red cell enzymopathies, these features are absent and there is often clinical or USS evidence of splenomegaly (the site of red cell breakdown).

In either case, review the blood film for diagnostic abnormalities:

- malaria parasites on thick and thin films (mandatory if recent travel to malaria endemic region)
- sickle cells – sickle cell anaemia

- red cell fragments – MAHA, e.g. haemolytic uraemic syndrome, thrombotic thrombocytopenic purpura; defective mechanical heart valve, march haemoglobinuria
- spherocytes – autoimmune haemolytic anaemia or hereditary spherocytosis
- Heinz bodies, bite cells – G-6-PD deficiency.

Discuss immediately with a haematologist if you suspect haemolytic uraemic syndrome or thrombotic thrombocytopenic purpura, e.g. AKI, neurological features, acute diarrhoeal illness. If spherocytes are present, perform a direct Coombs test to help differentiate autoimmune haemolytic anaemia from hereditary spherocytosis. If the cause is unclear, consider enzyme assays (G-6-PD or pyruvate kinase deficiency) and Hb electrophoresis (haemoglobinopathies) and refer to a haematologist.

Step 3 Seek evidence of bone marrow failure or haematological malignancy

Review the FBC and blood film for:

- deficiencies in other cell lines ($\downarrow$WBC, $\downarrow$platelets)
- $\uparrow$WBC, e.g. chronic myeloid leukaemia, chronic lymphocytic leukaemia
- atypical cells, e.g. blasts.

Examine for lymphadenopathy and splenomegaly, and refer for further investigation, e.g. bone marrow evaluation.

Look for evidence of a paraproteinaemia, e.g. multiple myeloma: send serum for protein electrophoresis and urine for measurement of Bence Jones protein. Discuss with a haematologist if these are positive or if there is clinical suspicion, e.g. bone pain, pathological fracture, lytic bone lesions, unexplained $\uparrow$Ca^{2+} or ESR.

Step 4 Consider chronic non-haematological disease

Consider chronic kidney disease as a potential cause for normocytic ($\downarrow$erythropoietin production) if GFR <60 mL/min/1.73 m^2, and especially if <30 mL/min/1.73 m^2. Measure ferritin and transferrin saturation to ensure that the patient is iron-replete (ferritin >100 ng/mL; transferrin saturation >20%) and discuss with a nephrologist.

The most common cause of normocytic anaemia is chronic inflammatory disease, e.g. rheumatoid arthritis, polymyalgia rheumatica, chronic infection or malignancy. Consider the diagnosis if:

- other causes of $\downarrow$Hb have been excluded (including iron, B$_{12}$, folate deficiency)
- there is no evidence of active bleeding
- anaemia is mild, e.g. Hb>80 g/L, and
- unexplained weight loss, fever, $\uparrow$ESR/CRP or $\downarrow$albumin – search for an underlying cause.

Step 5 Refer to a haematologist

Seek input from a haematologist if the cause of anaemia is still unclear, you suspect a serious or unusual haematological disorder or the patient fails to respond to therapy.

13

14 Fever

Fever (or pyrexia) is a body temperature >99th percentile of the healthy adult maximum; in clinical practice, a temperature ≥38°C is usually regarded as significant. Extreme fever (>41°C) is life threatening and tends to occur with gram negative bacteraemia, drug reactions, e.g. neuroleptic malignant syndrome, intracranial pathology (leading to central temperature dysregulation) or extreme environmental conditions. Pyrexia of unknown origin (PUO) is documented fever that persists without explanation for 2–3 weeks despite investigation.

Fever occurs most commonly as part of the acute phase response to infection. Sepsis is defined as 'life-threatening organ dysfunction due to a dysregulated host response to infection'*; it carries a significant mortality and must be recognized and managed quickly. Other causes of fever are malignancy, connective tissue disease, drug reactions, miscellaneous causes and fictitious fever.

*Singer M, Deutschman CS, Seymour CW, et al. The Third International Consensus Definitions for Sepsis and Septic Shock (Sepsis-3). JAMA. 2016 Feb 23;315(8):801-10.

Infection

Respiratory system

- Acute bronchitis.
- Pneumonia.
- Influenza.
- Empyema.
- Infective exacerbation of bronchiectasis/COPD.
- Tuberculosis (TB).

GI causes

- Gastroenteritis.
- Appendicitis.
- Biliary sepsis.
- Viral hepatitis.
- Diverticulitis.
- Intra-abdominal TB.
- Hepatic abscess.

Skin/soft tissue

- Cellulitis.
- Erysipelas.
- Necrotizing fasciitis.
- Pyomyositis.
- Infected pressure sore.
- Wound infection.

Musculoskeletal causes

- Septic arthritis (native and prosthetic joint).
- Osteomyelitis.
- Discitis.
- Epidural abscess.

Genitourinary tract

- Lower urinary tract infection (UTI), e.g. cystitis, prostatitis.
- Upper UTI (pyelonephritis).
- Perinephric collection.
- Pelvic inflammatory disease.
- Epididymo-orchitis.
- Syphilis.

CNS

- Meningitis (bacterial, viral, fungal, TB).
- Encephalitis.
- Cerebral abscess.

ENT

- Upper respiratory tract infection (RTI), e.g. tonsillitis.
- Otitis media.
- Quinsy.
- Dental abscess.

- Mumps/parotitis.
- Glandular fever (Epstein–Barr virus; EBV).
- Sinusitis.

Immunocompromised patients

- *Pneumocystis jiroveci (carinii)* pneumonia.
- Aspergillosis.
- TB.
- Atypical mycobacterial infection, e.g. *Mycobacterium avium intracellulare*.
- Cytomegalovirus (CMV) infection.
- Toxoplasmosis.
- Cryptococcal meningitis.
- *Nocardia* infection.
- Disseminated herpes/fungal infection.

Returning travellers

- Malaria.
- Typhoid.
- Infective diarrhoea, e.g. cholera, amoebiasis, *Shigella*.
- Amoebic liver abscess.
- *Strongyloides* infection.
- Schistosomiasis.
- Dengue.
- Chikungunya

Other infectious causes

- Leptospirosis.
- Brucellosis.
- Lyme disease.
- Q fever.
- HIV.
- Toxoplasmosis.
- Fungal infection.
- Measles, rubella.
- Herpes zoster infection (chickenpox or shingles).

Malignancy

- Haematological malignancy, including lymphoma, leukaemia, myeloma.

- Solid tumours, especially renal, liver, colon, pancreas.

Connective tissue disorders

- Giant cell arteritis/polymyalgia rheumatica.
- Rheumatoid arthritis.
- Systemic lupus erythematosus.
- Polymyositis.
- Polyarteritis nodosa.
- Wegener's granulomatosis.
- Churg–Strauss disease.
- Cryoglobulinaemia.
- Adult-onset Still's disease.

Drugs

- Drug fever (almost any drug).
- Antipsychotics (neuroleptic malignant syndrome).
- Anaesthetics (malignant hyperthermia).
- Cocaine, amphetamines, ecstasy.

Other causes

- Transfusion-associated.
- Thyrotoxicosis, thyroiditis.
- Phaeochromocytoma.
- Deep vein thrombosis (DVT)/pulmonary embolism (PE).
- Pancreatitis.
- Alcoholic hepatitis/delirium tremens.
- Rheumatic fever.
- Inflammatory bowel disease.
- Sarcoidosis.
- Atrial myxoma.
- Familial Mediterranean fever.
- Erythroderma/Stevens–Johnson syndrome.
- Fictitious (fever or apparent fever surreptitiously engineered by the patient).

14

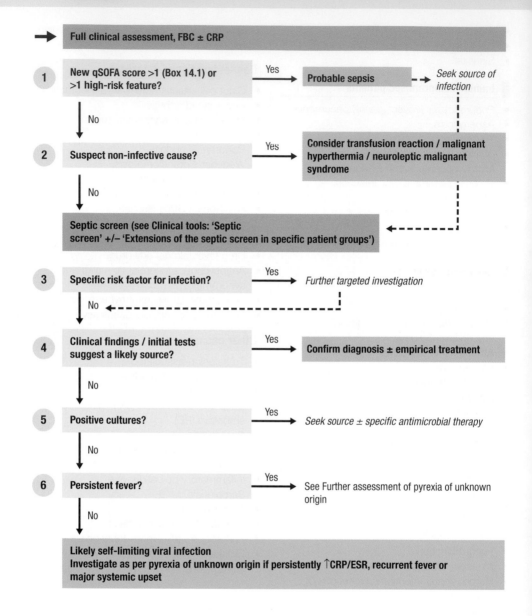

Full clinical assessment, FBC ± CRP

1 New qSOFA score >1 (Box 14.1) or >1 high-risk feature? — Yes → Probable sepsis ---→ *Seek source of infection*

No ↓

2 Suspect non-infective cause? — Yes → Consider transfusion reaction / malignant hyperthermia / neuroleptic malignant syndrome

No ↓

Septic screen (see Clinical tools: 'Septic screen' +/– 'Extensions of the septic screen in specific patient groups')

3 Specific risk factor for infection? — Yes → *Further targeted investigation*

No

4 Clinical findings / initial tests suggest a likely source? — Yes → Confirm diagnosis ± empirical treatment

No ↓

5 Positive cultures? — Yes → *Seek source ± specific antimicrobial therapy*

No ↓

6 Persistent fever? — Yes → See Further assessment of pyrexia of unknown origin

No ↓

Likely self-limiting viral infection
Investigate as per pyrexia of unknown origin if persistently ↑CRP/ESR, recurrent fever or major systemic upset

1 New qSOFA score >1 (Box 14.1) or >1 high-risk feature?

Unless you suspect a non-infective cause for fever (see step 2) use the qSOFA score (Box 14.1) to rapidly identify sepsis pending lab data/ABG/urine output trends: diagnose sepsis if qSOFA score >1 (assume baseline score of zero unless known pre-existing organ dysfunction). Also diagnose sepsis if >1 of the following features is present:

- Hypoxia (e.g. PaO_2/FiO_2 <53.3 KPa or supplemental O_2 required to maintain SpO_2 >94%)
- Hypotension (e.g. MAP <70 mmHg; SBP <100 mmHg or need for inotropes)
- GCS <15
- Oliguria: (e.g. not passed urine for ≥12 hours or urine output <0.5 ml/kg/hr)
- Serum creatinine >110 µmol/L or >50% rise from baseline.
- Bilirubin >20 µmol/L
- Platelets <150 × 10^9/L

Manage all patients with suspected sepsis in accordance with the Surviving Sepsis guidelines (http://www.survivingsepsis.org/GUIDELINES/Pages/default.aspx) while searching for a focus of infection – see Clinical tool: A septic screen (p. 142).

Assess haemodynamic status frequently (see Ch. 30) and manage as septic shock if there is persistent hypotension (mean arterial pressure [MAP] <65 mmHg) and ↑serum lactate (>2 mmol/L) despite adequate volume resuscitation.

2 Suspect non-infective cause for fever?

Most acute febrile illnesses are caused by infection, but the following conditions are

Box 14.1 qSOFA (quick SOFA) criteria

• Respiratory rate ≥ 22/min	1 point
• Altered mentation (e.g. GCS <15)	1 point
• Systolic blood pressure ≤ 100 mmHg	1 point

potentially life-threatening and important to recognize immediately; they may be overlooked if not specifically considered at the outset.

If the patient is receiving blood products, stop the transfusion, ensure the patient's ID matches that on the unit, and check that the ABO and RhD groups in the transfused blood are compatible with the patient. Contact the blood bank and seek immediate Haematology input if there is any suspicion of ABO incompatibility or other major transfusion reaction. Otherwise, monitor temperature and vital signs, and consider restarting the transfusion at a slower rate if observations are stable, the patient is systemically well and the rise in temperature is <1.5°C.

Suspect neuroleptic malignant syndrome if the patient has received neuroleptics, e.g. haloperidol, within the past 1–4 weeks and exhibits muscular rigidity, tremor and excessive sweating and/or altered mental status, especially in association with ↑CK.

If appropriate, ask the patient about recent use of cocaine, ecstasy or amphetamines; consider toxic hyperthermia if temperature is >39°C, especially if there are features of excessive sympathomimetic activity, e.g. ↑BP, ↑HR, dilated pupils, aggression, psychosis or serotonin syndrome, e.g. rigidity, hyper-reflexia. Measure CK, U+E, LFTs and coagulation, and monitor ECG, HR, BP and urine output, to identify complications such as rhabdomyolysis, acute renal failure, arrhythmia, disseminated intravascular coagulation and acute liver failure.

Assume malignant hyperthermia if the patient develops severe pyrexia with tachycardia ± rhabdomyolysis during administration of, or within 1–2 hours of exposure to, a volatile anaesthetic, e.g. halothane or succinylcholine.

Suspect heatstroke if the patient has had sustained exposure to very hot weather, e.g. during a heatwave or has been undertaking prolonged severe exertion in high temperatures.

In all of the above cases continue to evaluate for infection and other causes if there is any diagnostic doubt.

14

Clinical tool
A septic screen

The septic screen combines clinical assessment with laboratory analysis and imaging studies to identify a source of infection. It may also reveal non-infectious causes of pyrexia, e.g. malignancy. The full screen may not be required in all patients, especially if there is an obvious focus of infection.

General

- ≥2 sets of blood cultures, urinalysis, FBC, U+E, LFTs, CRP, CXR.

Respiratory

- Assess suspected RTI, e.g. new/worsening cough with purulent sputum or CXR consolidation as per page 123.
- Perform a pleural tap and send fluid for biochemical, microbiological and cytological analysis if unilateral pleural effusion (p. 129).
- If other respiratory features, e.g. haemoptysis, non-specific CXR hypoxia, consider further investigation, e.g. CT, bronchoscopy to exclude atypical infection, lung cancer and PE.

Abdominal

- Send stool samples for microscopy, culture and sensitivity testing ± *Clostridium difficile* toxin if acute diarrhoea.
- Investigate for inflammatory bowel disease, e.g. flexible sigmoidoscopy, if persistent bloody diarrhoea.
- Perform an urgent ascitic tap in any febrile patient with ascites; treat empirically as spontaneous bacterial peritonitis (SBP), pending culture, if >250 neutrophils/μL ascitic fluid. Consider TB and malignancy if fluid is exudative and initial cultures negative.

- If new-onset jaundice, arrange an abdominal USS and serology for viral hepatitis
  - Treat empirically for biliary sepsis and arrange surgical review if there is a cholestatic pattern of jaundice (p. 176) or USS shows dilated bile ducts.
  - Send blood and urine samples for leptospirosis culture and serology ± PCR if symptoms include purpura, ↓platelets or conjunctival congestion, or there has been recent exposure to potentially contaminated water, e.g. freshwater sports, sewage worker – liaise with the ID team.
- Check amylase and assess as described in Chapter 4 if acute abdominal pain with tenderness or guarding.
- If palpable abdominal mass investigate for infective, e.g. diverticular or appendiceal abscess, and non-infective, e.g. carcinoma, lymphoma, causes with USS or CT ± aspiration or biopsy.

Urinary tract

- Send an MSU if new-onset urinary tract symptoms, an indwelling urinary catheter or leucocytes/nitrites on urinalysis (bacterial UTI highly unlikely in the absence of either nitrites or leucocytes.)
- Arrange USS to exclude renal obstruction, calculus or a perinephric collection if loin pain or renal angle tenderness.
- Exclude urinary tract cancer ± inflammatory renal disease (see Ch. 16) if persistent haematuria (visible or non-visible) or loin pain with repeated negative MSU.
- Send swabs for *Neisseria gonorrhoeae* and *Chlamydia* if urethral or PV discharge.

Clinical tool—cont'd
A septic screen

Skin and soft tissue

- Send swabs from any wounds or sites discharging pus.
- Suspect cellulitis if there is an area of acutely hot, erythematous and painful skin; look for potential entry sites, e.g. peripheral cannulae, skin breaks.
- Seek immediate surgical assessment and give IV antibiotics if any features of severe necrotizing infection, e.g. rapid spread, crepitus, anaesthesia over lesion, major haemodynamic compromise or pain out of proportion with clinical findings.
- DVT may produce a low-grade fever – exclude as described on page 193 if acutely swollen limb.
- Consider investigation for osteomyelitis, e.g. bone scan, if persistent non-healing ulcer.
- Examine the whole body for rashes – seek urgent dermatology advice if blistering, mucosal involvement or pustules (see Ch. 27).

CNS

- Assume CNS infection, initially, if severe headache, meningism, purpuric rash, focal neurological signs, new-onset seizures or unexplained ↓GCS. Give immediate empirical treatment after blood cultures, arrange urgent neuroimaging and, if no contraindications (p. 170), perform lumbar puncture.
- If meningitis suspected, send a throat swab for Neisseria meningitidis PCR.

Cardiovascular

- Investigate for endocarditis (Box 14.2) with a transthoracic echocardiogram and ≥3 sets of blood cultures if new murmur, vasculitic/embolic phenomena or a predisposing cardiac lesion with no obvious alternative source of infection.
- Consider a transoesophageal echocardiogram if transthoracic images equivocal or persistent high clinical suspicion.

ENT

- Consider a throat swab for influenza during outbreaks or the autumn/winter season.
- Send a swab for Streptococcus pyogenes if pustular exudates.
- If parotitis or tender lymphadenopathy, consider a throat swab for mumps PCR and, if age-appropriate, check EBV serology (>95% of patients >35 years will have evidence of previous exposure).

Musculoskeletal

- If acutely swollen, painful joint, seek urgent orthopaedic assessment and perform diagnostic aspiration to exclude septic arthritis (see Ch. 20).
- If unexplained back pain with no other obvious source for fever, take ≥3 blood cultures and arrange spinal MRI to exclude discitis.

14

③ Specific risk factor for infection?

Infections other than those discussed above may need to be considered in patients returning to or entering the UK from abroad (especially from the tropics) and those who are immunocompromised or with IV drug use.

If the patient has come from an at-risk region for viral haemorrhagic fever and has unexplained bleeding, discuss urgently with the health protection team (before admission). Otherwise, complete a septic screen as per 'Clinical tool: Extensions to the septic screen in specific patient groups'. The prevailing strains and resistance patterns of common infections such as pneumonia may differ in other parts of the world, so seek input from an ID specialist at an early stage.

Immunocompromised patients may experience more severe sequelae from infection with common pathogens and are at greater risk of opportunistic infections, especially with mycobacteria, viruses and fungi. Follow the additional steps for immunocompromise (Clinical tool: Extensions to the septic screen in specific patient groups) if the patient has an acquired or congenital immunodeficiency (including HIV); is receiving treatment with high-dose steroids, immunosuppressants, DMARDs or anti-TNF drugs; or is neutropenic for any reason. More specific forms of immunocompromise include asplenia (↑susceptibility to encapsulated organisms and malaria) and the presence of indwelling vascular access devices or other prosthetic material. Test for HIV in patients who are at high risk or who present with an atypical infection or other indicators of HIV – see http://www.bhiva.org/documents/Guidelines/Testing/GlinesHIVTest08.pdf.

Ask about all forms of drug use in any patient presenting with unexplained fever. If there has been IV drug use, establish frequency, duration and sites of injection. Maintain awareness of any local/national outbreaks, as unusual organisms may be implicated, e.g. anthrax skin infections. Always consider the possibility of underlying blood-borne infection, e.g. hepatitis B or C, HIV. Discuss with the ID team if the patient is haemodynamically compromised or fails to improve on standard therapy.

Box 14.2 Modified Duke criteria for the diagnosis of infective endocarditis

Major criteria

Positive blood culture
- Typical organism from two cultures
- Persistent positive blood cultures taken >12 hours apart
- ≥3 positive cultures taken over >1 hour

Endocardial involvement
- Positive echocardiographic findings of vegetations
- New valvular regurgitation

Minor criteria

- Predisposing valvular or cardiac abnormality
- IV drug misuse
- Pyrexia ≥38°C
- Embolic phenomenon
- Vasculitic phenomenon
- Blood cultures suggestive – organism grown but not achieving major criteria
- Suggestive echocardiographic findings

Definite endocarditis: two major, or one major and three minor, or five minor

Possible endocarditis: one major and one minor, or three minor

Modified from Boon NA, Colledge NR, Walker BR, Hunter JAA. Davidson's Principles and Practice of Medicine, 20th edn. Edinburgh: Churchill Livingstone, 2006.

---

④ Clinical findings/initial tests suggest a likely source?

Following appropriate cultures, treat immediately with antibiotics according to the likely source and local guidelines in patients with severe sepsis. If no clear source is identified or the patient has neutropenia (especially if the neutrophil count is <1.0 × 10⁹/L) or other significant immunocompromise, provide empirical broad-spectrum antibiotic ± antifungal therapy. The choice of antimicrobials will depend on patient factors and local resistance patterns – discuss with Microbiology and other relevant specialties, e.g. Oncology, Haematology. Refine the antibiotic regimen in discussion with the Microbiology team on the basis of subsequent culture results.

Patients with recurrent fever, or fever in the absence of immunocompromise, neutropenia or haemodynamic disturbance can often wait for the results of cultures before antibiotic therapy is started. If there is a clear source of infection, start empirical antibiotic therapy and adjust as necessary in light of the culture results and sensitivity testing; otherwise, reassess daily whilst awaiting the full results of the septic screen.

5 Positive cultures?

Re-evaluate your initial diagnosis and treatment in the light of culture results.

Positive cultures may confirm a suspected source of infection, e.g. MSU, sputum and guide the most appropriate antibiotic therapy. On the other hand, blood cultures that yield an unexpected organism may challenge your working diagnosis and prompt re-evaluation for an alternative source, e.g. *Staphylococcus aureus* in suspected UTI.

In the patient with no obvious source of fever, positive blood cultures, especially in multiple bottles, confirm an infective aetiology and help to guide further investigation; for example, blood culture results are central to the diagnosis of infective endocarditis (see Box 14.2).

Persistently positive blood cultures despite appropriate antibiotic therapy suggest a deep-seated infection; the source must be identified and removed, e.g. debridement, drainage.

6 Persistent fever?

Acute fever is frequently a manifestation of self-limiting viral illnesses. In the absence of continuing pyrexia, ongoing symptoms or signs, or worrying investigation results, no further action is required.

Recurrent fever, especially with persistent elevation of inflammatory markers or significant constitutional upset, mandates further evaluation; if present, proceed to 'Further assessment of pyrexia of unknown origin'.

14

Clinical tool
Extensions to the septic screen in specific patient groups

Recent travel or residence abroad

- Document exactly where the patient has been, specific dates of travel and activities undertaken (including a sexual history). Ask about vaccinations/malaria prophylaxis prior to and during travel.
- Consult an ID specialist at an early stage for any returning traveller with unexplained fever.
- Exclude malaria if they are a recent traveller to an endemic region (http://www.cdc.gov/malaria/about/distribution.html) with three sets of blood films ± malaria antigen card:
  - use the antigen card to facilitate rapid diagnosis, particularly if acutely unwell, but also send films as the card may miss parasitaemia of <0.5% and is not accurate for speciation
  - take films over a 72-hour period, ideally after a fever spike, as this is when parasitaemia is highest
  - discuss any positive case immediately with an ID specialist and refer to the British Infection Society treatment guidance at http://www.journalofinfection.com/article/s0163-4453(16)00047-5/fulltext.
- If fever is accompanied by diarrhoea, isolate the patient and note all recent travel history on stool specimen requests. Discuss immediately with Microbiology and ID teams if any suspicion of cholera, e.g. refugee/aid worker in high-risk area.
- Send blood and stool cultures for typhoid if high fever, constitutional upset and recent travel to Asia (especially the Indian subcontinent), Africa (especially sub-Saharan) or Latin America. Discuss urgently with the ID team, especially if suggestive clinical features, e.g. rose-coloured spots over the trunk, relative bradycardia, constipation.
- Consider acute schistosomiasis if exposure to potentially infested water, e.g. freshwater swimming, rafting, water sports in Africa, South America or Asia, within the past 8 weeks, +/− eosinophilia, hepatosplenomegaly, RUQ tenderness, bloody diarrhoea or urticarial rash. Send blood for serology and discuss with an ID specialist.
- Arrange USS to exclude amoebic abscess if previous travel to the tropics and RUQ discomfort ± palpable liver.

- Check dengue fever serology if recent return from the tropics/subtropics and an acute febrile illness associated with a rash (generalized, blanching, macular in the initial stages), headache or severe aches and pains. Discuss immediately with the ID team if any suspicion of dengue haemorrhagic fever (epistaxis, GI bleeding, petechia, purpura, ↓platelets, coagulopathy) or dengue shock syndrome (↓BP, ↓capillary refill time, organ dysfunction).
- Send blood for Chikungunya serology/viral PCR if recent travel to an endemic region.

Immunocompromise

- In patients with HIV, check the most recent CD4 count and repeat if >3 months ago. Fungal and viral infections are more likely if CD4 count <200 but can occur at higher counts. Check compliance with anti-retroviral therapy/antimicrobial prophylaxis.
- Seek early advice from a respiratory specialist if there are respiratory symptoms or an abnormal CXR (especially cavitation) cavitation, or a high suspicion of *Pneumocystis* pneumonia due to any of the following features:
  - subacute, e.g. over 2–3 weeks, or progressive shortness of breath
  - non-productive cough
  - diffuse bilateral perihilar infiltrates on CXR or non-specific changes
  - unexplained hypoxaemia (including desaturation on exercise).
- Send sputum, for microscopy (acid-fast bacilli, fungal), histopathological analysis (*Pneumocystis*) and mycobacterial culture; if necessary, induce sputum by nebulized hypertonic saline in a negative-pressure environment and discuss need for other diagnostic procedures, e.g. bronchoalveolar lavage.
- If prominent GI symptoms, send blood for *Strongyloides* serology and consider investigation for CMV colitis, e.g. flexible sigmoidoscopy + biopsy and intra-abdominal TB, e.g. CT abdomen/pelvis ± targeted biopsy (samples must be sent in saline, not formalin, as acid-fast bacilli are destroyed).

Clinical tool—cont'd
Extensions to the septic screen in specific patient groups

- If CNS features, investigate as per the general septic screen but send blood for *Toxoplasma* serology, request CSF staining for *Cryptococcus* and TB, and biopsy any space-occupying lesion.
- Request a dermatology review and biopsy of any suspicious or unusual rashes, e.g. cutaneous T-cell lymphomas, Kaposi's sarcoma.
- Prolonged indwelling vascular access catheters, e.g. Hickman lines, tunnelled lines, carry a substantial risk of bacterial/fungal infection; suspect line infection in all cases where there is no clear alternative source, even if the entry point looks clean.
  - Take blood cultures from the line and, if feasible, remove sending the tip for culture.
  - Consider echocardiography to look for endocarditis in patients with confirmed bacteraemia – especially *S. aureus* or persistent fever.

- Discuss early with the relevant specialty if you suspect infection of prosthetic material, e.g. valve prosthesis, pacemaker and prosthetic joint.

IV drug use
- Take ≥3 sets of blood cultures prior to starting antibiotic therapy.
- Look at all new and old injection sites; if inflamed or tender, consider USS to exclude an underlying abscess.
- Arrange a Doppler USS to exclude DVT if there is any groin or leg swelling.
- Exclude ilio-psoas abscess by CT if there is groin or lower back pain with difficulty extending the leg.
- Arrange an echocardiogram ± transoesophageal echocardiography if there is no clear alternative source of fever or there is evidence of septic emboli on CXR (see Box 14.2).

14

Further assessment of pyrexia of unknown origin

Perform additional screening investigations (Box 14.3) in any patient with persistent unexplained fever. These may reveal a diagnosis or provide useful leads for further investigation.

- Discuss the significance of any positive serology with the ID/Microbiology team and a positive ANA, ENA or ANCA with the Rheumatology team.
- Biopsy any suspicious masses or lymphadenopathy (including bilateral hilar lymphadenopathy) detected clinically or radiologically.
- If an abscess is identified, request a surgical opinion regarding drainage.
- Discuss with Haematology and consider bone marrow examination if Bence Jones protein, paraproteinaemia or a significant blood film abnormality, e.g. atypical lymphocytes.
- Arrange muscle biopsy if ↑CK, to exclude inflammatory myositis.
- Perform a radioisotope bone scan to look for evidence of malignancy or osteomyelitis if persistent bony pain, ↑Ca^{2+}, ↑prostate-specific antigen or ↑alkaline phosphatase (with otherwise normal LFTs).
- If LFTs persistently deranged or hepatomegaly without an obvious cause, request a liver biopsy (with material for culture) to look for TB, sarcoidosis and granulomatous hepatitis.
- If persistent haematuria/proteinuria with negative MSU, discuss with the Renal team and consider renal biopsy to exclude glomerulonephritis.
- Use the Duke (see Box 14.2) and Jones criteria (Box 14.4) to confirm or refute a suspected diagnosis of endocarditis or rheumatic fever respectively.

Box 14.3 Further screening tests in pyrexia of unknown origin

Ensure that a full septic screen (see above) is carried out, plus:

Clinical

- Repeat a full clinical assessment, including travel, sexual, occupational and recreational history; lymph nodes, skin and eye examination; urinalysis; PR; breast and testicular examination.

Microbiological

- Serology for HIV, viral hepatitis (A–E), EBV, CMV, toxoplasmosis, Q fever, Lyme disease, brucellosis, syphilis, Chlamydia, Bartonella and Yersinia.
- Serology for leishmaniasis, amoebiasis, trypanosomiasis and schistosomiasis if there has been travel to the developing world.
- Tuberculin (Mantoux) test and three early morning urine specimens for TB microscopy and culture.
- Antistreptolysin O titre.

Biochemistry/immunology/haematology

- ANA, RF, ANCA.
- FBC with peripheral blood film, ferritin, LDH, CK, Ca^{2+}, plasma electrophoresis, TFTs, prostate-specific antigen (if male patient >50 years).
- Urine for Bence Jones protein.

Radiological

- CT chest/abdomen/pelvis.
- Echocardiogram.

Box 14.4 Jones criteria for the diagnosis of rheumatic fever

Major manifestations

- Carditis
- Polyarthritis
- Chorea
- Erythema marginatum
- Subcutaneous nodules

Minor manifestations

- Fever
- Arthralgia
- Previous rheumatic fever
- ↑ESR or CRP
- Leucocytosis
- First-degree atrioventricular block

PLUS

- Supporting evidence of preceding streptococcal infection: recent scarlet fever, raised antistreptolysin O or other streptococcal antibody titre, positive throat culture

N.B. Evidence of recent streptococcal infection is particularly important if there is only one major manifestation.

From Boon NA, Colledge NR, Walker BR, Hunter JAA. Davidson's Principles and Practice of Medicine, 20th edn. Edinburgh: Churchill Livingstone, 2006 (p. 617).

- Consider an ANCA-negative systemic vasculitis if palpable purpura, skin ulceration or livedo reticularis. Measure serum cryoglobulins (cryoglobulinaemic vasculitis); consider arteriography, e.g. renal, mesenteric or tissue biopsy if polyarteritis nodosa is suspected, e.g. eosinophilia, renal impairment, ↑BP, constitutional upset.
- If ↑ESR in a patient >50 years:
  - treat for giant cell arteritis and arrange temporal artery biopsy if there is headache, visual loss, scalp tenderness or an inflamed, thickened, pulseless or tender temporal artery
  - diagnose polymyalgia rheumatica if there is any proximal joint pain or stiffness – review the diagnosis if there is no response to systemic steroids within 72 hours.

- Suspect adult-onset Still's disease if microbiological and autoimmune investigations are consistently negative, and there are recurrent joint pains or a transient, non-pruritic, salmon-pink maculopapular rash that coincides with fever, especially if ↑↑↑ferritin.
- Review all drugs: discontinue one at a time for 72 hours and then reinstate if fever persists.
- If the cause remains unclear, consider a whole body PET scan to look for evidence of occult malignancy (e.g. lymphoma) or vasculitis, bone marrow biopsy or liver biopsy, and consider diagnoses of exclusion, e.g. Behçet's disease, familial Mediterranean fever, fictitious fever.

14

Haematemesis is the vomiting of blood from the upper GI tract. Bright red blood or clots imply active bleeding and are a medical emergency. Altered blood with a dark, granular appearance ('coffee-grounds') suggests that bleeding has ceased or has been relatively modest. *Melaena* is the passage of black tarry stools, usually due to acute upper GI bleeding (see 'Haematemesis' below), but occasionally due to bleeding within the small bowel or right side of the colon. *Haematochezia* is the passage of fresh red or maroon blood per rectum; it is usually due to colonic bleeding, but 15% of cases result from profuse upper GI bleeding.

Haematemesis

With major upper GI haemorrhage, resuscitation must take place alongside assessment. Diagnosis is secondary and will usually be established at upper GI endoscopy (UGIE). Many units have a major haemorrhage protocol with which you should be familiar.

Peptic ulcer

Peptic ulcer is the most common cause of upper GI bleeding (50%) and an important cause of massive haemorrhage. It is often accompanied by epigastric pain. Important aetiological factors include *Helicobacter pylori* infection (95% of duodenal, 75% of gastric ulcers) and NSAIDs/aspirin.

Gastritis/duodenitis

Gastritis/duodenitis (30%) is typically accompanied by dyspepsia, epigastric discomfort and nausea. Most commonly, it is due to excess alcohol consumption or NSAIDs/aspirin.

Oesophagitis

This is usually due to gastro-oesophageal reflux. There may be a history of heartburn, indigestion or painful swallowing.

Mallory–Weiss tear

This is a mucosal tear in the oesophago-gastric junction, following increased gastric pressure. 90% of these bleeds stop spontaneously. The history is characteristic: forceful retching with initially non-bloody vomit, followed by haematemesis.

Oesophageal/gastric varices

These are collateral veins that form in response to portal hypertension and allow portal blood to bypass the liver and enter the systemic circulation directly. The most common cause is hepatic cirrhosis. Segmental varices from portal vein thrombosis (pancreatitis) may occasionally occur. Patients typically present with massive upper GI bleeding.

Upper GI malignancy

There is often a background of weight loss, anorexia, early satiety or dysphagia; a palpable epigastric mass or signs of metastatic disease may rarely be evident.

Other uncommon causes

Congenital malformations of the vascular tree, e.g. Dieulafoy's lesion, can produce major haemorrhage. An aorto-duodenal fistula will usually present with massive haematemesis – suspect this if patient has had previous surgery for abdominal aortic aneurysm.

Rectal bleeding

The majority of patients have a benign cause. In acute rectal bleeding, assessment of bleeding severity and adequate resuscitation take precedence over diagnosis. The pattern of bleeding guides the location. Anorectal bleeding typically presents with intermittent episodes of minor, fresh, bright red bleeding during or after defecation, which is not mixed with the stools. Distal colon bleeding is darker red and may be partially mixed with the stools; proximal colon bleeding is dark red and fully mixed with stools. Remember that large volume upper GI or proximal colon bleeding can present with fresh bright red bleeding (and shock).

Perianal disorders

These are a common cause of rectal bleeding in all age groups. Bright red bleeding is often associated with other anorectal symptoms such as discomfort, mucus discharge or pruritus. Causes include haemorrhoids, fissure-in-ano, perianal Crohn's disease and anal cancer. Be aware that haemorrhoids can cause major bleeds. Always examine the anus of a patient presenting with rectal bleeding: diagnosis is made by PR examination and proctoscopy. Severe pain, especially during defecation, suggests anal fissure, and the patient will not tolerate PR examination. Always consider a concurrent proximal bleeding source.

Diverticular disease

Diverticular disease is the most common cause of severe acute rectal bleeding and typically occurs in older patients. Bleeding occurs due to erosion of a vessel in the neck of a diverticulum and is mostly fresh blood; it may be life-threatening but stops spontaneously in 75% of patients.

Colorectal carcinoma

Colorectal carcinoma is a common cancer in men and women. Recent weight loss, tenesmus, a change or alternating bowel habit or symptoms of colicky lower abdominal pain may be present. However, the presentation is frequently insidious with minimal symptoms. Polyps may also cause rectal bleeding. Diagnosis is made by colonic imaging (sigmoidoscopy/colonoscopy or CT colonography in patients who are unfit for endoscopic investigation.)

Inflammatory bowel disease

Colorectal inflammation in ulcerative colitis or Crohn's disease may cause rectal bleeding. The passage of frank blood ± mucus and tenesmus may occur in proctitis. Colitis produces bloody diarrhoea with intermittent cramping lower abdominal pain and, often, systemic upset. Endoscopy and biopsy of the lower bowel confirm the diagnosis; inflammatory markers (CRP, faecal calprotectin) provide a useful guide to disease activity. Perianal Crohn's disease is often associated with complex perianal fistulas.

Ischaemic colitis

Ischaemic colitis tends to occur in older patients, typically resulting in severe lower abdominal pain associated with rectal bleeding. It results from occlusion of the inferior mesenteric artery, which is usually due to situ thrombosis in atherosclerosis. (In contrast, acute embolus more commonly affects the superior mesenteric artery territory.)

Angiodysplasia (arteriovenous malformation)

These are degenerative vascular malformations and are an important cause of severe lower GI bleeding, predominantly in the elderly. Typical endoscopic features may be apparent but diagnosis is often challenging (CT angiography, labelled red cell scan) and bleeding frequently recurs.

15

Other causes

GI infections may cause bloody diarrhoea by causing local invasion of the mucosa, usually with systemic upset. Other small intestinal sources of rectal blood loss include Meckel's diverticulum (melaena) and intussusception ('currant jelly' bleeding) in young patients. Acute small bowel ischaemia may be associated with rectal bleeding but the predominant feature is severe abdominal pain and the patient is severely unwell. Small bowel tumours are rare and present with intermittent bleeding (may require capsule endoscopy).

Radiation proctocolitis should be considered in any patient with a history of pelvic radiation, e.g. for prostatic or gynaecological malignancy; most present within 2 years of radiotherapy.

Colonic ulcer is an uncommon cause of bleeding, usually related to use of NSAIDs. Rectal ulcers are poorly understood, typically occur in young adults and usually respond to conservative treatment (bulking agents and laxatives). Nicorandil is associated with oral, rectal and anal ulcers.

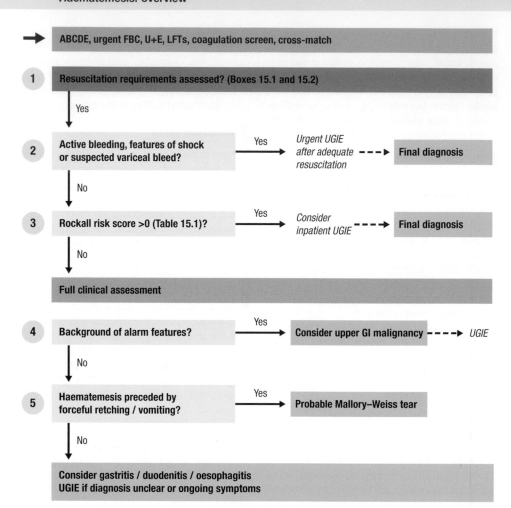

Box 15.1 Resuscitation in acute haemorrhage

First steps

- A+B before C: recheck airway frequently, especially if ↓GCS/vomiting. Give high concentration O_2
- Get help: one pair of hands is not enough. If necessary, call the medical emergency or cardiac arrest team

Secure IV access and monitoring

- 2 large bore cannulae in antecubital veins or equivalent
- Central venous cannulation, e.g. femoral line if peripheral access difficult
- Get expert help immediately if you cannot obtain adequate access
- Urgent FBC, U+E, LFTs, coagulation screen and cross-match (inform blood bank)
- Measure pulse, BP, RR, GCS and reassess peripheral perfusion every 10–15 min
- Insert urinary catheter; monitor hourly urine output

Resuscitate and reassess

Early shock features (see Box 15.2) or any ongoing blood loss:

- 0.5–1 L stat of IV crystalloid or colloid
- 2 units of red cells if Hb <8 g/dL, ongoing bleeding or >2 L IV crystalloid or colloid given

Reassess

- If advanced shock features or major blood loss on reassessment, resuscitate as per the adjacent column.
- Otherwise, continue with treatment and discuss with haematologist if any of the following:
  - known coagulopathy/anticoagulant therapy
  - INR >1 4
  - platelets <100 × 10⁹/L
  - fibrinogen <1 g/L
  - ≥4 L IV fluid in any form

Advanced shock features (see Box 15.2) or ongoing major blood loss:

- 1–2 L stat of IV crystalloid
- use red cells as soon as available
- consider O negative blood if significant delay in cross-matching (use group specific blood as soon as possible)

Reassess

- If ongoing advanced shock features or major blood loss, activate the major haemorrhage protocol: administer red cell concentrate (RCC) and fresh frozen plasma (FFP) and consider platelets and cryoprecipitate.
- Seek specialist input, e.g. ICU, GI, surgical, as appropriate and discuss haemostatic support, with haematologist.

Box 15.2 Clinical features of hypovolaemic shock

Early	Advanced
• HR >100 bpm	• Systolic BP <100 mmHg (or ↓40 mmHg from baseline)
• Capillary refill time (CRT) >2s	• HR >120 bpm
• Narrow pulse pressure	• RR >20 breaths/min
• ↓Postural BP	• Cold, mottled peripheries
• Pale, sweaty, anxious, thirsty	• Confused, lethargic, ↓GCS

1 **Resuscitation requirements assessed? (Boxes 15.1 and 15.2)**

Resuscitation is the top priority. Use Box 15.1 as a framework for evaluating resuscitation needs but tailor your assessment to the individual. Monitoring trends of the parameters in Box 15.2 provides far more information than a single 'snapshot' assessment and is essential for evaluating response to treatment. Do not rely exclusively on this framework and you should be aware that patients may respond differently to haemorrhage: young patients may compensate until blood loss is profound. Remember that heart rate may be misleading in patients on rate-limiting medications, e.g. beta-blockers, calcium channel blockers, or with fixed-rate pacemakers, and that compensatory vasoconstriction may not occur in patients on vasodilators. In patients who present with fresh, red haematemesis, the subsequent vomiting of 'coffee grounds' or passage of black tarry stools may simply be a manifestation of the original bleed, but further bright red haematemesis or haematochezia implies continued active bleeding.

15

2 Active bleeding, features of shock or suspected variceal bleed?

All patients with haematemesis accompanied by features of shock (see Box 15.2) or evidence of ongoing bleeding should have an urgent UGIE after adequate resuscitation. Variceal bleeds have a high mortality (30–50%) and usually require urgent UGIE following resuscitation and correction of coagulopathy. Assume variceal bleeding in any patient with known hepatic cirrhosis, clinical features of chronic liver disease (see Box 19.5, p. 176) or deranged LFTs with evidence of impaired hepatic synthetic function ($\uparrow$PT, $\downarrow$albumin).

3 Rockall risk score >0 (Table 15.1)?

In the absence of continued active bleeding, haemodynamic compromise or oesophageal varices, use a risk scoring system to guide the need for hospital admission and UGIE. The Rockall risk score comprises clinical (pre-endoscopic) and diagnostic (post-endoscopic) elements. A pre-endoscopic score of 0 predicts an extremely low risk of death (0.2%) and rebleeding (0.2%), but predicted mortality rises to 2.4% for a score of 1 and 5.6% for a score of 2. Admit patients with a pre-endoscopy Rockall score >0 for further assessment and observation; most need inpatient UGIE to calculate the full score and establish the diagnosis.

4 Background of alarm features?

Request UGIE to exclude upper GI malignancy if the patient has any of the following alarm features:

* weight loss
* anorexia or early satiety
* dysphagia
* epigastric mass
* lymphadenopathy
* jaundice
* age ≥50 years.

5 Haematemesis preceded by forceful retching/vomiting?

With a characteristic history of Mallory–Weiss tear, the diagnosis can often be made clinically, without the need for UGIE. In other cases, a diagnosis of gastritis and oesophagitis may be suggested by the history. Consider UGIE where there is no obvious explanation for symptoms or repeated haematemeses.

Table 15.1 Rockall risk score					
	Score				
Variable	**0**	**1**	**2**	**3**	
Age	<60 years	60–79 years	≥80 years		Pre-endoscopy: Initial score criteria
Shock	'No shock', systolic BP ≥100 mmHg, pulse <100 bpm	'Tachycardia', systolic BP ≥100 mmHg, pulse ≥100 bpm	'Hypotension', systolic BP <100 mmHg		
Comorbidity	No major comorbidity		Cardiac failure, ischaemic heart disease, any major comorbidity	Renal failure, liver failure, disseminated malignancy	
Diagnosis	Mallory–Weiss tear, no lesion identified and no stigmata of recent haemorrhage	All other diagnoses	Upper GI tract cancer		Post-endoscopy: Additional criteria for full score
Major stigmata of recent haemorrhage	None, or dark spot only		Blood in upper GI tract, adherent clot, visible or spurting vessel		

15

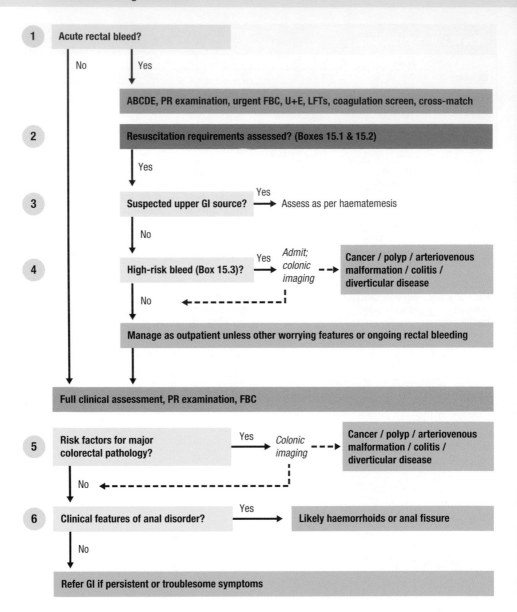

1   Acute rectal bleed?

Regard any prolonged, profuse or ongoing episode of bright red/maroon PR blood loss within the previous 24 hours as acute rectal bleeding. Assess patients with melaena in the same way as those with haematemesis (see above). Where the predominant problem is bloody diarrhoea, evaluate as described on page 93. In the absence of acute bleeding, proceed to step 5.

2   Resuscitation requirements assessed? (see Boxes 15.1 and 15.2)

Make adequate resuscitation your top priority. Evaluate and address resuscitation requirements as described for haematemesis, step 1.

3   Suspected upper GI source?

Assume, initially, that melaena reflects upper GI bleeding and assess as described for *haematemesis*.

Brisk bleeding from the upper GI tract may present with a fresh red PR bleed and implies severe, life-threatening haemorrhage. The diagnosis is straightforward if there is concomitant haematemesis but otherwise a high index of suspicion is essential. Proceed with a working diagnosis of lower GI bleeding in patients without haemodynamic instability but suspect an upper GI source in those with features of hypovolaemic shock. If present, seek senior GI input and consider UGIE as the first-line investigation following resuscitation, especially if there are any recent upper GI symptoms, e.g. epigastric pain, or known/suspected oesophageal varices.

4 High-risk bleed (Box 15.3)?

Consider non-admission or early discharge (with outpatient follow-up) if the patient has no high-risk features (see Box 15.2) or evidence of ongoing bleeding – especially if there is evidence of a benign anal disorder. Do not discharge a patient without making a clear decision as to the likely cause of bleeding. Admit any patient with risk factors for uncontrolled or recurrent bleeding (see Box 15.3). Once adequately resuscitated and clinically stable, arrange colonic imaging to establish the site and cause of bleeding. The majority of rectal bleeding settles with conservative management. Colonoscopy is most informative when the bleeding has stopped. CT angiography requires active ongoing bleeding of a sufficient rate to be detected.

Seek urgent senior surgical input in any patient with continued active bleeding, ongoing haemodynamic instability despite resuscitation or high transfusion requirements.

5 Risk factors for major colorectal pathology?

Refer the patient for urgent lower GI investigation (usually colonoscopy) to exclude colorectal cancer if any of the criteria in Box 15.4 is present.

Also consider lower GI endoscopic assessment if the patient has:

- systemic/extraintestinal features of inflammatory bowel disease (see Box 9.3, p. 91)
- a history of pelvic radiotherapy
- recent-onset, persistent bleeding when the patient is ≥50 years or has a strong family history of colorectal cancer, e.g. a first-degree relative <45 years at diagnosis, or two or more first-degree relatives.

6 Clinical features of anal disorder?

Perform careful rectal examination and proctoscopy in all patients to look for an anal disorder. Do not forget to look for anal cancer. If a benign anorectal pathology one is identified, provide reassurance but refer the patient for outpatient colorectal evaluation if there is diagnostic doubt or symptoms persist despite conservative management.

Arrange further GI investigation and/or referral in all patients without an obvious anorectal cause, in whom bleeding persists or recurs.

15

Box 15.3 Risk factors for adverse outcomes in acute lower GI bleeding

- Any haemodynamic instability
- Initial haematocrit <35% or need for red blood cell transfusion
- Any visualized red blood PR
- INR >1.4 or current anticoagulant use (warfarin, novel oral anticoagulants, aspirin/NSAID)
- Significant comorbidity, e.g. cardiorespiratory, renal, hepatic impairment or current hospital inpatient
- Age >60 years

Box 15.4 High-risk features for colorectal cancer in patients with rectal bleeding

- Rectal bleeding ≥4 weeks with change of bowel habit (↓ or ↑frequency or alternating bowel habit)
- Tenesmus
- Palpable rectal or abdominal mass
- Significant weight loss, e.g. ≥6 kg
- Previous excision of colorectal cancer or polyps
- History of inflammatory bowel disease
- Family history of colorectal cancer, polyps or inherited colorectal cancer syndromes
- Age >50 years without anal symptoms, e.g. discomfort, itching, lumps, prolapse

Haematuria, or blood in the urine, may be visible (macroscopic) or non-visible (microscopic), detected only by dipstick testing or urine microscopy. Visible haematuria strongly suggests significant urological disease and always requires further evaluation. Non-visible haematuria (defined in the UK as ≥1+ haematuria on 2 out of 3 urine dipstick tests) is a common incidental finding in asymptomatic patients and the challenge lies in differentiating benign causes from serious pathology.

It is important to differentiate haematuria from:
- contamination in menstruating women
- other causes of urine discolouration (Box 16.1).

Tumours

60% of renal cancers and 80% of bladder cancers present with haematuria. Both tumour types are rare below the age of 40. Associated features may include loin pain, abdominal mass and systemic upset (renal cancer) or lower urinary tract symptoms (LUTS), e.g. dysuria, frequency, urgency and hesitancy (bladder cancer). However, in the majority of cases, haematuria is the sole symptom and examination is normal. Risk factors are listed in Box 16.2. Around 12% of prostate cancers present with haematuria (more commonly microscopic).

Stones

Stones may cause obstruction anywhere along the urinary tract, though typically at sites of narrowing, e.g. the pelvi-ureteric junction, pelvic brim and vesico-ureteric junction. Those in the renal pelvis or bladder may remain asymptomatic for years and present incidentally with dipstick haematuria. Stones may be formed from calcium oxalate (80%, associated with hypercalciuria), from calcium phosphate (10% linked to renal tubular acidosis and hyperparathyroidism),

or other stone types (10%) comprising urate (excessive meat consumption or chemotherapy) and struvite (staghorn calculi, associated with chronic urinary tract infection) and cysteine (rare inherited disorders). Ureteric obstruction typically presents with renal 'colic' – acute, severe loin pain radiating to the groin ± genitalia that builds to a crescendo of intensity over a few minutes, often accompanied by restlessness (a key difference to peritonism where patients lie still), nausea and vomiting. The pain persists until obstruction is relieved. Visible haematuria may occur and dipstick is positive in 90% of cases.

Bacterial urinary tract infection

Women who are sexually active, pregnant, or are postmenopausal are prone to UTIs. UTIs in men <50 years old are uncommon. Sexually transmitted infections should be specifically investigated in this cohort. Common clinical features of lower UTI include frequency, dysuria, urgency, malodorous urine and visible or dipstick haematuria. In acute pyelonephritis (with ascending infection to the renal tract) there is typically loin pain, fever, rigors and significant systemic upset. UTI is likely if a dipstick test is positive for either nitrite or leucocyte esterase, but is unlikely if both are absent. A pure growth of >10^5 organisms/mL of fresh MSU confirms the diagnosis and permits sensitivity testing. A subset of patients (particularly women) develop recurrent UTIs. It is important to rule out renal tract stones (sources of chronic infection), incomplete bladder emptying (e.g. prostatic hypertrophy in men) and diabetes. Rarely, a renal tract malignancy may present with recurrent UTIs due to necrotic tissue with secondary infection.

Atypical infection

Urinary tuberculosis (TB) may cause visible haematuria ± other urinary tract symptoms,

Box 16.1 Causes of urine discolouration other than haematuria

Orange

- Concentrated normal urine, e.g. dehydration
- Conjugated bilirubin
- Rifampicin, isoniazid (also in tears/saliva/sweat), Senna
- Rhubarb, carrots
- Any cause of red urine

Red

- Myoglobinuria (rhabdomyolysis)
- Porphyrins
- Beetroot, blackberries
- Chlorpromazine, metronidazole, nitrofurantoin, warfarin
- Mercury and lead poisoning (rare)

Brown

- Conjugated bilirubin
- 'Muddy brown' urine – red cell casts in acute tubular necrosis (ATN)
- Homogentisic acid (in alkaptonuria or ochronosis)

Black (rare)

- Drugs: L-dopa
- Phenol and copper poisoning

Blue/Green

- Drugs/dyes, e.g. propofol, fluorescein, methylene blue
- Pseudomonal urine infection

Box 16.2 Risk factors for urinary tract cancer

- Smoking
- Occupational exposure to chemicals/dyes (benzenes, aromatic amines)
- Irritative voiding symptoms
- Previous pelvic irradiation
- Cyclophosphamide exposure
- Schistosomiasis – increases risk of bladder squamous cell carcinoma (rather than transitional cell carcinoma)
- Chronic inflammation of other causes

pulmonary manifestations and constitutional upset. Urinalysis is positive for WBC but routine culture is negative. Diagnosis requires a fresh early morning urine sample for acid-/alcohol-fast bacilli and TB culture. Painless visible haematuria toward the end of voiding is the most common initial presenting feature of *Schistosoma haematobium* infection, most commonly acquired in Egypt/East Africa, e.g. by swimming in freshwater lakes. Clues to diagnosis include travel history and eosinophilia. Non-visible haematuria is also common in bacterial endocarditis.

Renal disease

Haematuria may occur as a result of disorders that disrupt the glomerular basement membrane (glomerulonephritis). Associated features include proteinuria, hypertension, oedema and renal failure. Those most likely to result in haematuria include anti-glomerular basement membrane disease (Goodpasture's syndrome), small-vessel vasculitis, e.g. Wegener's granulomatosis, post-streptococcal glomerulonephritis, SLE and immunoglobulin A (IgA) nephropathy. In IgA nephropathy there may be intermittent episodes of visible haematuria coinciding with upper respiratory tract infections. Diagnosis of glomerular disease is made by renal biopsy. Inherited renal disorders, such as Alport's syndrome and adult polycystic kidney disease, may also present with visible or non-visible haematuria.

Other causes

- Trauma: direct urethral trauma; blunt or penetrating abdominal/pelvic injury.
- Iatrogenic: renal biopsy, transurethral resection of prostate, cystoscopy, urinary catheterisation.
- Vascular: arterio-venous malformations; renal vein thrombosis.
- Coagulopathy.
- Renal cysts.
- Acute tubular necrosis.
- Thin basement membrane disease (common, benign, often familial).
- Loin pain-haematuria syndrome.
- Extreme exertion, e.g. distance running.

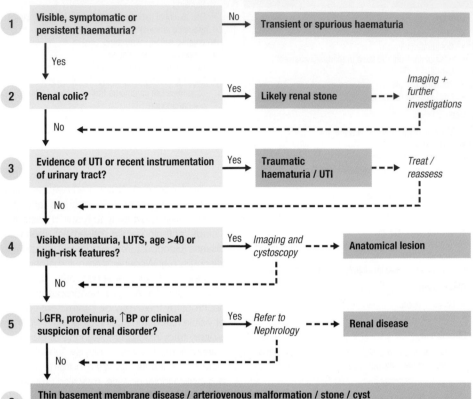

Full clinical assessment, urinalysis, U+E

1 Visible, symptomatic or persistent haematuria? — No → Transient or spurious haematuria

Yes

2 Renal colic? — Yes → Likely renal stone ----→ *Imaging + further investigations*

No

3 Evidence of UTI or recent instrumentation of urinary tract? — Yes → Traumatic haematuria / UTI ----→ *Treat / reassess*

No

4 Visible haematuria, LUTS, age >40 or high-risk features? — Yes *Imaging and cystoscopy* ----→ Anatomical lesion

No

5 ↓GFR, proteinuria, ↑BP or clinical suspicion of renal disorder? — Yes *Refer to Nephrology* ----→ Renal disease

No

6 Thin basement membrane disease / arteriovenous malformation / stone / cyst
Monitor regularly for new or recurrent visible haematuria / lower urinary tract symptoms / proteinuria / ↓GFR

1 Visible, symptomatic or persistent haematuria?

Consider other causes of urine discoloration (see Box 16.1) that may mimic visible haematuria. Use dipstick testing (at least 1+) on a freshly voided sample to detect non-visible haematuria; send urine for microscopy only in uncertain cases, e.g. suspicion of myoglobinuria. Ask specifically about episodes of visible haematuria in any patient with a positive dipstick test. Repeat dipstick testing at a later date if the test was performed during menstruation, shortly after strenuous exercise or following urinary catheterization.

Evaluate further for haematuria as described below if the patient has:
- visible haematuria
- non-visible haematuria with loin pain or LUTS
- 2 out of 3 positive dipstick tests for haematuria at different times.

2 Renal colic?

The combination of haematuria and renal colic (see above) suggests ureteric obstruction, usually from a stone or, less commonly, from clots or sloughed renal papilla. Confirm the presence and position of a stone with a CT of the kidneys, ureters and bladder (CT KUB). Dipstick the urine for infection (nitrites and leucocytes). Observe closely for decreased urine output and symptoms of infection. Perform further investigations to establish an underlying cause, e.g. chemical composition of stone; plasma calcium/phosphate/ uric acid. Refer to Urology for further management.

3 Evidence of UTI or recent instrumentation of urinary tract

Refer to Urology if visible haematuria follows surgical or invasive procedures of the renal tract, e.g. renal biopsy, ureteroscopy, transurethral resection of prostate, or abdominal/pelvic/ genital trauma.

The absence of leucocytes and nitrites on dipstick effectively excludes UTI in most cases. If dipstick testing is positive or there is strong clinical suspicion, send a midstream urine sample for culture; treat confirmed infection then recheck for non-visible haematuria.

Consider infective endocarditis if there is fever, splinter haemorrhages, predisposing lesion or new murmur.

Do not attribute haematuria to anticoagulation or antiplatelet treatment alone without further investigation.

4 Visible haematuria, LUTS, age >40 or high-risk features?

In the absence of renal colic and following treatment/exclusion of transient causes of haematuria, you must exclude cancer if any of the following features is present:
- visible haematuria
- LUTS
- age >40 years
- high-risk features for urinary tract cancer (see Box 16.2).

Refer such patients to Urology for further investigation, e.g. renal USS ± IVU or CT urogram and cystoscopy.

5 ↓GFR, proteinuria, ↑BP or clinical suspicion of renal disorder?

Refer to a nephrologist for further evaluation ± renal biopsy if any of the following features is present:
- proteinuria, e.g. albumin : creatinine ratio ≥30
- renal impairment (GFR <60 mL/min)
- ↑BP in a patient <40 years
- connective tissue disease, e.g. SLE
- family history of Alport's syndrome/adult polycystic kidney disease
- episodes of visible haematuria coinciding with upper urinary tract infections.

6 Likely benign cause. Monitor periodically.

Isolated microscopic haematuria is common and usually due to benign disease, e.g. thin basement membrane disease. Provided that the above causes have been excluded, reassure patients that further investigation is not necessary but continue to monitor (e.g. annually) for features such as new urinary tract symptoms, visible haematuria, proteinuria or renal impairment.

16

Haemoptysis, coughing up blood, requires thorough evaluation to exclude serious pathology such as lung cancer, tuberculosis (TB) and pulmonary embolism (PE); many patients will require detailed imaging and specialist assessment. Massive haemoptysis (>500 mL/24 hours) may be life-threatening.

Respiratory tract infections

Respiratory tract infections (RTIs) are the most common cause of haemoptysis. They typically cause blood-stained purulent sputum rather than frank blood, and have associated features such as cough, fever and dyspnoea. In acute bronchitis, mucosal inflammation can rupture superficial blood vessels; patients with chronic obstructive pulmonary disease may have haemoptysis during an infective exacerbation. Pneumonia may cause frank haemoptysis, especially with invasive bacteria, e.g. *Staphylococcus aureus*, *Klebsiella* spp. or fungi; patients are usually profoundly unwell. Mycetoma, lung abscess and TB may cause massive haemoptysis. More commonly, TB produces chronic cough with small haemoptyses, fever, night sweats, weight loss and characteristic CXR changes.

Lung tumours

Haemoptysis is common in primary bronchial tumours but rare in secondary lung tumours. Risk factors are smoking (especially ≥40 pack-years) and age >40 years; repeated small haemoptyses or blood-streaked sputum for ≥2 weeks strongly suggests malignancy. Massive haemoptysis may occur with erosion of tumour into a large vessel. Weight loss, recent-onset cough, finger clubbing and lymphadenopathy are well-recognized features. CXR may show a variety of abnormalities (Box 17.1) but is sometimes normal.

Pulmonary embolism

Frank haemoptysis occurs due to pulmonary infarction, usually accompanied by sudden-onset dyspnoea and pleuritic pain. A pleural rub or signs of deep vein thrombosis (DVT) are present in a minority of cases. CXR may show a wedge-shaped peripheral opacity or pleural effusion, but is most often normal.

Bronchiectasis

There is typically a background of chronic cough with copious foul-smelling purulent sputum. Finger clubbing and coarse inspiratory crackles may be evident on examination.

Other causes

Pulmonary oedema may cause pink, frothy sputum but dyspnoea is almost always the dominant complaint. Other causes include pulmonary hypertension (especially associated with mitral stenosis), coagulopathies, foreign body inhalation, chest trauma, Wegener's granulomatosis and Goodpasture's syndrome.

Box 17.1 **The CXR in lung cancer**

Common abnormalities on CXR in patients with lung cancer include:

- a discrete mass (see Fig. 17.1) or cavitating lesion (see Fig. 17.2)
- collapse of a lobe secondary to tumour obstruction (see Figs 17.3 and 17.4)
- unilateral hilar enlargement or pleural effusion (see Fig. 12.6, p. 119)
- consolidation (see Figs 12.3 and 12.4, p. 118) that fails to resolve or recurs in the same lobe.

In a substantial proportion of cases, the CXR is normal.

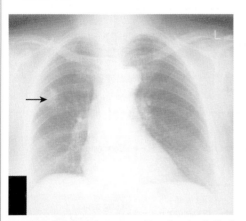

Fig. 17.1 A solitary lung mass. (From Douglas G, Nicol F, Robertson C. Macleod's Clinical Examination, 12th edn. Edinburgh: Churchill Livingstone, 2009.)

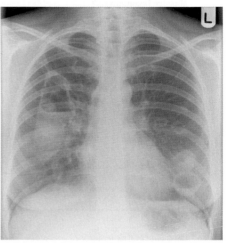

Fig. 17.2 A cavitating lung lesion. (From Corne J, Pointon K. Chest X-ray Made Easy, 3rd edn. Edinburgh: Churchill Livingstone, 2010.)

17

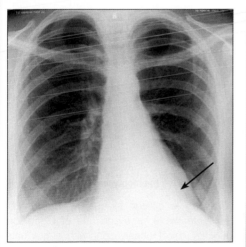

Fig. 17.3 Left lower lobe collapse. The changes in left lower lobe collapse may be subtle and easily overlooked; note the triangular opacification behind the heart, giving the appearance of an unusually straight left heart border. (From Boon NA, Colledge NR, Walker BR. Davidson's Principles & Practice of Medicine, 20th edn. Edinburgh: Churchill Livingstone, 2006.)

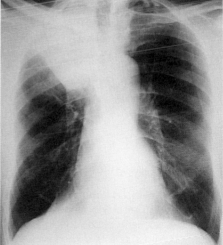

Fig. 17.4 Right upper lobe collapse. Note the right upper zone opacification, loss of volume in the right lung field and tracheal deviation. (From Corne J, Pointon K. Chest X-ray Made Easy, 3rd edn. Edinburgh: Churchill Livingstone, 2010.)

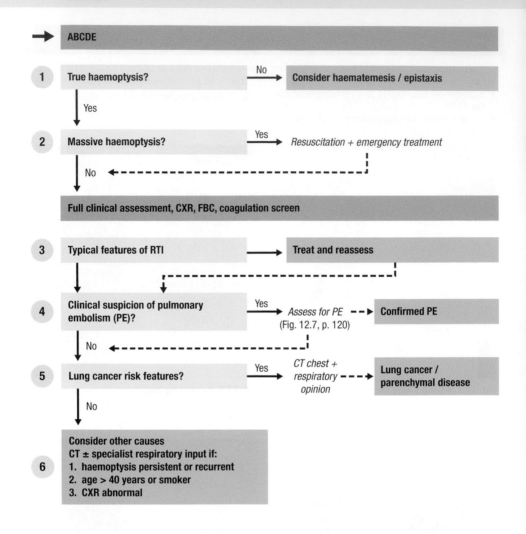

➡ **ABCDE**

1 | **True haemoptysis?** — No → **Consider haematemesis / epistaxis**

↓ Yes

2 | **Massive haemoptysis?** — Yes → *Resuscitation + emergency treatment*

↓ No ⇠ -

Full clinical assessment, CXR, FBC, coagulation screen

3 | **Typical features of RTI** ⟶ **Treat and reassess**

↓

4 | **Clinical suspicion of pulmonary embolism (PE)?** — Yes → *Assess for PE (Fig. 12.7, p. 120)* - - ▶ **Confirmed PE**

↓ No ⇠ - - - - - - - - - - - - - - - - -

5 | **Lung cancer risk features?** — Yes → *CT chest + respiratory opinion* - - ▶ **Lung cancer / parenchymal disease**

↓ No

6 | **Consider other causes**
CT ± specialist respiratory input if:
1. **haemoptysis persistent or recurrent**
2. **age > 40 years or smoker**
3. **CXR abnormal**

---

1 | **True haemoptysis?**

A clear history of blood being coughed up or mixed with sputum reliably indicates haemoptysis.

Blood that suddenly appears in the mouth without coughing suggests a nasopharyngeal origin; ask about nosebleeds and look for epistaxis or a bleeding source within the mouth.

Blood originating from the GI tract is typically dark, acidic (test pH) and may contain food particles; blood that is frothy, alkaline and bright red or pink suggests a respiratory source.

2 | **Massive haemoptysis?**

Bleeding is difficult to quantify clinically but estimate the volume and rate of blood loss, e.g. by direct observation, with a graduated container. The major risk is asphyxiation through flooding of alveoli or airway obstruction. Use the ABCDE approach (Chapter 2) and seek immediate anaesthetic help if any of the following is present:

- large blood volume, e.g. >50 mL in 1 hour

- airway compromise
- haemodynamic instability.

3 Typical features of RTI?

Haemoptysis for <1 week with purulent sputum and/or fever suggests acute RTI; assess as described on page 123 and arrange follow-up review after treatment to ensure that haemoptysis has resolved. Also arrange a follow-up CXR within 6 weeks for any patient with radiographic consolidation to ensure resolution.

4 Clinical suspicion of pulmonary embolism?

PE is easily forgotten and easily missed. Physical and CXR findings are unreliable so maintain a high index of suspicion. Consider PE and assess as shown in Fig. 12.7 (p. 120) if haemoptysis is acute and accompanied by any of the following:

- rapid-onset pleuritic pain or dyspnoea
- symptoms or signs of DVT
- specific risk factors, e.g. active malignancy, recent surgery
- new-onset frank haemoptysis with no other obvious cause (e.g. no typical features of RTI).

5 Lung cancer risk features?

You must exclude lung cancer, even if another diagnosis appears more likely, in any patient with persistent haemoptysis (>2 weeks) and:

- history of cigarette smoking
- weight loss, finger clubbing, Horner's syndrome, cervical lymphadenopathy
- mass, cavitating lesion, persistent consolidation/collapse or unilateral hilar adenopathy/pleural effusion on CXR (see Box 17.1).

Thoracic CT is a useful first-line investigation and may reveal a tumour or other cause for haemoptysis, e.g. bronchiectasis; but refer the patient to a respiratory specialist (urgently if smoker >40 years) for further assessment ± bronchoscopy even if CT is normal.

6 Consider other causes/ further investigation

Perform a coagulation screen in any patient on anticoagulant therapy, with a history of bleeding disorder or with evidence of bleeding elsewhere, or if there is no clear alternative cause.

Chronic cough with daily mucopurulent sputum production or persistent coarse inspiratory crackles suggests bronchiectasis – confirm the diagnosis with high-resolution thoracic CT.

Consider TB if any of the following features is present:

- prior residence in an endemic area
- immunosuppression (HIV, malnutrition, general debility)
- suggestive clinical features, e.g. night sweats, fever, weight loss
- suggestive CXR findings, e.g. a cavitating lesion (see Fig. 17.2), persistent consolidation, miliary TB.

If suspected, obtain ≥3 sputum samples for acid-fast bacilli and mycobacterial culture, and seek expert respiratory input.

Exclude Goodpasture's syndrome and Wegener's granulomatosis if there is evidence of renal involvement, e.g. haematuria, proteinuria, ↓GFR: check for anti-glomerular basement membrane and anti-PR3 (c-ANCA) antibodies and seek renal input.

Arrange an ECG if the patient has:

- a history of rheumatic fever
- exertional dyspnoea, orthopnoea, paroxysmal nocturnal dyspnoea
- signs of mitral stenosis, e.g. loud S1, low-pitched mid-diastolic murmur
- signs of pulmonary hypertension, e.g. loud P2, right ventricular heave.

If the cause is still unclear, consider CT and specialist respiratory input – especially if >40 years, smoking history, ongoing symptoms or any CXR abnormality.

17

18 Headache

Headache is extremely common and usually benign. The challenge is to identify the small minority of patients with serious underlying pathology and those with disorders that respond to specific treatments.

Subarachnoid haemorrhage (SAH)

The headache is typically of sudden onset (reaches maximal intensity within a few seconds), occipital and very severe. Distress and photophobia are common but neck stiffness may take hours to develop. Large bleeds may be complicated by ↓GCS, seizure or focal neurological signs. Most cases are evident on CT but LP is required in suspected cases with normal CT.

Benign thunderclap headache mimics the headache of SAH but investigation reveals no evidence of an intracranial vascular disorder. It may be associated with coitus or exercise.

Other vascular causes

Intracerebellar haemorrhage: typically presents with acute-onset headache, nausea, vomiting, dizziness and ataxia ± ↓GCS.

Spontaneous intracerebral or intraventricular haemorrhage: the onset of headache is usually over minutes to hours accompanied by a focal neurological deficit ± ↓GCS.

Chronic subdural haematoma: may present insidiously with headache +/− confusion and/or balance problems. The headache may be exacerbated by straining, bending or exercise. At least one quarter of patients have no clear history of head trauma so have a high index of suspicion, particularly in older patients or those taking anticoagulants.

Cerebral venous thrombosis: headache is common but variable, e.g. 'thunderclap', throbbing, 'band-like', as are associated features, e.g. nausea, vomiting, seizures, cranial nerve palsies, hemiparesis, ataxia and ↓GCS.

Vertebrobasilar dissection: may cause acute-onset occipital/posterior neck pain with brainstem signs and symptoms.

Meningitis

Classically presents with headache, fever and meningism. The onset of headache is typically over hours rather than sudden. Viral meningitis is usually self-limiting, with headache the most prominent clinical feature. Bacterial meningitis is life-threatening; presenting features include ↓GCS, signs of shock (see Box 30.1, p. 267), purpuric rash (see Fig. 27.13, p. 244) and focal neurological signs. LP (see Clinical tool, p. 170) is helpful in the diagnosis but must not delay IV antibiotics therapy. Beware atypical presentations in immunocompromised, pregnant or alcoholic patients.

Migraine

Recurrent severe headaches lasting several hours to a few days, usually accompanied by photophobia, phonophobia and nausea ± vomiting. In one-third there are associated focal neurological features – an 'aura' (Box 18.1). The headache is typically intense, throbbing and unilateral. The patient usually prefers to lie in a quiet, darkened room. Triggers include cheese, chocolate, alcohol and oral contraceptives. A first attack aged >40 years is uncommon.

Cluster headache

This refers to severe, unilateral, retro-orbital headache with restlessness, agitation and ipsilateral lacrimation, conjunctival injection and rhinorrhoea. Attacks are short-lived (15–90 minutes) but occur frequently and repeatedly (often at the same time each day) in 'clusters' lasting days to weeks; these are separated by months without symptoms. The male to female ratio is 5 : 1.

> **Box 18.1 What constitutes a migraine aura?**
>
> Auras are focal neurological phenomena that precede or accompany a migrainous headache. They occur in 20–30% of patients, usually developing gradually over 5–20 minutes and lasting <60 minutes. Most are visual but they may also be sensory or motor. Common examples include:
> - 'fortification spectra': shimmering zigzag lines that move across the visual field
> - flashing lights or spots
> - temporary loss of vision
> - numbness/dysaesthesia on one side of the body
> - expressive dysphasia.

Temporal arteritis (giant cell arteritis)

A large-vessel vasculitis, closely associated with polymyalgia rheumatica, more common in women and unusual in patients <50 years. Clinical features include localized headache (temporal/occipital), scalp tenderness, jaw claudication, visual loss, constitutional upset (malaise, night sweats, pyrexia, weight loss), and an abnormal temporal artery (inflamed, tender, non-pulsatile). ESR/CRP are almost always raised. The potential for rapid-onset irreversible visual loss necessitates urgent treatment with steroids. Temporal artery biopsy may confirm the diagnosis but should not delay steroid treatment.

Acute glaucoma

Acute glaucoma, an ophthalmological emergency, occurs due to a sudden increase in intraocular pressure. The typical patient is long-sighted, middle-aged or elderly, and presents with periorbital pain (± frontal headache), nausea and vomiting, blurred vision with halos around lights and conjunctival injection. Urgent ophthalmology referral is mandatory.

Raised intracranial pressure

May occur as a primary disorder (idiopathic intracranial hypertension) especially in overweight young women taking the oral contraceptive pill, or secondary to an intracranial space-occupying lesion. In the latter case, there may be focal neurological signs, change in personality or new-onset seizures. Headache tends to be worse in the morning and on lying flat, coughing or straining. There may be associated vomiting, often without nausea +/− papilloedema.

Sinusitis

This causes a dull, throbbing headache associated with facial pain over the sinuses. It tends to be worse on bending forward. There are invariably associated nasal symptoms, e.g. congestion or discharge. Sinusitis lasting >8 weeks requires CT to confirm the diagnosis.

Medication overuse headache

A common cause of chronic frequent headache (often daily) caused by excessive use of analgesics, ergotamines or triptans. Treatment of choice is withdrawal of the overused medication.

Tension headache

The headache is usually bilateral (often generalized or frontal) and described as 'dull', 'tight' or 'pressing' in nature. Unlike migraine, nausea and photophobia are uncommon and the patient can often continue with normal activities.

Other causes

- Carbon monoxide poisoning.
- Hypercapnia.
- Drugs: vasodilators, e.g. nitrates, 'recreational' drugs, e.g. solvents.
- Trigeminal neuralgia (brief, repetitive episodes of intense shooting/stabbing/'electric shock'-like pain in II and III divisions of trigeminal nerve).
- Trauma: extradural haemorrhage, subdural haemorrhage, concussion.

18

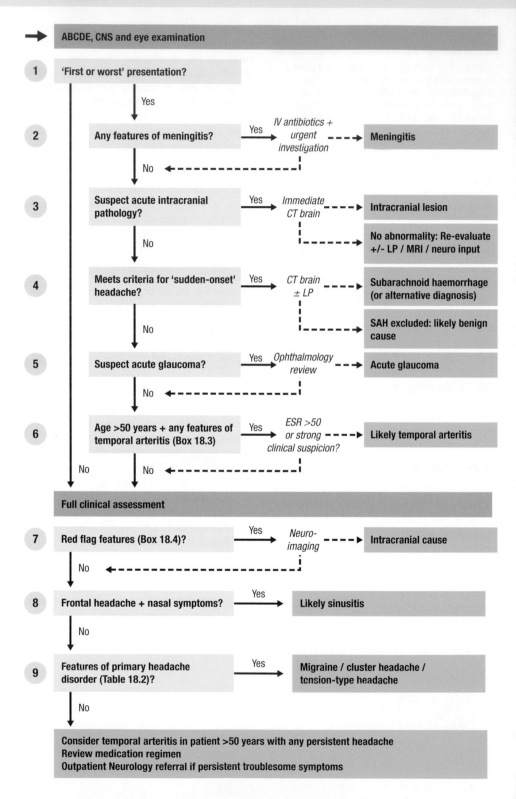

1 'First or worst' presentation?

Acute severe pathology is less likely in patients with recurrence of a longstanding problem than in patients with a first presentation of headache. However, patients with a pre-existing headache disorder, e.g. migraine, may also present acutely with another diagnosis such as SAH. If a patient with chronic headaches presents with a new headache that is markedly different in severity or character to normal, assess it as new-onset headache.

2 Any features of meningitis?

Identifying patients with bacterial meningitis is the top priority to allow rapid, potentially life-saving, antibiotic treatment. Patients may lack classical features but, in almost all cases, there will be at least one of:

- fever (≥38° C)
- rash (not always petechial)
- signs of shock (see Box 30.1, p. 267)
- acute-onset headache, e.g. over hours with meningism (Box 18.2).

SAH may also present with severe headache and meningism, but is less likely if the headache onset was not sudden (see below).

If you suspect meningitis, take blood cultures and throat swabs and give IV antibiotics immediately. If there are no contraindications, perform LP for CSF analysis (see Clinical tool). If you suspect raised intracranial pressure, perform CT prior to LP. It is difficult to distinguish viral from early bacterial meningitis clinically, so manage as bacterial meningitis pending CSF analysis.

3 Suspect acute intracranial pathology?

Arrange immediate neuroimaging to exclude life-threatening intracranial pathology, e.g. haemorrhage or space-occupying lesion with mass effect, if any of the following is present:

- ↓GCS
- focal neurological signs
- new-onset seizures
- history of recent head injury
- anticoagulation or coagulopathy.

Box 18.2 Meningism?

Meningism (neck stiffness, photophobia, positive Kernig's sign) denotes irritation of the meninges. To test for neck stiffness, lie the patient supine with no pillow, place your fingers behind their head and gently attempt to flex the head until the chin touches the chest (Fig. 18.1A); firm resistance to passive flexion and rigidity in the neck muscles indicate neck stiffness. To test for Kernig's sign, flex one of the patient's legs at the hip and knee with your left hand placed over the medial hamstrings. Extend the knee with your right hand maintaining the hip in flexion (Fig. 18.1B). Resistance to extension by spasm in the hamstrings ± flexion of the other leg indicates a positive test.

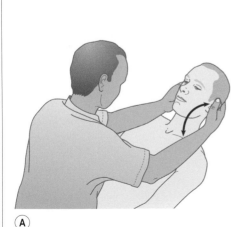

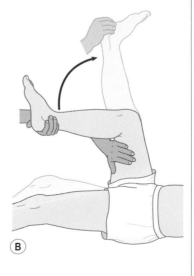

(A)   (B)

Fig. 18.1 Testing for meningeal irritation.

18

Clinical tool
LP and CSF interpretation

Contraindications to LP

- Infected skin over the needle entry site.
- Radiological evidence of raised intracranial pressure.
- Clinical suspicion of raised intracranial pressure: ↓GCS, focal neurological signs, papilloedema, new seizures.
- Coagulopathy or platelets <50×10^9/L.
- Severe agitation and restlessness.

CSF interpretation

Routine interpretation of CSF results includes (Table 18.1):
- opening pressure (supine position)
- protein
- glucose (always compare with blood glucose)
- cell count.

Additional tests, e.g. culture, PCR, oligoclonal bands, may be required in some circumstances.

Additional points to consider

- Early bacterial meningitis may be mistaken for viral meningitis as there is a predominance of lymphocytes in the CSF. If there is any possibility of bacterial meningitis, treat the patient with antibiotics pending further investigation, e.g. blood/CSF culture.
- If there is a ↑lymphocyte count, send CSF for viral PCR, including herpes and enterovirus.
- Symptoms and signs in tuberculous meningitis are often mild or obscure – consider it if the patient has immunocompromise or is from an endemic TB region, especially if the CSF results suggest the diagnosis (see above). If suspected, send CSF for acid-fast bacilli and mycobacterial PCR and culture.
- Non-infective disorders can produce a lymphocytic picture, including lupus, sarcoidosis and malignant meningitis. Check autoantibodies and discuss with Rheumatology if there are any other suggestive features.
- A difficult procedure may result in a 'traumatic tap', i.e. red cells in the CSF. This can complicate interpretation of the WBC. A rule of thumb is that 1 white cell per 1000 red cells is normal. However, if the CSF picture is unclear, then the clinical history must be taken into account.

Table 18.1 Interpretation of CSF results

Condition	Opening pressure	CSF protein (mg/L)	CSF glucose (mmol/L)	Lymphocytes (× 10⁶/L)	Neutrophils (× 10⁶/L)	Red cells (× 10⁶/L)
Normal	5–18 cm H₂O	200–450	>60% of blood glucose 3–5	<5	0	0
Bacterial meningitis	↑ or normal	↑	<50% of blood glucose	↑: usually <neutrophils but may be predominant cell type in early stages	≥1 is +ve Usually >100 May be 0 in very early stages	0
Viral meningitis	↑ or normal	↑ or normal	<60% of blood glucose but >50%	>5 is +ve Usually >50	0	0
TB meningitis	↑	↑↑: may be >1000	<30% of blood glucose	100% >50	0	0
Subarachnoid haemorrhage	↑	↑	>60% of blood glucose	0; if ↑red cells, then 1 white cell per 1000 red cells is normal	0	↑: often in thousands
Late subarachnoid haemorrhage	↑ or normal	↑	>60% blood glucose	0	0	0 but +ve for xanthochromia (haem breakdown product)
Vasculitis	↑	↑: may be >100	>60% of blood glucose	0 Occasionally ↑ as a cause of aseptic meningitis	0	0

18

LP may be required to exclude meningitis or SAH if CT does not yield a diagnosis and no alternative cause is apparent, e.g. toxicity, metabolic derangement. Review the presentation and, if appropriate, evaluate for seizure (p. 276), coma (see Ch. 7) or 'Limb weakness' (see Ch. 22). Seek urgent Neurology input if the cause remains unclear.

4 **Meets criteria for 'sudden-onset' headache?**

Exclude SAH in any patient with a severe 'first or worst' headache that reaches peak intensity within 5 min of onset and persists for >1 hour.

Headache in SAH may not be instantaneous in onset but almost always reaches maximal intensity within 5 min and rarely resolves in <1 hour. In these circumstances, no clinical features can reliably rule out the diagnosis so neuroimaging ± CSF analysis is mandatory. CT has almost 100% sensitivity for SAH when performed within 6 hours on a contemporary multi-slice scanner and reported by a qualified radiologist. Beyond 6 hours, if the CT is normal, then LP, at least 12 hours from the onset of headache, must be performed to look for xanthochromia; its absence effectively excludes SAH. The major differential diagnosis is benign thunderclap headache; however, all sudden-onset severe headaches should, ideally, be discussed with a neurologist.

5 **Suspect acute glaucoma?**

Acute glaucoma is sight-threatening. Request urgent Ophthalmology review if the patient has acute-onset headache (especially frontal or periorbital) accompanied by any of the following features:

- conjunctival injection
- clouding of the cornea
- irregular/non-reactive pupil
- ↓visual acuity or blurred vision
- sees coloured 'halos' around lights.

6 **Age >50 years + any features of temporal arteritis (Box 18.3)?**

Suspect temporal arteritis in patients >50 years with new-onset headache and any features shown in Box 18.3. Check ESR and CRP urgently; ESR >50 mm/hour makes the diagnosis

---

Box 18.3 Features suggesting temporal arteritis

- Pain localized to temporal or occipital region
- Inflamed, thickened, pulseless or tender temporal artery
- Scalp tenderness
- Jaw claudication
- Visual loss (may be temporary initially)
- Constitutional symptoms: fever, malaise, fatigue, night sweats, weight loss
- Symptoms of polymyalgia rheumatica (proximal pain, stiffness, etc.)

Box 18.4 Red flag features

- New-onset headache/change in headache in patients over 50 years
- Focal CNS signs, ataxia or new cognitive or behavioural disturbance
- Persistent visual disturbance
- Headache that changes with posture or wakes the patient up
- Headache brought on by physical exertion
- Papilloedema
- New-onset headache in a patient with HIV, active malignancy or immunocompromised

---

highly likely. In these circumstances, or where clinical suspicion is high, e.g. >2 features from Box 18.3, start steroid therapy immediately. A prompt response to steroids essentially confirms the diagnosis, though, ideally, temporal artery biopsy should be performed within 2 weeks of starting steroids.

7 **Red flag features (Box 18.4)?**

Regardless of headache duration, you must exclude serious underlying intracranial pathology if any features in Box 18.4 are present. Arrange CT brain ± MRI and, if normal, seek input from a neurologist. Consider benign intracranial hypertension in patients with features of ↑intracranial pressure but no mass on neuroimaging.

8 **Frontal headache + nasal symptoms?**

Whilst frontal headache may raise the suspicion of sinusitis, the diagnosis should only be made when there are associated nasal symptoms. Look for at least two of:

- nasal blockage/congestion
- rhinorrhoea/discharge

Table 18.2 Diagnostic criteria for headache			
	Migraine	Cluster	Tension-type
Episodes	≥5 headache episodes meeting the following criteria, or ≥2 episodes associated with typical aura (see Box 18.1)	≥5 episodes of headache with:	≥10 episodes of headache with the following criteria:
1.	Headache duration of 4–72 hours	Severe, unilateral orbital, supraorbital or temporal pain lasting 15–180 minutes	Duration 30 minutes to 7 days
2.	≥2 of: Unilateral location Pulsating quality Moderate to severe intensity Disabling[1]	Frequency of attacks: 1 per 2 days to 8 per day	≥2 of: Bilateral location Pressing or tightening (non-pulsating) quality Mild to moderate intensity Non-disabling[2]
3.	≥1 of: Nausea ± vomiting, Photophobia + phonophobia	≥1 of: Restlessness/agitation or Ipsilateral facial signs[3]	None of: Photophobia Phonophobia Nausea Vomiting

[1]Aggravation by or causing avoidance of routine physical activity, e.g. walking or climbing stairs.
[2]Not aggravated by or causing avoidance of routine physical activity, e.g. walking or climbing stairs.
[3]Conjunctival injection, lacrimation, nasal congestion, rhinorrhoea, forehead and facial sweating, miosis, ptosis, eyelid oedema.Modified from Headache Classification Committee of the International Headache Society (IHS) 2013. The International Classification of Headache Disorders, 3rd edn (beta version). Cephalalgia. 33(9):629–808.

18

- loss of smell
- facial pressure or tenderness.

Further investigation is not necessary in acute sinusitis but refer the patient to ENT if there are chronic symptoms.

9 Features of primary headache disorder (Table 18.2)?

Primary headache disorders, e.g. tension headache, migraine are responsible for most headaches.

Diagnosis relies on associated features and patterns of presentation (see Table 18.2). By definition, they cannot be diagnosed on the basis of a single episode. However, where the presentation is typical, it may be reasonable to class a case as a likely first presentation of a primary headache disorder. Where a recurrent headache does not fit neatly into a diagnostic category, refer to a neurologist.

Jaundice describes the yellow pigmentation of skin, sclerae and mucous membranes that results from accumulation of bilirubin within tissues. This may result from ↑red cell breakdown (haemolysis), ↓uptake/conjugation by the liver (hepatocellular dysfunction) or impaired biliary drainage (cholestasis). Jaundice is often further classified according to the anatomic location of the lesion: pre-hepatic – haemolysis; hepatic – hepatocellular dysfunction and/or intrahepatic bile duct obstruction; post-hepatic – extrahepatic bile duct obstruction. It is important to remember that patients may have more than one aetiology (e.g. alcoholic hepatitis on a background of cirrhosis due to chronic hepatitis C infection).

Pre-hepatic causes of jaundice

Haemolytic disorders (Box 19.1) cause accumulation of unconjugated bilirubin in plasma due to ↑red cell destruction. LFTs are otherwise normal, but there may be anaemia with evidence of haemolysis on blood tests and film. Clinical features of pre-hepatic jaundice include normal coloured urine and dark stools. Biochemically there is an unconjugated hyperbilirubinaemia.

Hepatic causes of jaundice

Problems with conjugation

Gilbert's syndrome is a benign congenital condition affecting 2–5% of the population. Decreased glucuronyl transferase activity limits bilirubin conjugation and therefore excretion into the bile, causing mild jaundice during periods of fasting or intercurrent illness. There are no other clinical/biochemical features of liver disease.

Acute liver injury

Toxic, infective, autoimmune, metabolic and vascular liver insults may lead to acute hepatitis. Jaundice results from impaired bilirubin transport across hepatocytes. There may also be obstruction of biliary canaliculi due to inflammation and oedema. There is typically a disproportionate increase in ALT and AST relative to ALP and GGT. Extensive liver damage may cause *acute liver failure*, characterized by jaundice, encephalopathy (Table 19.1) and coagulopathy (typically INR >1.5) in the absence of pre-existing liver disease. Causes of acute liver failure are shown in Box 19.2.

Potential causes of acute drug-induced liver injury are listed in Box 19.3. LFTs may take months to normalize after drug cessation, especially with cholestatic injury.

Acute alcoholic hepatitis may occur in individuals without chronic liver disease following intensive binge drinking and presents with jaundice, constitutional upset, tender hepatomegaly and fever.

In acute viral hepatitis, jaundice is usually preceded by a 1–2-week prodrome of malaise, arthralgia, headache and anorexia. Hepatitis A–E viruses are responsible for most cases; less common causes include cytomegalovirus (CMV), Epstein–Barr virus (EBV) and herpes simplex. Diagnosis is confirmed by serology. Recovery occurs over 3–6 weeks in most cases, but chronic infection develops in up to 10% of patients with hepatitis B and 80% with hepatitis C.

A rare cause of infective jaundice is icteric leptospirosis (Weil's disease), a severe illness characterized by deep jaundice, fever, bleeding, e.g. epistaxis, haematemesis, renal failure and, often, a purpuric rash.

Autoimmune hepatitis most often presents with established cirrhosis but 25% of cases manifest as an acute hepatitis with jaundice and constitutional symptoms. It is more common in females (ratio 3:1), and there is an association with other autoimmune conditions. Serum immunoglobulin (IgG) levels are raised and serum autoantibodies may be present.

Table 19.1 West Haven grading of hepatic encephalopathy

Stage	Alteration of consciousness
0	No change in personality or behaviour No asterixis
1	Impaired concentration and attention span Sleep disturbance, slurred speech, asterixis, agitation or depression
2	Lethargy, drowsiness, apathy or aggression Disorientation, inappropriate behaviour, slurred speech
3	Confusion and disorientation, bizarre behaviour Drowsiness or stupor Asterixis usually absent
4	Comatose with no response to voice commands Minimal or absent response to painful stimuli

Box 19.2 Causes of acute liver failure

Drugs/toxins

- Paracetamol overdose[1]
- Anti-tuberculous drugs
- Ecstasy
- Halothane
- *Amanita phalloides*
- Carbon tetrachloride

Infection

- Acute viral hepatitis (A, B, E)[1]
- Cytomegalovirus (CMV), Epstein–Barr virus (EBV)

Vascular

- Shock/ischaemic hepatitis
- Budd–Chiari syndrome

Other

- Wilson's disease
- Autoimmune hepatitis
- Acute fatty liver of pregnancy
- Extensive malignant infiltration

[1]Denotes common cause.

Box 19.1 Causes of haemolysis

Hereditary

- Erythrocyte membrane defects
  - Hereditary spherocytosis
  - Hereditary elliptocytosis
- Erythrocyte enzyme defects
  - Glucose-6-phosphate dehydrogenase deficiency
- Haemoglobinopathies
  - Thalassaemia
  - Sickle cell

Acquired

- Immune
  - Autoimmune haemolytic anaemia
  - Alloimmune: haemolytic transfusion reaction, haemolytic disease of the newborn
- Fragmentation syndromes
  - Microangiopathic haemolytic anaemia, e.g. haemolytic uraemic syndrome/thrombotic thrombocytopenic purpura
  - Mechanical heart valves
- Drugs, e.g. dapsone
- Infections, e.g. malaria
- Paroxysmal nocturnal haemoglobinuria

Box 19.3 Drugs causing acute hepatotoxicity

Acute hepatitis

- Paracetamol (in overdose)
- Cocaine, ecstasy
- Aspirin, NSAIDs
- Halothane
- Anti-tuberculous therapy: pyrazinamide, isoniazid, rifampicin
- Antifungals: ketoconazole
- Antihypertensives: methyldopa, hydralazine, dronedarone

Cholestasis/cholestatic hepatitis

- Antibiotics: penicillins, e.g. flucloxacillin, co-amoxiclav, ciprofloxacin, macrolides, e.g. erythromycin
- Chlorpromazine
- Azathioprine
- Oestrogens (including the oral contraceptive pill)
- Amitriptyline
- Carbamazepine
- ACE inhibitors
- Cimetidine/ranitidine
- Sulphonamides

19

Box 19.4 Causes of cirrhosis

- Chronic alcohol excess
- Chronic viral hepatitis (hepatitis B or C)
- Non-alcoholic fatty liver disease (NAFLD)
- Autoimmune hepatitis
- Cholestatic
  - Primary sclerosing cholangitis
  - Primary biliary cirrhosis
  - Secondary biliary cirrhosis
- Metabolic
  - Hereditary haemochromatosis
  - Wilson's disease
  - Alpha$_1$-antitrypsin deficiency
  - Cystic fibrosis
- Venous obstruction
  - Cardiac failure
  - Budd–Chiari syndrome
- Drugs, e.g. methotrexate
- Cryptogenic

Box 19.5 Stigmata of chronic liver disease

- Spider naevi
- Digital clubbing
- Palmar erythema
- Loss of axillary/pubic hair
- Parotid swelling
- Gynaecomastia
- Testicular atrophy

Modified from Headache Classification Committee of the International Headache Society (IHS) 2013. The International Classification of Headache Disorders, 3rd edn (beta version). Cephalalgia. 33(9):629–808.

Wilson's disease, an inherited disorder of copper metabolism, can present with acute hepatitis, and occasionally causes acute liver failure. A ↓serum caeruloplasmin is highly suggestive.

Hepatic vein thrombosis (Budd–Chiari syndrome) typically presents with upper abdominal pain, hepatomegaly and marked ascites due to liver outflow venous congestion.

Cardiac failure may cause hepatic injury due to vascular congestion with resultant jaundice and ↑ALT.

Ischaemic hepatitis ('shock liver') may result from impaired hepatic perfusion in a patient with shock; the ALT is usually markedly raised.

Cirrhosis

Chronic liver injury from any cause (Box 19.4) results in extensive hepatocellular loss, fibrosis and disturbance of the normal hepatic architecture. Hepatocellular insufficiency leads to jaundice, coagulopathy and ↓albumin. Portal hypertension and consequent porto-systemic shunting of blood result in oesophageal varices and hepatic encephalopathy (see Table 19.1). Portal hypertension, ↓albumin and generalized salt and water retention, due to haemodynamic and endocrine abnormalities, lead to ascites. There may be characteristic 'stigmata' on examination (Box 19.5).

Hepatic tumours

Malignant infiltration by primary or, more commonly, metastatic tumours may cause jaundice due to intrahepatic duct obstruction or extensive replacement of liver parenchyma. Common associated features include cachexia, malaise, RUQ pain (stretching of the liver capsule) and hepatomegaly.

Post-hepatic/biliary causes of jaundice

Jaundice due to biliary obstruction is associated with a pronounced rise in ALP and GGT (produced in the biliary epithelium). Clinical features may include pale stools, dark urine and itch. A raised PT may occur due to vitamin K malabsorption from the GI tract.

Gallstones

Gallstones are the most common cause of extrahepatic cholestasis; the onset of jaundice is relatively rapid, may be intermittent and is typically accompanied by epigastric/RUQ pain. Cholecystitis is diagnosed on abdominal USS by an inflamed gallbladder (thick-walled) containing gallstones. A dilated common bile duct on USS implies extrahepatic biliary obstruction and may be due to gallstones lodged in the common bile duct (choledocholithiasis). The presence of RUQ pain, fever and rigors suggests bacterial infection proximal to the obstruction (ascending cholangitis) and requires prompt antibiotics and decompression (ERCP).

Mirizzi's syndrome arises from extrinsic compression of the common hepatic duct by a large stone within the gallbladder, with features of obstructive jaundice.

Benign strictures

Benign strictures may result from trauma, particularly during biliary surgery or as a consequence of inflammation within the biliary tree, e.g. recurrent cholangitis, pancreatitis.

Autoimmune

In primary biliary cirrhosis, there is progressive destruction of the intrahepatic bile ducts. Ninety percent of patients are female. Pruritus usually precedes jaundice. The presence of anti-mitochondrial antibodies is diagnostic. Primary sclerosing cholangitis causes inflammation, fibrosis and strictures of the intrahepatic and extrahepatic biliary tree. It is more common in men and 75% of patients have ulcerative colitis.

Malignancy

Painless jaundice may represent a malignant cause of obstructive jaundice. Cancer of the head of the pancreas typically presents with insidious, progressive jaundice due to extrinsic compression of the common bile duct, often with marked weight loss, nausea and anorexia. Pain may be absent in the early stages.

Cholangiocarcinoma is a malignant tumour of the intra-hepatic or extrahepatic biliary tree that most commonly presents with painless jaundice, often with pruritus.

Other important causes of malignant extrinsic biliary compression include duodenal ampullary tumours and enlarged lymph nodes at the porta hepatis.

19

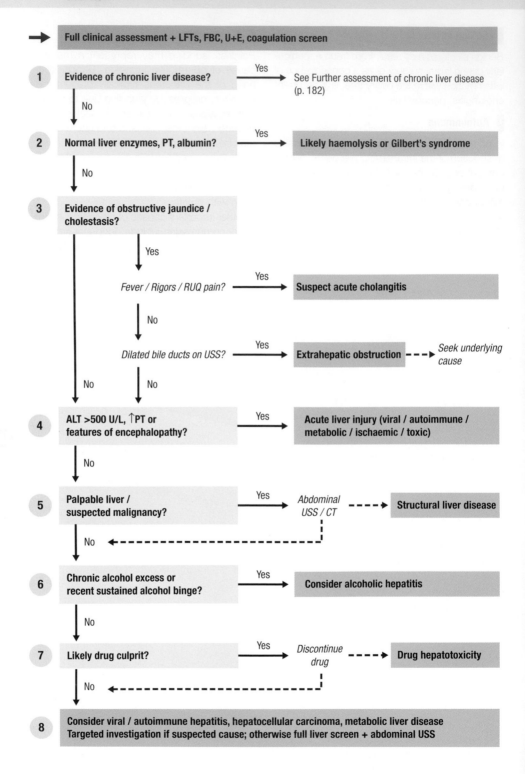

Full clinical assessment + LFTs, FBC, U+E, coagulation screen

1 Evidence of chronic liver disease? — Yes → See Further assessment of chronic liver disease (p. 182)

No

2 Normal liver enzymes, PT, albumin? — Yes → **Likely haemolysis or Gilbert's syndrome**

No

3 Evidence of obstructive jaundice / cholestasis?

Yes

Fever / Rigors / RUQ pain? — Yes → **Suspect acute cholangitis**

No

Dilated bile ducts on USS? — Yes → **Extrahepatic obstruction** - - - → *Seek underlying cause*

No   No

4 ALT >500 U/L, ↑PT or features of encephalopathy? — Yes → **Acute liver injury (viral / autoimmune / metabolic / ischaemic / toxic)**

No

5 Palpable liver / suspected malignancy? — Yes → *Abdominal USS / CT* - - - → **Structural liver disease**

No

6 Chronic alcohol excess or recent sustained alcohol binge? — Yes → **Consider alcoholic hepatitis**

No

7 Likely drug culprit? — Yes → *Discontinue drug* - - - → **Drug hepatotoxicity**

No

8 Consider viral / autoimmune hepatitis, hepatocellular carcinoma, metabolic liver disease
Targeted investigation if suspected cause; otherwise full liver screen + abdominal USS

1 Evidence of chronic liver disease?

In the absence of an established diagnosis, look for signs of chronic liver disease, particularly physical stigmata (see Box 19.5) and evidence of complications of cirrhosis, e.g. portal hypertension.

- Multiple spider naevi, in the absence of pregnancy/pro-oestrogenic drugs, strongly suggest chronic liver disease. The other stigmata lack specificity individually but are helpful in combination.
- Ascites, especially in association with dilated, superficial periumbilical veins ('caput medusae'), is a useful pointer to portal hypertension but may have other causes in jaundiced patients, e.g. intra-abdominal malignancy or right heart failure with hepatic congestion. The rapid onset of ascites, jaundice, hepatomegaly and abdominal pain suggests acute Budd–Chiari syndrome.
- Hepatic encephalopathy (see Table 19.1) and synthetic dysfunction (see below) may occur in acute liver failure but are highly suggestive of chronic liver disease when they occur against a background of previous clinical/biochemical evidence of liver disturbance.
- Abdominal USS can demonstrate morphologic features of cirrhosis, e.g. coarse echotexture, ↑nodularity and provide supportive evidence of portal hypertension (splenomegaly, reversed flow in the portal vein). In difficult cases, biopsy may be required to confirm the diagnosis and suggest the aetiology.

Evaluate any patient with jaundice and a background of established or suspected cirrhosis as described in 'Further assessment of chronic liver disease' (p. 182).

2 Normal liver enzymes, PT, albumin?

If there are no features of haemolysis or chronic liver disease, jaundice is mild (bilirubin <100 µmol/L) and LFTs are otherwise normal, the likely diagnosis is Gilbert's syndrome.

Consider haemolysis if features of liver disease are absent and blood results suggest ↑red cell breakdown (e.g. ↓Hb, ↑LDH, ↓haptoglobin,

red cell fragments on blood film) ± evidence of ↑red cell production (e.g. ↑reticulocytes, polychromasia). Further assessment is described on page 136.

3 Evidence of obstructive jaundice/cholestasis?

A rise in ALP/GGT out of proportion to ALT/AST suggests that jaundice is due to impaired biliary excretion, especially if accompanied by pale stools/dark urine. If there are features of sepsis, take blood cultures, give IV antibiotics, arrange urgent abdominal USS and discuss with the surgical team. Otherwise, perform USS to look for bile duct dilatation (indicating extrahepatic obstruction) and an underlying cause, e.g. gallstones.

If USS does not show dilated bile ducts, proceed to step 4.

If USS shows dilated bile ducts but does not reveal the underlying cause, arrange further imaging. MRCP provides excellent definition of the biliary tree – request it if you suspect gallstones (acute or recurrent RUQ pain), or if there is a past history of biliary pathology. CT allows better visualization of the pancreas – arrange if jaundice is painless with an insidious, progressive onset, especially in the elderly, to exclude pancreatic cancer. ERCP also provides useful diagnostic information but is more often undertaken subsequently to allow removal of gallstones or stenting of the ducts.

4 ALT >500 U/L, ↑PT or features of encephalopathy?

Identify patients with acute liver failure

Look for features of acute liver failure in all jaundiced patients without pre-existing liver disease or extrahepatic biliary obstruction, especially if there is evidence of extensive hepatocellular injury (↑↑ALT).

Hepatic encephalopathy (see Table 19.1) may be subtle; look closely for ↓concentration/alertness, mild disorientation, behavioural changes and reversal of the sleep/wake cycle. Test specifically for constructional apraxia, e.g. ask the patient to draw a five-pointed star or clock face, and asterixis (Fig. 19.1). Exclude hypoglycaemia and other

19

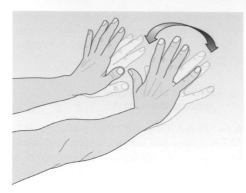

Fig. 19.1 Examining for asterixis. Asterixis (hepatic flap) is a repetitive, jerky tremor of the outstretched hands resulting in transient loss of extensor muscle tone at the wrist. It is due to metabolic brainstem dysfunction and is common in ventilatory failure, hepatic encephalopathy, renal failure and cardiac failure. (From Douglas G, Nicol F, Robertson C. Macleod's Clinical Examination, 12th edn. Edinburgh: Churchill Livingstone, 2009.)

metabolic abnormalities and consider CT brain to exclude intracranial pathology, especially if there are focal neurological abnormalities. EEG may assist the diagnosis.

An ↑PT (in the absence of anticoagulation, pre-existing coagulopathy or extensive cholestasis) indicates ↓hepatic synthetic function; measure in all patients with jaundice – daily if there is ↑↑ALT or worsening jaundice. If ↑, do not correct unless there is major haemorrhage.

Seek cause of acute liver injury

Enquire about alcohol and paracetamol intake, all recent drugs (prescribed or otherwise) and possible exposure to environmental/occupational toxins, e.g. carbon tetrachloride. Check viral serology (IgM antibodies to hepatitis B core antigen (HBc), hepatitis A virus (HAV), hepatitis E virus (HEV) CMV and EBV), serum caeruloplasmin, autoantibodies (ANA, ASMA, LKM) and gamma-globulins, and perform a full toxicology screen. Arrange abdominal USS to exclude Budd–Chiari syndrome and extensive malignant infiltration.

Repeatedly monitor and reassess patients with acute liver failure

Monitor closely in ICU or a high dependency unit (HDU) for complications including:

- hypoglycaemia
- hyperkalaemia

Box 19.6 King's College Hospital criteria for liver transplantation in acute liver failure

Paracetamol overdose

- H⁺ >50 nmol/L (pH <7.3) at or beyond 24 hours following the overdose

  or
- Serum creatinine >300 μmol/L plus PT >100 seconds (INR > \6.5) plus encephalopathy grade 3 or 4

Non-paracetamol cases

- PT >100 seconds (INR >6.5)

  or
- Any three of the following:
  - jaundice to encephalopathy time >7 days
  - age <10 or >40 years
  - indeterminate (non-A, non-B hepatitis) or drug-induced causes
  - bilirubin >300 μmol/L
  - PT >50 seconds (INR >3.5)

Creatinine of 300 μmol/L ≅ 3.38 mg/dL. Bilirubin of 300 μmol/L ≅ 17.6 mg/dL.

Modified from O'Grady JG, Alexander GJ, Hayllar KM, Williams R, 1989. Early indicators of prognosis in fulminant hepatic failure. Gastroenterology. 97(2):439–445.

- metabolic acidosis
- renal failure (develops in >50%, often necessitating haemofiltration)
- cerebral oedema with ↑intracranial pressure
- bacterial or fungal infection.

Use the King's College criteria (Box 19.6) to identify patients who may require transplantation. Liaise early and closely with a specialist liver unit to enable timely transfer if necessary.

5   Palpable liver/suspected malignancy?

Consider abdominal USS or CT to exclude malignant or other structural liver disease if the patient has:

- clinical evidence of hepatomegaly
- known malignancy with metastatic potential
- a palpable abdominal/rectal mass or lymphadenopathy
- ascites in the absence of chronic liver disease
- unexplained weight loss/cachexia/lymphadenopathy.

Any abnormal lesions identified may require biopsy for a tissue diagnosis.

6 Chronic alcohol excess or recent sustained alcohol binge?

Establish alcohol intake in all jaundiced patients. Be tactful but persistent. Start with a general enquiry before quantifying typical weekly intake. In addition to the total number of drinks, consider the alcohol content (ask about brand if necessary) and, for spirits, the measure per drink. Screen for potential problem drinking (see Box 2.1, p. 11). Seek a collateral history from relatives and friends, and observe closely for features of alcohol withdrawal if you suspect covert alcohol abuse.

Suspect alcoholic hepatitis in any patient with longstanding excessive consumption, e.g. >40 units/week or recent binge drinking (e.g. >100 units/week), or who develops severe withdrawal symptoms after 24–48 hours in hospital. Helpful supporting features include tender hepatomegaly and an AST:ALT ratio of >1. Once the diagnosis is made, calculate the Glasgow alcoholic hepatitis score to assess prognosis and guide treatment.

7 Likely drug culprit?

Enquire about ALL drugs taken within the preceding 6 weeks including over-the-counter, e.g. NSAIDs, paracetamol and herbal remedies. Box 19.2 contains some common causes of hepatotoxicity but there are many others; consult with a pharmacist or review the literature if uncertain. Wherever possible, discontinue any suspected drug culprit and observe the effect on bilirubin and LFTs. Liver biochemistry may take months to normalize, so consider further investigations (see below) in the interim unless clinical suspicion of drug toxicity is very high,

e.g. the patient recently started co-amoxiclav or anti-tuberculous therapy.

8 Consider other causes. Targeted investigation or full liver screen

If the cause remains uncertain, screen for viral, autoimmune, hereditary and metabolic conditions (Box 19.7), arrange an abdominal USS if not already performed and confirm alcohol intake. If there is fever, purpura, ↓platelets, conjunctival congestion or recent exposure to potentially contaminated water (e.g. freshwater sports, sewage worker), send blood and urine samples for leptospiral culture, serology ± PCR (liaise with the microbiology laboratory) and consider empirical antibiotic treatment. Liver biopsy may be required if jaundice persists without a clear cause and potential drug culprits have been removed.

Box 19.7 Screening investigations in jaundice/ suspected liver disease

Serology

- Hepatitis B surface antigen (HBsAg), Hepatitis C antibodies HCV Ab (+ IgM antibodies to HBc, HAV, HEV, CMV and EBV if acute)

Metabolic

- Ferritin, alpha$_1$-antitrypsin level, caeruloplasmin

Autoimmune

- AMA, ASMA, ANA, LKM, immunoglobulins

Other

- Abdominal USS, alpha-fetoprotein, paracetamol level, toxicology screen

19

Further assessment of chronic liver disease

Step 1 Establish the underlying cause

Try to determine the underlying aetiology in all new presentations of cirrhosis or in situations where the cause is unclear. Assess alcohol intake and perform screening investigations as listed in Box 19.7. Exclude treatable causes (e.g. Wilson's disease, haemochromatosis). Consider referral for liver biopsy if the cause remains uncertain.

Step 2 Look for evidence of complications/decompensation

Assess all patients with known or suspected cirrhosis for complications. Evaluate for hepatic encephalopathy and examine for ascites, oedema, jaundice and malnutrition. Measure albumin and PT to assess hepatic synthetic function, as well as bilirubin, U+E (hyponatraemia, hepatorenal syndrome) and FBC (anaemia, thrombocytopenia). Consider investigation for pulmonary complications such as pleural effusion, hepatopulmonary syndrome and pulmonary hypertension in patients with breathlessness, cyanosis or $\downarrow$SpO$_2$. If not already done screen for oesophageal varices with UGIE and for hepatocellular carcinoma with 6–12-monthly abdominal USS; USS will also detect small-volume ascites and splenomegaly.

Step 3 Seek precipitants of decompensation

Patients with cirrhosis have limited hepatic metabolic reserve and many factors can precipitate acute decompensation including spontaneous bacterial peritonitis, other intercurrent infection, surgery, alcohol excess, hepatotoxic drugs and hepatocellular carcinoma.

In a cirrhotic patient who develops jaundice, coagulopathy or encephalopathy:

- perform a full sepsis screen (see Clinical tool, p. 142), including an ascitic tap for microscopy and culture if ascites is present
- review all drugs and alcohol intake

- ensure that an abdominal USS has been performed within the last 6 months.

Additionally, in patients with encephalopathy:

- seek evidence of upper GI bleeding (stool evaluation, $\downarrow$Hb, $\uparrow$urea)
- look for and correct constipation (PR examination, stool chart)/dehydration/electrolyte disturbance
- minimize use of opioids and other sedative drugs.

In cases of worsening ascites, evaluate salt and water intake and compliance with diuretics, exclude spontaneous bacterial peritonitis and consider Budd–Chiari syndrome.

Step 4 Assess prognosis

Use the Child–Pugh classification (Table 19.2) to assess prognosis in patients with cirrhosis. Other poor prognostic factors include $\uparrow$creatinine and $\downarrow$Na$^+$, a small liver and variceal haemorrhage. Consider referral to a transplant centre for patients with Child–Pugh grade B or C. Absolute contraindications to transplantation include metastatic malignancy, active sepsis, cholangiocarcinoma and active alcohol or IV drug abuse.

Table 19.2 Child–Pugh classification of cirrhosis			
Score	1	2	3
Bilirubin (μmol/L)	<34	34–50	>50
Albumin (g/L)	>35	28–35	<28
Ascites	None	Mild	Marked
Encephalopathy	None	Mild	Marked
Prolongation of PT (seconds)	<4	4–6	>6
Child A = Score <7: 1-year survival 82% Child B = Score 7–9: 1-year survival 62% Child C = Score >9: 1-year survival 42%			

This chapter relates primarily to acute swelling of the knee, hip, elbow, shoulder and ankle. Swelling may arise from periarticular structures (bursae, tendons, muscles) or the joint. Conditions affecting the joint itself usually cause diffuse swelling, warmth, tenderness and restriction in both active and passive movement. In contrast, bursitis/tendinopathies cause localized tenderness and swelling in the area of the joint but with minimal restriction in joint movement. Pain is limited to certain planes of movement and is worse with active rather than passive movement.

Periarticular conditions

Bursitis is most commonly caused by repetitive movement, particularly if pressure is applied over the bursa during the process. Symptoms may arise after unaccustomed activity. Less often it may result from infection, rheumatoid disease or gout. Common sites of bursitis are pre-/infrapatellar (knee), olecranon (elbow), trochanteric (hip) and subacromial (shoulder).

Tendinopathies and *enthesopathies* (where the tendon attaches to the bone) are usually caused by overuse or by repetitive minor trauma. Other causes include infection and systemic conditions, e.g. rheumatoid disease, gout/pseudogout, Reiter's disease, ankylosing spondylitis. Tenderness over the tendon, with discomfort aggravated by movement, is usual and crepitus may be detected. Common sites for enthesopathies are the elbow (lateral and medial epicondyles) and knee. Osgood-Schlatter disease (inflammation of the patellar tendon at the tibial tuberosity) is a common disorder in adolescents experiencing rapid growth spurts.

Articular conditions

Septic arthritis

Septic arthritis may lead to irreversible cartilage and joint destruction, and so should be identified or excluded early. Haematogenous spread is the usual route of infection, but local skin or bone infection may occur. Common organisms are *S. aureus*, *N. gonorrhoeae* and *Salmonella* spp. Risk factors include a prosthetic joint, skin infection, joint surgery, diabetes mellitus, increasing age, immunocompromise and IV drug use. Pain, swelling, tenderness and erythema develop over a few hours. The joint is often held in slight flexion with the patient extremely reluctant to move it. Fever and ↑WBC/CRP may be present but are unreliable features, particularly in patients taking steroids or NSAIDs and in the immunosuppressed.

Trauma

Trauma may result in haemarthrosis if there is injury to a vascular structure within the joint (a fracture or ligamentous injury) or to a traumatic effusion, e.g. from a meniscal tear in the knee.

Any local penetrating injury predisposes to infection and requires urgent surgical debridement and washout.

Crystal arthropathy

The two most common forms are gout (uric acid) and pseudogout (calcium pyrophosphate).

A past history of gout, alcohol excess, diuretic use and renal stones are risk factors, as are conditions that cause high cell turnover (polycythaemia, lymphoma, psoriasis). In acute gout the metatarso-phalangeal joint of the great toe is most frequently affected, followed by the ankle, knee, small joints of the feet/hands, wrist and elbow. Onset is often sudden and exquisitely painful. The affected joint is hot, red and swollen, with shiny overlying skin.

Reactive arthritis

Reactive arthritis is an autoimmune, non-purulent arthritis that arises as a result of infection elsewhere in the body, typically within 4 weeks of GI or GU infection (*Chlamydia, Campylobacter, Yersinia, Salmonella, Shigella*). The swelling may appear suddenly or develop over a few days following an initial spell of joint stiffness in the joints. The disorder most commonly affects men between 20–50 years old and typically lasts for 2–6 months. The most commonly affected joints are lower limb large joints and sacroiliac joints. The classic triad of reactive arthritis comprises non-infectious urethritis, conjunctivitis/anterior uveitis and arthritis. However, this is found only in a minority of patients.

Polyarthropathy presenting as monoarthropathy

Osteoarthritis commonly affects the hands, feet, spine and the large weight-bearing joints, such as the hips and knees. Acute single-joint exacerbations may follow minor trauma. It usually evolves insidiously over months to years but may present with an acute exacerbation. Other polyarthopathies such as rheumatoid arthritis (RA) or psoriatic arthritis may occasionally present with disproportionate or isolated swelling of a single joint but definitive diagnosis of RA requires involvement of more than one joint (Table 20.1).

Bone cancer and secondary deposits

Any bone tumour near a joint can potentially cause swelling, although pain is usually the presenting feature. The most common cancers to metastasize to bone are those of the breast, lung, kidney, prostate and thyroid. Most lesions are visible on X-ray. Be careful to investigate patients who present with joint swelling following (minor) trauma that fails to settle as this may be a presentation of bone malignancy.

Table 20.1 The 2010 American College of Rheumatology/European League Against Rheumatism classification criteria for rheumatoid arthritis

Criterion	Score[1]
A. Joint involvement	
1 large joint	0
>1 large joints	1
1–3 small joints (± involvement of large joints)	2
4–10 small joints (± involvement of large joints)	3
10 joints (at least 1 small joint)	5
B. Serology	
Negative RF and negative ACPA	0
Low-positive RF or low-positive ACPA	2
High-positive RF or high-positive ACPA	3
C. Acute-phase reactants	
Normal CRP and normal ESR	0
Abnormal CRP or abnormal ESR	1
D. Duration of symptoms	
<6 weeks	0
≥6 weeks	1

[1]A score of ≥6/10 indicates definite RA.
ACPA – Anti-citrullinated protein antibody.
Source modified from Aletaha D, Neogi T, Silman AJ et al. 2010. Rheumatoid arthritis classification criteria: an American College of Rheumatology/European League Against Rheumatism collaborative initiative. Arthritis Rheum. 62(9):2582–2591.

20

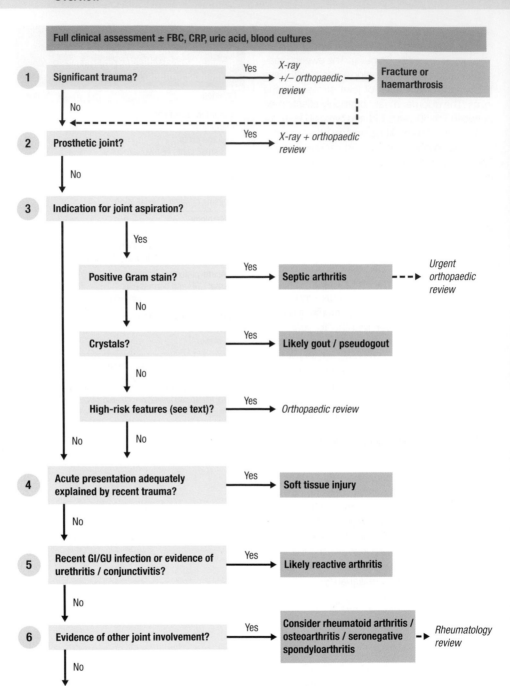

Full clinical assessment ± FBC, CRP, uric acid, blood cultures

1 Significant trauma? — Yes → *X-ray +/– orthopaedic review* → **Fracture or haemarthrosis**

No ↓

2 Prosthetic joint? — Yes → *X-ray + orthopaedic review*

No ↓

3 Indication for joint aspiration?

Yes ↓

Positive Gram stain? — Yes → **Septic arthritis** ⇢ *Urgent orthopaedic review*

No ↓

Crystals? — Yes → **Likely gout / pseudogout**

No ↓

High-risk features (see text)? — Yes → *Orthopaedic review*

No   No

4 Acute presentation adequately explained by recent trauma? — Yes → **Soft tissue injury**

No ↓

5 Recent GI/GU infection or evidence of urethritis / conjunctivitis? — Yes → **Likely reactive arthritis**

No ↓

6 Evidence of other joint involvement? — Yes → **Consider rheumatoid arthritis / osteoarthritis / seronegative spondyloarthritis** ⇢ *Rheumatology review*

No ↓

7 Consider periarticular cause, haemarthrosis, rheumatic fever or monoarticular presentation of oligo- or polyarthritis (see Step 6)

1 Significant trauma?

Perform plain X-rays if the patient has a history of recent trauma. If a fracture is identified, refer to an orthopaedic specialist.

Suspect haemarthrosis if severe joint swelling arises within 30–60 minutes of injury or occurs in a patient with impaired coagulation. Aspiration of a tense, traumatic haemarthrosis may help alleviate pain – consult an orthopaedic specialist and correct any coagulation abnormalities prior to aspiration (under strict aseptic technique).

In the absence of a coagulation abnormality, swelling that develops 24 hours or more after joint injury is likely to represent a traumatic effusion.

2 Prosthetic joint?

In patients with a swollen/tender prosthetic joint, perform an X-ray and consult an orthopaedic specialist. Do not aspirate a prosthetic joint without prior orthopaedic consultation because of the risk of introducing infection. Aspiration of prosthetic joints is typically undertaken by orthopaedic specialists in a sterile operating theatre environment.

3 Indication for joint aspiration?

Take blood for FBC, CRP, urate and blood cultures, but note that a normal WBC, and CRP do not exclude septic arthritis. Strongly consider plain X-rays if not undertaken already.

Perform joint aspiration (using strict aseptic technique) with urgent Gram stain and microscopy, followed by culture and sensitivity, in any patient with an acutely swollen, painful, warm joint in the absence of trauma, if you suspect septic arthritis. Aspiration of the knee is relatively simple but the other joints, especially the hip and ankle, require expert technique – seek orthopaedic help. Never aspirate through infected overlying tissues.

A joint aspirate that shows organisms on Gram stain is diagnostic of septic arthritis but is only positive in 30–50% of cases. Elevated WBC detected in joint aspirate suggests infection (Table 20.2), even if the Gram stain fails to demonstrate organisms – seek expert advice.

Crystal-induced arthropathy is suggested by the microscopic identification of monosodium urate in gout or calcium pyrophosphate dehydrate (CPP) in pseudogout crystals (see Table 20.2). However, this does not rule out a superimposed infection.

In the absence of crystals or a positive Gram stain, seek orthopaedic review if the aspirate is bloody or there is any ongoing suspicion of septic arthritis, e.g. typical clinical presentation, inflammatory aspirate (see Table 20.2) or immunocompromised patient.

4 Acute presentation adequately explained by recent trauma?

A significant proportion of acute large joint swellings in the context of trauma, with a normal X-ray, are soft tissue injuries with variable degrees of ligamentous/cartilaginous/tendinous injury. If the history is diagnostic, and joint examination features are consistent with a soft tissue injury, and the X-ray is reassuring, manage the patient conservatively. Consider referral to physiotherapy if there are specific concerns regarding joint function and tissue injury.

20

Table 20.2 Features of inflammatory and non-inflammatory joint aspirates

	Non-inflammatory synovial aspirate	Inflammatory synovial aspirate
Macroscopic features		
Volume	Small	Large
Appearance	Clear, straw coloured	Cloudy or opaque due to pus, red due to blood
Viscosity	High (hyaluronate present)	Low (hyaluronate breakdown)
Microscopic features		
Cellularity	Low	High (turbid fluid)
WBC	Low	High (infection, RA, gout) *(neutrophil predominance suggests bacterial infection, eosinophilia suggests RA, tuberculosis, arthritis, Lyme disease)*
Crystals	Absent	Gout: negatively birefringent MSU crystals Pseudogout: positively birefringent CPP crystals
Glucose	Slightly lower than serum	Significantly lower than serum in infection
Protein	Normal	Elevated
Gram stain	No organisms	Assess for bacterial species
Microbiological culture	Negative	Bacterial growth if present

5 Recent GI/GU infection or evidence of urethritis/conjunctivitis?

In a young patient with non-traumatic acute arthritis in whom septic arthritis has been excluded, the presence of any of the following features is highly suggestive of reactive arthritis:

- diarrhoea
- urinary frequency
- dysuria or urgency
- urethral discharge within the preceding 6 weeks (typically 1–3 weeks)
- genital ulceration or circinate balanitis
- symptoms/signs of conjunctivitis or iritis, e.g. pain, irritation, tearing, discharge or redness.

6 Evidence of other joint involvement?

Examine all joints carefully, looking for evidence of swelling and/or tenderness; note the distribution and symmetry of additional joint involvement.

The diagnostic criteria for RA are shown in Table 20.1. Consider a seronegative arthritis if there is prominent axial involvement/sacroiliitis or a history/clinical features of inflammatory bowel disease or psoriasis.

Unless the diagnosis is clearly osteoarthritis, refer for specialist rheumatological assessment.

7 Consider other causes

Use USS to detect/assess effusions of the hip and shoulder joints and periarticular conditions – tendinopathies, bursitis and muscle haematoma. Always consider spontaneous haemarthrosis in patients with coagulopathy (including those on anticoagulation or with haemophilia). Evaluate for rheumatic fever if there is a flitting arthritis associated with other characteristic features (see Box 14.4, p. 148). Seek Rheumatology advice if you suspect a monoarticular presentation of RA (see Table 20.1), osteoarthritis or seronegative arthritis.

The predominant cause of leg swelling is oedema – the abnormal accumulation of fluid within the interstitial space. Oedema may result from:

- ↑hydrostatic pressure in the venous system due to ↑intravascular volume or obstruction
- ↓plasma proteins, mainly albumin, that retain fluid within the vascular compartment (↓'oncotic' pressure), *or*
- obstruction to lymphatic drainage: 'lymphoedema'.

Unilateral oedema usually indicates localized pathology, e.g. venous or lymphatic obstruction. Bilateral oedema may be due to a local cause but more often represents the combination of generalized fluid overload and gravity. Oedema is frequently multifactorial, so search for additional causes, even if you identify a possible culprit.

Generalized oedema

Cardiogenic causes

Cardiogenic lower limb oedema is typically accompanied by other signs of volume overload ± structural heart disease (Fig. 21.1). In congestive cardiac failure (CCF), salt and water retention due to persistent neurohormonal activation leads to an ↑ in intravascular volume. High systemic venous hydrostatic pressure may also be caused by high right ventricular filling pressures if there is concomitant right heart failure. In CCF, right heart failure may reflect involvement of the right ventricle (RV) in the underlying disease process (e.g. dilated cardiomyopathy) but is more often due to chronically high left sided filling pressures which leads in turn to pulmonary hypertension.

In the absence of left heart disease, right heart failure may arise from other causes of pulmonary hypertension (e.g. chronic lung disease, thromboembolism or primary pulmonary vascular disease), pericardial disease (e.g. constriction, tamponade) or primary right heart pathology (e.g. pulmonary/tricuspid valve disease, RV infarction, arrhythmogenic RV cardiomyopathy).

Renal failure

In advanced renal failure, ↓salt and water excretion results in fluid retention and ↑systemic venous hydrostatic pressure. Chronic renal failure and heart failure commonly co-exist (cardiorenal syndrome) and may both contribute to generalized oedema.

Hypoalbuminaemia

Hypoalbuminaemia produces oedema by ↓plasma oncotic pressure. Causes include nephrotic syndrome (↑albumin loss in urine); chronic liver disease (↓hepatic synthesis of albumin); systemic inflammatory processes (leakage of albumin from the intravascular space due to increased capillary permeability ± persistent synthesis of 'acute-phase proteins' such as CRP in preference to albumin); protein-losing enteropathy (leakage of albumin into the gut due to lymphatic obstruction or mucosal disease); and advanced malnutrition.

Iatrogenic causes

Box 21.1 lists drugs that cause oedema.

Idiopathic cyclic oedema

Idiopathic cyclic oedema commonly affects women, most frequently of child-bearing age. Bilateral leg oedema progresses through the day and is most prominent in the evening. The aetiology is unclear.

Local causes of oedema

Deep vein thrombosis

Deep vein thrombosis (DVT) causes local oedema due to physical obstruction of venous drainage.

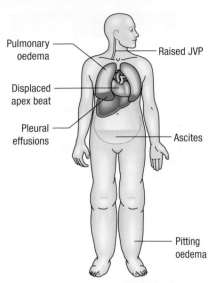

Pulmonary oedema

Raised JVP

Displaced apex beat

Pleural effusions

Ascites

Pitting oedema

Fig. 21.1 Clinical features of heart failure.

Box 21.1 Drugs causing oedema

- Calcium channel blockers
- IV fluids
- Corticosteroids
- Mineralocorticoids (fludrocortisone)
- Thiazolidinediones ('glitazones')
- Withdrawal of diuretics
- NSAIDs
- Oestrogens
- Progestogens
- Testosterone
- Growth hormone

Clinical features are notoriously unreliable; D-dimer and/or Doppler ultrasound are integral to diagnosis. Rarely, bilateral or inferior vena caval thrombosis may cause bilateral swelling.

Chronic venous insufficiency

The most common cause of chronic unilateral and bilateral leg swelling. Incompetent valves in the deep and perforating veins impair venous return with a rise in hydrostatic pressure. There may be varicose veins and characteristic skin changes (Box 21.2). Dependent/gravitational oedema is a variant of this condition, to be considered if immobility is an issue, e.g. post-stroke patients.

Box 21.2 Skin changes in chronic venous insufficiency

- Haemosiderin pigmentation
- Atrophy
- Hair loss
- Varicose eczema
- Induration and fibrosis of subcutaneous tissues
- Ulceration

Pelvic mass

A pelvic mass may obstruct local venous drainage and increase hydrostatic pressure by compressing pelvic veins. With ovarian tumours, oedema is usually unilateral. Bilateral oedema is common in pregnancy because of ↑blood volume and bilateral venous compression by the gravid uterus but the diagnosis is usually obvious; suspect DVT if there is a sudden increase in leg swelling, particularly in the third trimester.

Lymphoedema

Causes include malignancy (lymphatic invasion or lymphoma), previous lymph node surgery or radiotherapy, filariasis and congenital lymphatic abnormalities. Early lymphoedema may be indistinguishable from other forms of oedema but with progression it becomes firm and non-pitting with characteristic skin changes (see below).

Other causes

Compartment syndrome (↑pressure, vascular compromise and tissue injury within a fascial compartment), *rupture of a Baker's cyst* (a swelling of the semi-membranous bursa at the back of the knee) or *gastrocnemius*, *superficial thrombophlebitis* and *cellulitis* may all present with an acutely painful, swollen leg.

Lipoedema is not true oedema but an accumulation of excess subcutaneous fat. There is typically bilateral symmetrical leg swelling that is non-pitting and spares the dorsum of the feet. *Pretibial myxoedema* is an abnormal dermal accumulation of connective tissue components in Graves' disease. It causes areas of non-pitting oedema on the anterior or lateral aspects of the legs, with pink/purple plaques or nodules. Most patients will have evidence of Graves' ophthalmopathy.

21

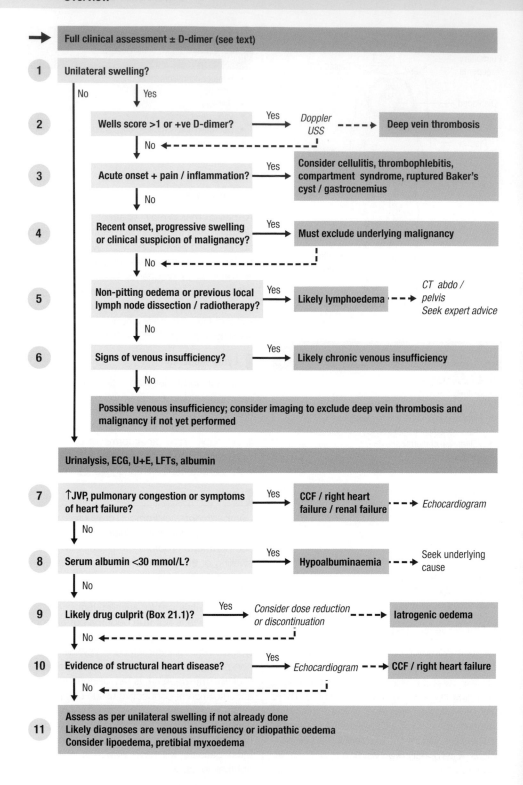

➡ **Full clinical assessment ± D-dimer (see text)**

1 **Unilateral swelling?**

No   Yes

2 **Wells score >1 or +ve D-dimer?**   Yes → *Doppler USS* - - - - → **Deep vein thrombosis**

No ← - - - - - - - - - - - - - - -

3 **Acute onset + pain / inflammation?**   Yes → **Consider cellulitis, thrombophlebitis, compartment syndrome, ruptured Baker's cyst / gastrocnemius**

No

4 **Recent onset, progressive swelling or clinical suspicion of malignancy?**   Yes → **Must exclude underlying malignancy**

No ← - - - - - - - - - - - - - - - -

5 **Non-pitting oedema or previous local lymph node dissection / radiotherapy?**   Yes → **Likely lymphoedema** - - → *CT abdo / pelvis Seek expert advice*

No

6 **Signs of venous insufficiency?**   Yes → **Likely chronic venous insufficiency**

No

Possible venous insufficiency; consider imaging to exclude deep vein thrombosis and malignancy if not yet performed

Urinalysis, ECG, U+E, LFTs, albumin

7 **↑JVP, pulmonary congestion or symptoms of heart failure?**   Yes → **CCF / right heart failure / renal failure** - - → *Echocardiogram*

No

8 **Serum albumin <30 mmol/L?**   Yes → **Hypoalbuminaemia** - - → Seek underlying cause

No

9 **Likely drug culprit (Box 21.1)?**   Yes → *Consider dose reduction or discontinuation* - - - - → **Iatrogenic oedema**

No ← - - - - - - - - - - - - - - -

10 **Evidence of structural heart disease?**   Yes → *Echocardiogram* - - → **CCF / right heart failure**

No ← - - - - - - - - - - - - - - - -

11 **Assess as per unilateral swelling if not already done**
Likely diagnoses are venous insufficiency or idiopathic oedema
Consider lipoedema, pretibial myxoedema

1 Unilateral swelling?

Examine both limbs for evidence of swelling and pitting. If there is bilateral lower limb swelling, even if asymmetrical, go to step 7.

2 Wells score >1 or +ve D-dimer?

Consider DVT in any patient with unilateral limb swelling, even without apparent risk factors or other signs or symptoms. Pre-test clinical prediction tools, e.g. Wells score (Table 21.1), can guide further investigation. Evaluate for bilateral DVT in any patient with risk factors and bilateral leg swelling.

- If Wells score is ≥2, DVT is likely – arrange a Doppler USS scan to confirm/refute the diagnosis.
- If Wells score is <2, perform a D-dimer blood test. If negative, DVT is excluded; if positive, arrange a Doppler USS scan.

Table 21.1 Wells score (deep vein thrombosis)

Clinical feature	Score
Active cancer (treatment within last 6 months or palliative)	+1 point
Paralysis, paresis or recent plaster immobilization of leg	+1 point
Recently bedridden >3 days or major surgery under general/regional anaesthesia in previous 12 weeks	+1 point
Local tenderness along distribution of deep venous system	+1 point
Entire leg swollen	+1 point
Calf swelling >3 cm compared to asymptomatic leg (measured 10 cm below tibial tuberosity)	+1 point
Pitting oedema confined to symptomatic leg	+1 point
Collateral superficial veins (non-varicose)	+1 point
Alternative diagnosis at least as likely as DVT, e.g. cellulitis, thrombophlebitis	−2 points

Source: Wells PS et al. 1997. Value of assessment of pretest probability of deep-vein thrombosis in clinical management. Lancet. 350(9094):1795–1798.

- Arrange Doppler USS in all pregnant patients with suspected DVT, as exclusion by D-dimer has not been validated in this group.

3 Acute onset + pain/inflammation?

Consider *cellulitis* if swelling is accompanied by a discrete area of erythema, heat, swelling and pain ± fever or ↑WBC/CRP; negative blood cultures/skin swabs do not rule out the diagnosis. In *superficial thrombophlebitis*, signs are localized, with redness and tenderness along the course of a vein, which may be firm and palpable.

A *ruptured Baker's cyst* may be clinically indistinguishable from DVT; USS will reveal the diagnosis and exclude DVT.

Consider *gastrocnemius muscle rupture* in patients with sudden onset of pain during sporting activity ± pain on muscle palpation (maximal at the medial musculotendinous junction) – USS may be helpful.

Consider *compartment syndrome* if unilateral limb swelling is accompanied by any of the features in Box 21.3; if suspected, check CK (rhabdomyolysis) and arrange urgent orthopaedic review.

21

Box 21.3 Features of compartment syndrome

Clinical context

Lower limb fracture, trauma, crush injury, vascular injury
Drug overdose or ↓GCS

Symptoms

Pain (especially if increasing or deep/aching)
Paraesthesia/numbness[1]
Paresis/paralysis[1]

Signs

Pain on passive muscle stretching
Tense, firm or 'woody' feel on palpation
↓Capillary refill or absent distal pulses[1]
Muscle contracture[1]

Investigations

↑↑CK

[1]Numbness, paraesthesia, paralysis, absent pulse and contracture are late features; their absence does not exclude the diagnosis.

4 Recent onset, progressive swelling or clinical suspicion of malignancy?

A pelvic or lower abdominal mass may produce leg swelling by compressing the pelvic veins or lymphatics. Exclude underlying malignancy if any of the following is present:

- weight loss
- previous pelvic cancer
- postmenopausal or intermenstrual PV bleeding
- a palpable mass or local lymphadenopathy
- any new-onset, progressive, unilateral leg swelling with no clear alternative explanation.

Perform a rectal ± vaginal examination, check a PSA level (males) and arrange imaging with USS (transabdominal or transvaginal) or CT as appropriate.

5 Non-pitting oedema or previous local lymph node dissection/radiotherapy?

Distinguish lymphoedema from other causes of swelling, as it is unlikely to respond to conventional treatments and should prompt consideration of an underlying malignancy (new or recurrent). Consider the diagnosis if any of the following is present:

- previous pelvic malignancy, local radiotherapy or lymph node dissection
- known or family history of congenital lymphatic anomaly
- oedema that is firm and non-pitting
- inability to pinch the dorsal aspect of skin at the base of the second toe (Stemmer sign)
- thickening of overlying skin with warty or 'cobblestone' appearance.

If you suspect lymphoedema, seek expert advice and consider CT of the pelvis and abdomen to look for evidence of underlying malignancy.

6 Signs of venous insufficiency?

Suspect chronic venous insufficiency if any of the following is present:

- characteristic skin changes (Box 21.2)
- prominent varicosities in the affected limb
- previous DVT or vein stripping/harvesting in the affected limb

- longstanding pitting oedema with diurnal variation in a patient >50 years.

If none of these is present, reconsider the need to exclude underlying DVT and malignancy, and assess as described for bilateral leg swelling to look for a cause of generalized oedema.

7 ↑JVP, pulmonary congestion or symptoms of heart failure?

↑JVP signifies high central venous pressure (due to volume overload and/or ↑cardiac filling pressures) and therefore implies a cardiogenic/renal cause for bilateral pitting oedema rather than local venous obstruction or low oncotic pressure. Assume CCF if patients also have suggestive symptoms (orthopnoea, paroxsmal nocturnal dyspnoea, recent-onset exertional dyspnoea), a background of LV dysfunction, myocardial infarction or left sided valve disease or (irrespective of the JVP) clinical or CXR features of pulmonary congestion. Bear in mind the possibility of right heart failure secondary to pulmonary hypertension (or less commonly right heart disease) in patients with severe chronic lung disease or clear lung fields. In either case, arrange an echocardiogram to assess cardiac structure and function including LV/RV size and function, valvular function and pulmonary artery pressure. Even in the absence of ↑JVP or obvious pulmonary congestion, consider CCF and arrange an echocardiogram in patients with recent-onset exertional or nocturnal dyspnoea since these signs can be challenging to detect or subtle.

Consider renal impairment as a cause or contributor to fluid retention if GFR<30; see 'Further assessment of renal failure' (p. 230) and seek renal advice if new presentation, major change from baseline or severe oliguria.

8 Serum albumin <30 mmol/L?

Hypoalbuminaemia may cause or contribute to oedema, particularly when <25 g/L. Search for an underlying cause.

Screen for nephrotic syndrome by urinalysis, looking for proteinuria. If the test is positive, collect a 24-hour urine sample; >3 g protein/24 hours confirms the diagnosis.

Suspect ↓hepatic synthetic function if there are deranged LFTs or features of chronic liver disease (Box 19.5, p. 176) and PT is prolonged.

A persistent acute-phase response (resulting in ↓albumin synthesis) may occur in chronic infection, inflammatory illness or occult malignancy. Suspect this if the patient has a persistently ↑CRP/ESR, recurrent pyrexia, lymphadenopathy, constitutional upset (fever, sweats, malaise, weight loss) or local signs or symptoms, e.g. palpable mass, active synovitis – investigate as for fever/pyrexia of unknown origin (p. 148).

Consider protein-losing enteropathy and seek GI advice if there is a history or symptoms of GI disorder. Malnutrition must be prolonged and severe to cause a significant decrease in serum albumin and is a diagnosis of exclusion.

9 Likely drug culprit (see Box 21.1)?

Drug causes are listed in Box 21.1. Where feasible, review after trial discontinuation.

10 Evidence of structural heart disease?

Bilateral lower limb oedema is less likely to have a cardiogenic cause if there are no accompanying signs or symptoms of heart failure. However, in the absence of any clear alternative cause, consider echocardiography if there are any pointers toward underlying structural heart disease including:

- a past history of MI, cardiac surgery, valvular disease, pulmonary embolism or chronic lung disease (e.g. COPD, obstructive sleep apnoea)
- Heart murmur, S3, displaced apex beat or parasternal heave
- Cardiomegaly on CXR
- Significant ECG abnormality, e.g. Q waves, left or right bundle branch block; see Box 6.1, p. 51.

11 Assess as per unilateral swelling. Likely venous insufficiency or idiopathic oedema

If there is bilateral swelling, first return to step 1 and assess for 'unilateral' causes, e.g. bilateral DVT.

Venous insufficiency is the likeliest cause in patients >50 years or in those with skin changes/predisposing factors. Idiopathic cyclic oedema is a common cause in women of child-bearing age (mechanism not understood) but consider an echocardiogram to exclude pulmonary hypertension. Gravitational oedema may occur with longstanding immobility.

If pitting is absent, consider lipoedema or pretibial myxoedema.

21

Limb weakness may be focal or generalized. Diagnosis relies on careful clinical assessment, complemented, in most cases, by appropriate brain or spinal imaging. Current stroke management mandates urgent evaluation of unilateral limb weakness. However, focal limb weakness can be caused by many non-stroke pathologies and these should not be overlooked in the rush to definitive management.

Stroke

Stroke is the most common cause of unilateral limb weakness. Patients typically present with sudden onset of weakness of the arm, leg or facial muscles, on one side. Symptoms persist for >3 hours and often do not resolve. An initial flaccid paresis progresses to upper motor neuron (UMN) weakness days later. There may be associated signs of cortical dysfunction (Box 22.1) or other sensory, visual or coordination problems. Aside from rare examples, such as those affecting certain areas of the brainstem, symptoms and signs are consistently unilateral.

Transient ischaemic attack (TIA)

TIAs are temporary, focal, ischaemic insults to the brain. Symptoms and signs usually last for at least 10 minutes and are comparable to stroke but resolve entirely without permanent neurological sequelae. The traditional definition of TIA describes a syndrome lasting less than a day, but this does not correlate with modern knowledge of stroke – symptoms >3 hours are likely to show permanent ischaemic damage to the brain on advanced imaging. With rare exceptions, TIAs do not cause loss of consciousness.

Space-occupying lesions

Space-occupying lesions, e.g. tumour, abscess, chronic subdural haematoma, can cause symptoms and signs mimicking stroke but the onset is typically more gradual and progressive. There may be features of raised ICP or clues to the underlying pathology, e.g. malignancy, or a source of septic emboli such as infective endocarditis.

Spinal cord lesions

Transverse lesions produce bilateral UMN limb weakness (para/tetraparesis), with loss of all sensory modalities below the spinal cord level and disturbance of sphincter function. Unilateral lesions (Brown–Séquard syndrome) cause ipsilateral UMN weakness and loss of proprioception below the cord level, with contralateral loss of pain and temperature sensation.

Causes may be compressive lesions, e.g. intervertebral disc prolapse, trauma, vertebral metastases or intrinsic pathology, e.g. transverse myelitis, glioma, spinal infarct, vitamin B_{12} deficiency. Circumferential pain across or sensory loss below a thoracic or lumbar dermatome suggests cord compression (but is not always present) – the level should correlate with neurological examination of the lower limbs. Saddle anaesthesia, bilateral leg pain, urinary retention and reduced anal tone suggest cauda equina syndrome, and should prompt urgent imaging.

Peripheral nerve lesions

Lower motor neuron (LMN) weakness may result from generalized disease of peripheral nerves (peripheral neuropathy), or from lesions affecting a plexus (plexopathy), spinal root (radiculopathy) or single nerve (mononeuropathy). In peripheral neuropathy, the longest nerves tend to be affected first, leading to a 'glove-and-stocking' pattern of weakness and sensory loss; in the other lesions, weakness and sensory loss reflect the muscles/skin regions innervated by the affected nerve(s) or nerve root.

Motor neuron disease

A chronic degenerative condition that presents with gradual, progressive weakness and a combination of UMN and LMN signs. There may

---

Box 22.1 Signs of cortical dysfunction

- Visual field defect
- Dysphasia
- Dyspraxia
- Neglect
- Sensory or visual inattention.

---

be bulbar involvement but sensory features are absent.

Other causes

Encephalitis may cause limb weakness as part of a constellation of central neurological symptoms including confusion, seizures and altered consciousness. Multiple sclerosis can present with almost any pattern of UMN limb weakness, though paraparesis secondary to transverse myelitis is most typical. Transient focal limb weakness can occur immediately after a focal seizure (Todd's paresis). Migraine occasionally causes limb weakness (hemiplegic migraine) but this is a diagnosis of exclusion. Myasthenia gravis causes 'fatigability' of limb muscles. Generalized muscle weakness may result from congenital/inflammatory myopathy, e.g. polymyositis, endocrine or metabolic disturbance, e.g. Cushing's syndrome, hypokalaemia, or drugs/toxins, e.g. corticosteroids, alcohol; it is also a common, non-specific presentation of acute illness in frail, elderly patients.

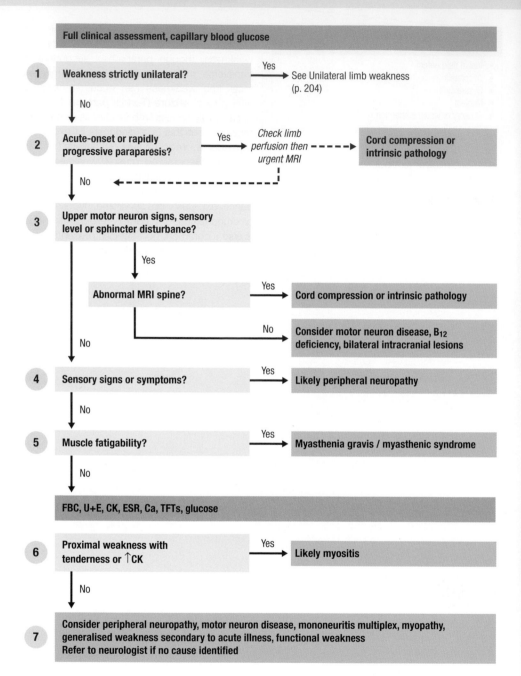

Full clinical assessment, capillary blood glucose

1 Weakness strictly unilateral? —Yes→ See Unilateral limb weakness (p. 204)

No ↓

2 Acute-onset or rapidly progressive paraparesis? —Yes→ *Check limb perfusion then urgent MRI* ----→ Cord compression or intrinsic pathology

No ↓

3 Upper motor neuron signs, sensory level or sphincter disturbance?

↓ Yes

Abnormal MRI spine? —Yes→ Cord compression or intrinsic pathology

No → No → Consider motor neuron disease, B12 deficiency, bilateral intracranial lesions

4 Sensory signs or symptoms? —Yes→ Likely peripheral neuropathy

No ↓

5 Muscle fatigability? —Yes→ Myasthenia gravis / myasthenic syndrome

No ↓

FBC, U+E, CK, ESR, Ca, TFTs, glucose

6 Proximal weakness with tenderness or ↑CK —Yes→ Likely myositis

No ↓

7 Consider peripheral neuropathy, motor neuron disease, mononeuritis multiplex, myopathy, generalised weakness secondary to acute illness, functional weakness
Refer to neurologist if no cause identified

1 Weakness strictly unilateral?

Assess power in all four limbs and grade according to the MRC scale (Table 22.1). Ask about any pre-existing limb weakness that predates the current presentation, e.g. old stroke, and whether it has changed recently. In any rapid-onset weakness, perform a CBG; if <3.0 mmol/L, send blood for lab glucose measurement but treat immediately with IV dextrose and then reassess.

If the current presentation of limb weakness is confined to one side of the body assess as per *unilateral limb weakness* (this includes patients with contralateral facial weakness). Otherwise, continue on the current diagnostic pathway, even if signs are markedly asymmetrical.

2 Acute-onset or rapidly progressive paraparesis?

In any patient with sudden-onset or rapidly progressive paraparesis or tetraparesis:

- immobilize the cervical spine pending imaging, if there is suspicion of recent trauma
- discuss immediately with a vascular surgeon if weakness is accompanied by features of acute limb ischaemia, e.g. pain; cold/pale/mottled skin; absent pulses
- otherwise, arrange urgent spinal imaging, usually MRI, to exclude cord compression or traumatic injury.

If MRI confirms a compressive lesion, discuss with a neurosurgeon or oncologist, depending on the clinical context and likely cause.

If MRI excludes cord compression (and does not yield a definitive alternative diagnosis), consider spinal stroke if the onset of weakness was very sudden, especially if accompanied by severe back pain. Examine for sparing of proprioception and vibration sense, and look specifically for MRI changes of spinal infarction. Otherwise, seek urgent neurological review and continue to assess as described below.

3 Upper motor neuron signs, sensory level or sphincter disturbance?

Bilateral weakness associated with UMN signs (↑tone, brisk reflexes, extensor plantar response), a sensory level (Fig. 22.1) and/or bladder/bowel dysfunction suggests myelopathy.

- Arrange an MRI spine to exclude cord compression and structural intrinsic spinal disease, e.g. syringomyelia, glioma, abscess.
- If neither is present, check whether the patient has had previous radiotherapy (post-radiation myelopathy) and measure plasma vitamin B_{12} levels to exclude subacute combined degeneration of the cord.
- Suspect transverse myelitis if the MRI shows evidence of inflammatory change and the time from first onset of symptoms to maximal weakness was between 4 hours and 21 days – refer to a neurologist for further evaluation, e.g. CSF analysis, autoimmune and infective screen.
- Suspect motor neuron disease (amyotrophic lateral sclerosis) if weakness is slowly progressive and sensory features are absent, especially if there are associated LMN signs, e.g. fasciculation, or bulbar involvement.

Table 22.1 Medical Research Council (MRC) power rating	
Grade	Findings on examination
1	No movement, not even muscle flicker
2	Flicker of muscle contraction only
3	Movement possible only when action of gravity is removed and against no resistance
4	Can move against gravity but not completely against full active resistance
5	Normal power against full active resistance

Box 22.2 Symptoms and signs suggestive of raised intracranial pressure
- Severe headache
- ↓GCS
- VI nerve palsy or unilateral pupillary dilatation
- Vomiting
- Bradycardia/systolic hypertension
- Papilloedema

22

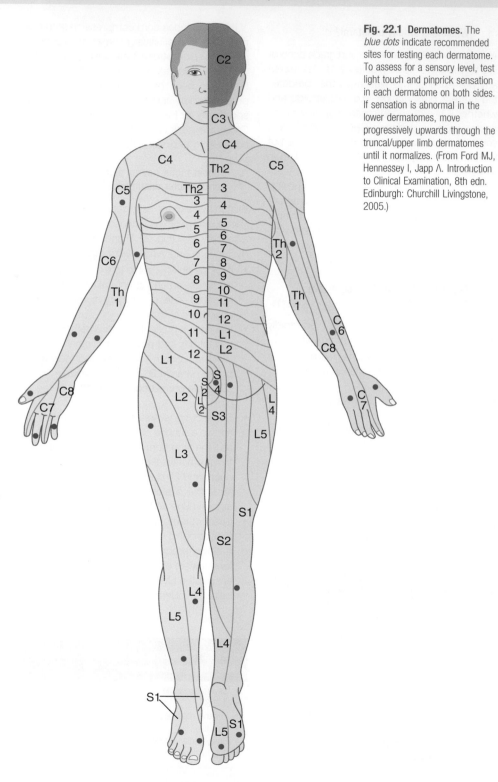

Fig. 22.1 Dermatomes. The *blue dots* indicate recommended sites for testing each dermatome. To assess for a sensory level, test light touch and pinprick sensation in each dermatome on both sides. If sensation is abnormal in the lower dermatomes, move progressively upwards through the truncal/upper limb dermatomes until it normalizes. (From Ford MJ, Hennessey I, Japp Λ. Introduction to Clinical Examination, 8th edn. Edinburgh: Churchill Livingstone, 2005.)

Consider brain imaging to exclude bilateral intracranial lesions, e.g. cerebral emboli/metastases, venous stroke, demyelination, in any patient with bilateral UMN limb weakness and:

- no evidence of myelopathy, i.e. normal MRI spine, no sensory level/sphincter disturbance), or
- associated cortical signs (see Box 22.1), features of ↑ICP (Box 22.2), cranial nerve lesions or cerebellar involvement.

Consider CT angiography of the Circle of Willis to exclude basilar artery thrombosis in patients with bilateral but asymmetrical neurology associated with drowsiness and change in behaviour with a normal CT brain (seek expert advice). Obtain specialist neurological input in any suspected case of motor neuron disease or multiple sclerosis, or if the cause remains unclear.

4 Sensory signs or symptoms?

In the absence of UMN signs, sphincter dysfunction or a sensory level, the combination of bilateral or generalized limb weakness with sensory disturbance is usually due to peripheral neuropathy.

Table 22.2 Clinical features of Guillain–Barré syndrome

Remember these as the five 'A's:

Acute course:	Time from onset to maximal weakness = hours to 4 weeks
Ascending weakness:	Initially in legs, progressing to arms ± respiratory/bulbar/facial muscles At presentation 60% have weakness in all four limbs; 50% have facial weakness
Areflexia:	Absence of tendon reflexes helps to distinguish Guillain–Barré syndrome from myelopathy
Associated sensory symptoms:	Distal numbness, tingling or pain often precedes weakness Loss of proprioception more common than pain and temperature
Autonomic involvement:	Sinus tachycardia, postural hypotension, impaired sweating often present Urinary retention and constipation are later features

Consider Guillain–Barré syndrome if distal lower limb numbness or tingling is followed by rapidly ascending weakness and absent tendon reflexes (Table 22.2).

- Measure urinary porphyrins to exclude acute intermittent porphyria.
- Confirm the diagnosis with nerve conduction studies and LP (↑CSF protein with normal cell count and glucose).
- Check and monitor vital capacity for evidence of respiratory depression.
- Refer early to a neurologist for further evaluation.

Slowly progressive limb weakness that is more marked distally with a 'glove-and-stocking' pattern of sensory loss strongly suggests a sensorimotor peripheral neuropathy, e.g. chronic inflammatory demyelinating polyneuropathy, hereditary sensorimotor neuropathy.

- Arrange nerve conduction studies to confirm peripheral nerve disease and differentiate demyelination from axonal degeneration.
- Investigate for an underlying cause, e.g. serum protein electrophoresis, HIV test, urinary porphyrins, fasting blood glucose.

Consider spinal imaging to exclude bilateral radiculopathy if sensory loss and motor signs follow a nerve root distribution (see Table 22.4).

5 Muscle fatigability?

22

Consider myasthenia gravis if the history or examination findings suggest fatigable muscle weakness: initially normal muscle power that rapidly weakens with sustained or repeated activity. Ocular and bulbar muscles tend to be affected before limb muscles.

Ask about the effect of exercise and other activities on weakness.

- Enquire specifically about diplopia during reading, weakening of the voice and difficulty in chewing/swallowing after the first few mouthfuls of food.
- Examine for ptosis.
- Observe patients as they hold their arms above their head for a sustained period.
- Listen while the patient counts to 50.

In suspected cases, consider a Tensilon test if rapid confirmation is required, e.g. myasthenic crisis or severe global weakness; otherwise, check for anti-acetylcholine receptor antibodies, arrange a thoracic CT to exclude thymoma and seek expert neurological input.

Tendon reflexes are normal in myasthenia gravis. If muscle fatigability is accompanied by absent tendon reflexes that can be elicited following sustained muscle contraction, consider Lambert–Eaton myasthenic syndrome, a paraneoplastic syndrome – check for serum antibodies to voltage-gated calcium channels, arrange electrophysiological studies and screen for an underlying malignancy.

6 Proximal weakness with tenderness or ↑CK

Suspect myositis if symmetrical proximal muscle weakness is accompanied by ↑CK. If the patient is taking statins reassess after a period of discontinuation. Otherwise, send an autoantibody screen, including anti-synthetase antibodies, e.g. anti Jo-1 (associated with polymyositis); exclude other toxic causes, e.g. cocaine; and arrange muscle biopsy.

Even if the CK is normal, consider further investigation with muscle biopsy in any patient with symmetrical proximal muscle weakness associated with aching, tenderness, pyrexia or ↑ESR.

7 Consider other causes

Advanced myopathy may cause a degree of muscle wasting and diminished tendon reflexes but suspect an LMN lesion if there is flaccidity, absent reflexes and/or fasciculation.

- Consider Guillain–Barré syndrome if there is new-onset, progressive limb weakness: the features in Table 22.2 distinguish from other causes. If suspected, confirm with LP and nerve conduction studies.
- Suspect lumbosacral plexopathy if there is severe pain and progressive weakness/wasting of quadriceps with absent knee reflexes – arrange imaging to exclude malignant infiltration of the plexus and check fasting blood glucose to exclude diabetes mellitus (diabetic amyotrophy).
- Exclude other causes of motor neuropathy – check serum lead and urinary porphyrins and arrange nerve conduction studies.
- If nerve conduction studies are normal, the most likely diagnosis is motor neuron disease (progressive muscular atrophy) – arrange electromyography and refer the patient to a neurologist.

In patients with a 'patchy' pattern of weakness, examine to exclude multiple discrete peripheral nerve lesions (Fig. 22.2), i.e. mononeuritis

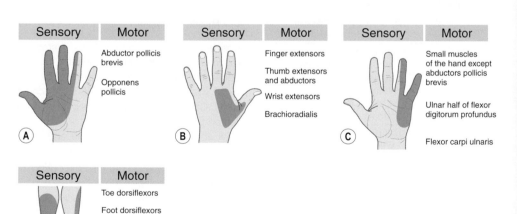

Fig. 22.2 Clinical signs in peripheral nerve lesions. [A] Median nerve. [B] Radial nerve. [C] Ulnar nerve. [D] Common peroneal nerve. (From Douglas G, Nicol F, Robertson C. Macleod's Clinical Examination, 12th edn. Edinburgh: Churchill Livingstone, 2009.)

multiplex; if suspected, arrange neurophysiological assessment and investigate for an underlying malignant, vasculitic or infiltrative disorder.

In patients with proximal muscle weakness ± wasting and no associated neurological abnormality, screen for underlying metabolic, nutritional, endocrine and drug-related causes.

- Enquire about alcohol intake.
- Consider trial discontinuation of any potentially causative medication, e.g. statin, fibrate.
- Check for an underlying biochemical disorder, e.g. $\downarrow K^+$, $\uparrow Ca^{2+}$.
- Look for clinical/biochemical features of diabetes, Cushing's syndrome, Addison's disease, thyroid disorders and acromegaly.
- Check 25(OH) cholecalciferol alongside serum calcium, alkaline phosphatase and

parathyroid hormone, if osteomalacia considered. At risk groups include the elderly, cirrhotic, malnourished patients and ethnic minority groups, but this is overall a more common problem than is recognized.

Assess frail, elderly patients with generalized weakness as described in Ch. 24.

Consider a functional aetiology if there are no objective features of organic disease and the severity or pattern of weakness is inconsistent – especially if the patient has a background of other functional disorders, e.g. irritable bowel syndrome, fibromyalgia.

Refer for specialist neurological evaluation if the cause remains unclear.

22

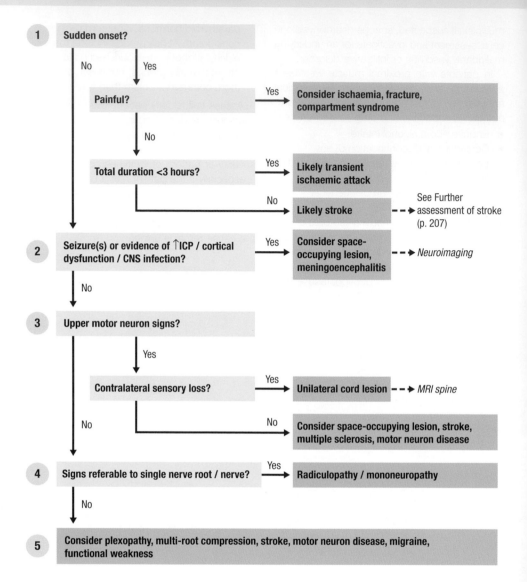

1 Sudden onset?

No · Yes

Painful? — Yes → Consider ischaemia, fracture, compartment syndrome

No

Total duration <3 hours? — Yes → Likely transient ischaemic attack

No → Likely stroke ---▶ See Further assessment of stroke (p. 207)

2 Seizure(s) or evidence of ↑ICP / cortical dysfunction / CNS infection? — Yes → Consider space-occupying lesion, meningoencephalitis ---▶ *Neuroimaging*

No

3 Upper motor neuron signs?

Yes

Contralateral sensory loss? — Yes → Unilateral cord lesion ---▶ *MRI spine*

No · No → Consider space-occupying lesion, stroke, multiple sclerosis, motor neuron disease

4 Signs referable to single nerve root / nerve? — Yes → Radiculopathy / mononeuropathy

No

5 Consider plexopathy, multi-root compression, stroke, motor neuron disease, migraine, functional weakness

1 Sudden onset?

Evaluate weakness as 'sudden-onset' if it reaches maximal intensity within a few minutes from the first appearance of symptoms.

If there is painful weakness of a single limb, consider vascular and orthopaedic causes:

- compare pulses, colour, temperature and capillary refill with the unaffected limb – seek immediate vascular review if there is any suspicion of acute limb ischaemia
- request an X-ray of the limb if there is any history of trauma
- measure CK and request an urgent orthopaedic review if there are features of compartment syndrome (see Box 21.3, p. 193).

Consider post-ictal weakness (Todd's paresis) if the history suggests seizure activity immediately prior to the onset of weakness – arrange rapid neuroimaging unless the cause of seizures is already established, the post-ictal phase is known to include limb weakness and the weakness is improving.

Acute non-neurological illness or hypotension may exacerbate established limb weakness from an old stroke – suspect this if the current weakness is confined to the same territory as a previously documented persistent neurological deficit and there are other clinical/laboratory features to suggest acute systemic illness, but maintain a low threshold for further neuroimaging.

In the absence of the above causes, sudden-onset unilateral weakness is highly likely to represent a stroke or TIA. If symptoms persist for >3 hours, then proceed, in the first instance, to 'Further assessment of stroke' (p. 207).

Diagnose TIA if symptoms have resolved completely and lasted <3 hours.

- Evaluate for risk factors and sources of embolism as described under 'Further assessment of stroke'.
- Assess the risk of impending stroke using the ABCDD score (Table 22.3).
  - Admit or arrange next-day specialist referral for any patient with >1 TIA in a week or an ABCDD score ≥4 for urgent control of risk factors and carotid Doppler USS.

Table 22.3 ABCDD score in TIA

	1	2
Age	≥60	
Blood pressure	Systolic ≥140 or diastolic ≥90	
Clinical features	Speech disturbance, no weakness	Unilateral weakness
Duration of attack	10–59 minutes	≥60 minutes
Diabetes	Yes	

- Otherwise, consider discharge with appropriate secondary prevention and specialist follow-up within a week.
- Arrange neuroimaging prior to discharge in any patient taking warfarin.

2 Seizure activity or evidence of ↑intracranial pressure/cortical dysfunction/CNS infection?

New-onset seizures, signs of cortical dysfunction (see Box 22.1) or evidence of ↑ICP (see Box 22.2) suggest underlying brain pathology.

- Arrange prompt neuroimaging (usually CT brain) to identify the cause.
- Seek anaesthetic review prior to scanning if GCS <8 or signs of airway compromise.
- See page 276 for further assessment of seizures.
- In all cases, seek expert neurological advice and consider further investigation with LP ± MRI if CT fails to reveal an underlying cause.

Consider meningoencephalitis if there is onset of limb weakness over hours accompanied by fever, meningism (Box 18.2, p. 169), purpuric rash or features of shock (Box 30.1, p. 267). If meningoencephalitis is suspected, obtain blood cultures, give empirical IV antibiotics/antivirals and arrange urgent CT brain; thereafter, perform an LP for CSF analysis unless contraindicated (p. 170).

22

3 Upper motor neuron signs?

A UMN pattern of weakness indicates a lesion proximal to the anterior horn cell; progressive onset of weakness suggests a space-occupying lesion whilst a rapid onset favours a vascular or inflammatory cause.

Exclude a unilateral cord lesion if there is dissociated sensory loss (ipsilateral proprioception/vibration; contralateral pain/temperature) or a clear sensory level. Otherwise, arrange neuroimaging; CT is the usual first-line modality but consider MRI if CT is inconclusive, especially if there are brainstem features, e.g. contralateral cranial nerve palsies or cerebellar signs.

Consider an atypical presentation of motor neuron disease (usually bilateral) if neuroimaging fails to reveal a cause and sensory features are absent, especially if there are associated LMN signs.

4 Signs referable to single nerve root/nerve?

In the absence of UMN signs, suspect a radiculopathy if clinical signs are referable to a single nerve root (Table 22.4), or a mononeuropathy if they correspond to a single peripheral nerve (see Fig. 22.2). If radiculopathy is suspected, consider a spinal MRI, particularly if weakness is progressive.

5 Consider other causes

Perform 2 lesion or demyelination in any patient presenting with hemiparesis, even if there are no obvious UMN features; if results are normal, consider hemiplegic migraine.

If weakness is confined to a single limb, consider multi-level root compression (see Table 22.4) or plexopathy, e.g. lumbosacral plexopathy (see above) or brachial plexopathy.

Otherwise, consider mononeuritis multiplex (see above), an atypical presentation of motor neuron disease (usually bilateral) or functional weakness.

Seek expert neurological input in any case where the diagnosis remains unclear.

Table 22.4 Clinical signs of nerve root compression			
Root	Weakness	Sensory loss (see Fig. 22.1)	Reflex loss
C5	Elbow flexion (biceps), arm and shoulder abduction (deltoid)	Upper lateral arm	Biceps
C6	Elbow flexion (brachioradialis)	Lower lateral arm, thumb, index finger	Supinator
C7	Elbow (triceps), wrist and finger extensors	Middle finger	Triceps
L4	Inversion of foot	Inner calf	Knee
L5	Dorsiflexion of hallux/toes	Outer calf and dorsum of foot	
S1	Plantar flexion	Sole and lateral foot	Ankle

Further assessment of stroke

Step 1 Assess eligibility for thrombolysis/mechanical clot retrieval

If facilities are available, refer immediately to stroke team for consideration of thrombolysis/mechanical clot retrieval in any patient with a potentially disabling stroke whose first onset of symptoms occurred within the last 4.5 hours (potentially longer time frame if mechanical clot retrieval available). Where the time of onset is uncertain, e.g. symptoms present on awakening, define it as the last time the patient was known to be well. Assess rapidly for contraindications (Box 22.3) in conjunction with the on-call stroke team. In patients who meet clinical eligibility criteria, arrange immediate CT brain to exclude haemorrhagic stroke.

Step 2 Classify stroke according to clinical and radiological findings

Arrange neuroimaging to differentiate haemorrhagic stroke from ischaemic stroke and to exclude non-stroke pathology, e.g. space-occupying lesion. Perform a CT brain urgently if

- the patient is eligible for thrombolysis (see above)
- coagulation is impaired
- ↓GCS
- symptoms include a severe headache
- there is a rapidly progressive neurological deficit
- cerebellar haemorrhage is suspected (to exclude obstructive hydrocephalus).

Otherwise, perform CT within 12 hours of presentation. Irrespective of CT findings, use the Bamford classification (Box 22.4) to categorize stroke.

Box 22.3 Contraindications to thrombolysis[1]

- Seizure at stroke onset
- Symptoms suggestive of subarachnoid haemorrhage
- Prior intracranial haemorrhage
- Intracranial tumour
- Stroke or serious head trauma within last 3 months
- Arterial puncture at a non-compressible site or LP within 1 week
- Active haemorrhage
- Suspected acute pericarditis or aortic dissection
- Systolic BP >185 mmHg or diastolic BP >110 mmHg
- INR >1.7, thrombocytopenia or bleeding disorder
- Pregnancy

[1]Most are relative contraindications – seek guidance from the on-call stroke team if the patient is otherwise eligible.

Step 3 Evaluate for risk factors/underlying cause

In any patient with ischaemic stroke, identify modifiable risk factors for vascular disease, including hypertension, hypercholesterolaemia, smoking and diabetes; arrange Doppler USS to determine the presence and severity of carotid stenosis unless the affected territory is within the posterior circulation or the patient is unfit for vascular surgery.

Suspect a cardiac source of cerebral embolism if the patient has

- current or previous evidence of atrial fibrillation
- a recent myocardial infarction
- clinical features suggesting endocarditis, e.g. fever and new murmur
- ≥2 cerebral infarcts (especially in different territories)
- other systemic embolic events, e.g. lower limb ischaemia.

Consider further investigation with transthoracic and, in selected cases, transoesophageal echocardiography.

Investigate for an unusual cause of stroke in younger patients without vascular risk factors.

- Perform a vasculitis and thrombophilia screen.
- Request a bubble-contrast echocardiography to detect a right-to-left shunt, e.g. patent foramen ovale that would permit 'paradoxical embolism' from the venous circulation.
- Consider MRA to exclude carotid/vertebral artery dissection.

Box 22.4 Bamford classification of stroke

This separates stroke into four clinical presentations that relate to the affected vascular territory and correlate with prognosis.

TACS (total anterior circulation stroke)

- All three of:
  1. weakness/sensory deficit affecting 2 out of 3 of face/arm/leg
  2. homonymous hemianopia
  3. cortical dysfunction, e.g. dysphasia, apraxia

PACS (partial anterior circulation stroke)

- Two out of three of the TACS criteria, or cortical dysfunction alone

LacS (lacunar stroke)

- Causes limited motor/sensory deficits with *no* cortical dysfunction

PoCS (posterior circulation stroke)

- Causes a variety of clinical syndromes, including homonymous hemianopia, cerebellar dysfunction and the brainstem syndromes

22

Low back pain is defined as posterior pain between the lower rib margin and the buttock creases; it is acute if the duration is <6 weeks, persistent if it lasts for 6 weeks to 3 months, and chronic if it is present for >3 months. In 90% of patients no specific underlying cause is found – the pain is thought to originate from muscles and ligaments, and is termed 'mechanical'.

Radicular pain ('*sciatica*') originates in the lower back and radiates down the leg in the distribution of ≥1 lumbosacral nerve roots (typically L4–S2) ± a corresponding neurological deficit (radiculopathy).

A thorough history and examination, supplemented where necessary by spinal imaging, is critical to identify patients with low back pain who have serious and/or treatable pathology.

Mechanical back pain

This is by far the most common cause of low back pain. The pain tends to be worse during activity, relieved by rest, and is not associated with sciatica, leg weakness, sphincter disturbance, claudication or systemic upset. An acute episode is often precipitated by bending, lifting or straining. In most cases, the pain resolves after a few weeks but recurrence or persistent low-grade symptoms are relatively common. Risk factors for developing chronic, disabling pain include depression, job dissatisfaction, disputed compensation claims and a history of other chronic pain syndromes.

Lumbar disc herniation

This is the most common cause of sciatica. It predominantly affects young and middle-aged adults, often following bending or lifting. Symptoms may be exacerbated by sneezing, coughing or straining. The diagnosis is largely clinical and most cases resolve within 6 weeks. Imaging is needed for patients with persistent pain and/or neurological deficit.

Lumbar spine stenosis

Narrowing of the lumbar spinal canal typically occurs in patients >50 years as a result of degenerative spinal changes and may cause lumbosacral nerve root compression. Patients often have longstanding, non-specific low back pain before developing dull or cramping discomfort in the buttocks and thighs precipitated by prolonged standing/walking and eased by sitting or lying down (neurogenic claudication).

Vertebral trauma and fracture

This most commonly follows a fall, road traffic accident or sporting injury, but may occur with minimal or no trauma in patients with osteoporosis or spinal conditions, e.g. ankylosing spondylitis. A patient with localized low back pain following trauma requires imaging to evaluate instability and involvement of the spinal canal/cord.

Spondyloarthritides (inflammatory back pain)

These chronic inflammatory joint diseases include ankylosing spondylitis and psoriatic arthritis, and predominantly affect the sacroiliac joints and axial skeleton; they have a strong genetic association with HLA-B27. Ankylosing spondylitis typically presents in early adulthood with an insidious onset of progressive back pain and stiffness over months to years.

Spinal tumour

Vertebral metastases from breast, lung, prostate or renal cancer are far more common than primary vertebral or other spinal tumours. The spine is frequently involved in patients with multiple myeloma. Red flag features (see Box 23.1) may suggest the diagnosis, which is best confirmed with MRI.

- New-onset pain in a patient >55 years
- Active or previous cancer
- Constant, unremitting or night pain
- Focal bony tenderness
- Unexplained weight loss
- Fever, sweats, malaise, anorexia

Box 23.2 Factors that increase the risk of spinal infection

- Diabetes mellitus
- General debility
- Indwelling vascular catheters
- IV drug abuse
- Previous TB infection
- Immunosuppression, e.g. HIV infection, chronic steroid therapy

Spinal infections

Pyogenic vertebral osteomyelitis, epidural abscess, 'discitis' or vertebral tuberculosis (TB) may produce severe, progressive pain, often with localized tenderness and reduced range of movement. Typical associated features include fever, sweats, malaise and ↑WBC/inflammatory markers. Risk factors for spinal infection are shown in Box 23.2. MRI is sensitive for detecting infection and differentiating from tumour.

Cauda equina syndrome

Compression of the collection of nerve roots at the base of the spine due to central disc prolapse, trauma or haematoma may lead to irreversible neurological damage and needs emergency referral for decompression. Diagnosis is best confirmed by MRI.

Other causes

- Spondylolisthesis (forward slippage of one vertebra on another): may cause back and radicular pain, and occasionally requires operative decompression.
- Pelvic pathology, e.g. prostate cancer, pelvic inflammatory disease.
- Renal tract pathology, e.g. stones, cancer, pyelonephritis.
- Abdominal aortic aneurysm.
- Shingles.
- Pregnancy.

23

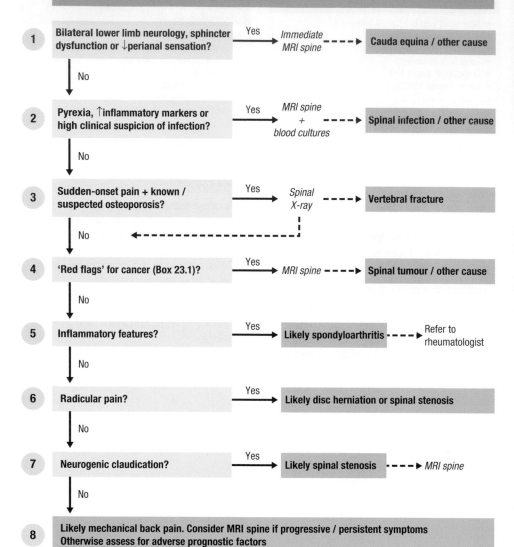

Full clinical assessment + lumbar spine examination

1   Bilateral lower limb neurology, sphincter dysfunction or ↓perianal sensation? — Yes → *Immediate MRI spine* ┄┄► Cauda equina / other cause

No

2   Pyrexia, ↑inflammatory markers or high clinical suspicion of infection? — Yes → *MRI spine + blood cultures* ┄┄► Spinal infection / other cause

No

3   Sudden-onset pain + known / suspected osteoporosis? — Yes → *Spinal X-ray* ┄┄► Vertebral fracture

No

4   'Red flags' for cancer (Box 23.1)? — Yes → *MRI spine* ┄┄► Spinal tumour / other cause

No

5   Inflammatory features? — Yes → Likely spondyloarthritis ┄┄► Refer to rheumatologist

No

6   Radicular pain? — Yes → Likely disc herniation or spinal stenosis

No

7   Neurogenic claudication? — Yes → Likely spinal stenosis ┄┄► *MRI spine*

No

8   Likely mechanical back pain. Consider MRI spine if progressive / persistent symptoms
Otherwise assess for adverse prognostic factors

Clinical tool
Examination of the lumbar spine

- Look for abnormal posture (scoliosis/loss of lordosis) from the back and side when the patient is standing.
- Feel for tenderness over the bony prominences and paraspinal muscles.
- Observe extension, flexion and lateral flexion of the lumbar spine (Fig. 23.1).
- Assess spinal flexion using Schober's test: locate the line between the posterior superior iliac crests (L3/L4 interspace); mark two points 10 cm above and 5 cm below this line. Ask the patient to bend forward as far as possible, with the knees extended. Lumbar flexion is restricted if the points separate by <5 cm.

- Test for sciatic nerve root compression (Fig. 23.2): with the patient supine, slowly flex the hip to 90° with the knee fully extended; limitation of flexion by pain radiating down the back of the leg to the foot (increased by dorsiflexing the ankle) indicates L4/L5/S1 nerve root tension (usually due to L3/4, L4/5 or L5/S1 lumbar disc herniation).
- Test for femoral nerve root compression (Fig. 23.3): with the patient prone, flex the knee to 90°; then, if pain-free, slowly extend the hip. Pain radiating from the back down the front of the leg to the knee indicates L2/L3/L4 nerve root tension.

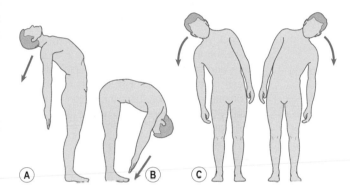

Fig. 23.1 Movements of the spine. A Extension. B Flexion. C Lateral flexion. (From Ford MJ, Hennessey I, Japp A. Introduction to Clinical Examination, 8th edn. Edinburgh: Churchill Livingstone, 2005.)

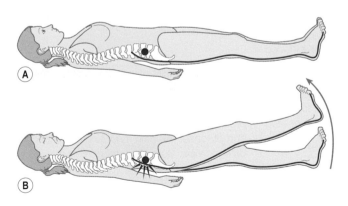

Fig. 23.2 Stretch test – sciatic nerve roots A Neutral; nerve roots slack. B Straight leg raising limited by tension of root over prolapsed disc. (From Ford MJ, Hennessey I, Japp A. Introduction to Clinical Examination, 8th edn. Edinburgh: Churchill Livingstone, 2005.)

23

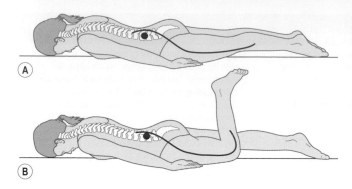

Fig. 23.3 Stretch test – femoral nerve. ⒜ Patient prone and free from pain because femoral roots are slack. ⒝ When femoral roots are tightened by flexion of the knee +/− extension of the hip pain may be felt in the back. (From Ford MJ, Hennessey I, Japp A. Introduction to Clinical Examination, 8th edn. Edinburgh: Churchill Livingstone, 2005.)

① Bilateral lower limb neurology, sphincter dysfunction or ↓perianal sensation?

Ask specifically about:

- change in urinary frequency
- any new difficulty in starting or stopping micturition
- a change in the sensation of toilet paper when wiping after defecation
- episodes of urinary/faecal incontinence.

If there is any suspicion of bowel/bladder dysfunction, perform a PR examination to assess anal tone and measure bladder volume immediately after voiding by bedside USS or catheterisation; >200 mL suggests urinary retention.

Enquire also about weakness or unusual sensations, e.g. numbness, tingling in the lower limbs; examine the legs carefully for reduced power, diminished reflexes and sensory disturbance, and test perianal sensation.

Arrange immediate MRI spine to exclude cauda equina syndrome in any patient with low back pain (irrespective of its characteristics) associated with any of:

- urinary or faecal incontinence
- urinary retention (significant post-void residual urine or ↑bladder volume with no urge)
- altered perianal sensation/↓anal tone
- bilateral lower limb neurological signs or symptoms.

Request emergency orthopaedic/neurosurgical review if the MRI confirms cauda equina compression.

② Pyrexia, ↑inflammatory markers or high clinical suspicion of infection

Check WBC, CRP and ESR and perform spinal X-rays if the patient has risk factors for spinal infection (see Box 23.2), localized spinal tenderness or a history of night sweats, shivers or constitutional upset. Take three blood cultures and arrange urgent MRI spine if any of the following is present:

- pyrexia >37.9°C
- ↑WBC/CRP/ESR
- high clinical suspicion in a patient with an indwelling vascular catheter, IV drug abuse or immunosuppression
- X-ray features suggestive of osteomyelitis
- A known focus of infection, e.g. abscess, cellulitis.

③ Sudden-onset pain + known/suspected osteoporosis?

Perform plain X-rays to look for lumbar compression fractures if the patient has new and abrupt onset of pain and known/suspected osteoporosis. Suspect osteoporosis if:

- long-term systemic steroids have been taken
- >65 years of age with loss of height, kyphosis or previous radial/hip fracture.

Seek an alternative cause if the X-ray reveals no fracture or one that does not correspond to the level of pain. Consider further investigation if there are any red flag features, other than age (see below).

4 'Red flags' for cancer (Box 23.1)?

Investigate for vertebral metastases, e.g. radio-isotope bone scan if the patient has a history of active or previous lung/prostate/breast/renal/thyroid cancer. Perform a breast examination and myeloma screen, measure PSA (in males), Ca^{2+} and ALP, and consider MRI spine in any other patient with 'red flag' features.

5 Inflammatory features?

Check ESR/CRP and perform plain spinal X-rays if gradual onset of low back pain and stiffness.

Refer to rheumatology for further evaluation of possible inflammatory back pain if there are X-ray features of spondylitis, e.g. squaring of the vertebral bodies/sacroiliitis or >1 of the following:

- morning stiffness lasting >30 minutes
- improvement of symptoms with exercise but not rest
- nocturnal back pain that arises in the second half of the night
- radiation of pain into the buttocks
- restricted lumbar spine movements
- sacroiliac tenderness
- ↑ESR/CRP with no alternative explanation.

6 Radicular pain?

Pain is 'radicular' if it radiates to the lower limb beyond the knee with any of:

- dermatomal distribution (see Fig. 22.1, p. 200)
- evidence of radiculopathy
- positive sciatic or femoral stretch test (Figs 23.2 and 23.3).

Suspect lumbar disc herniation in acute-onset radicular pain, especially if the nerve stretch test is positive. In the absence of red flags or other concerning features, reassess after 6–12 weeks of analgesia ± physiotherapy.

Suspect lumbar spinal stenosis if the patient is >50 years with a slow progressive onset of symptoms and/or features of neurogenic claudication (see below).

Consider referral for further investigation if:

- persistent pain
- evidence of >1 nerve root involvement
- major disability
- suspected lumbar spinal stenosis.

7 Neurogenic claudication?

Consider neurogenic claudication if low back pain is accompanied by bilateral thigh or leg discomfort, e.g. burning, cramping, tingling, that arises during walking or on standing and is rapidly relieved by sitting, lying down or bending forward.

Evaluate first for vascular claudication if the patient has a history of atherosclerotic disease, >1 vascular risk factor, e.g. diabetes mellitus, smoking, ↑BP, ↑cholesterol or signs of peripheral arterial disease, e.g. diminished pulses, femoral bruit, trophic skin changes. Check the ankle: brachial pressure index (ABPI) and request a vascular opinion if <1.0.

If neurogenic claudication is still suspected, consider MRI spine to confirm the presence of lumbar spinal stenosis, especially if symptoms are disabling.

8 Likely mechanical back pain. Consider MRI spine if progressive/persistent symptoms

Refer to orthopaedics if neurological dysfunction or spinal deformity. In the absence of neurological, structural, infective, red flag or radicular features, provide reassurance and analgesia, recommend that the patient stays active and reassess after a period of 6–12 weeks. If pain persists, look for features of depression and explore other potential psychosocial factors. Spinal imaging is unlikely to be helpful but seek specialist input if there are persistent or progressive disabling symptoms.

23

Patients may present with falls, difficulty mobilizing or complete immobility. Younger patients can usually be rapidly categorized into an underlying aetiology, but evaluation of elderly patients is more complex. Normal physiological changes of ageing – increased body sway, reduced muscle bulk (sarcopenia) and impaired reaction time – increase the likelihood of mobility problems. Moreover, mobility problems may be self-reinforcing, as reduced activity leads to loss of muscle function and confidence. A thorough, systematic approach is essential to identify adverse consequences of immobility, serious underlying pathology and potentially reversible contributing factors.

Accidental trip

Some falls are the unavoidable consequence of a trip or stumble. In the absence of significant injury, recurrent mobility problems or other concerns, these patients do not require detailed assessment. However, many elderly patients exhibit post hoc rationalization of their fall ('I must have tripped on the carpet'), so falls should only be classified as accidental if there is unequivocal evidence for this.

'Secondary' mobility presentations

Immobility and instability may occur as a consequence of other specific problems such as dizziness, joint pains or focal limb weakness. In these cases, assessment should focus, initially, on the underlying primary problem to determine the cause. Some patients with apparent falls may actually be experiencing blackouts and, again, this necessitates a different diagnostic approach.

Acute illness or drug reaction

In elderly/frail patients, a sudden decline in mobility (acute fall, inability to mobilize) may be the principal manifestation of any acute medical, surgical or psychiatric illness or a side-effect of certain medications (Box 24.1). In those with chronic underlying mobility problems, a relatively minor insult may lead to a major deterioration in mobility.

Multifactorial mobility problems

In patients with recurrent falls or other chronic mobility problems, there is often no single identifiable cause but rather multiple contributing factors, e.g. muscle weakness, balance disorder, polypharmacy, cognitive impairment, arthritis, ↓visual acuity, hearing loss. A comprehensive and multidimensional approach to assessment is essential.

Box 24.1 Drugs associated with increased risk of falls

- Alcohol
- Anticonvulsants
- Antidepressants
- Antihypertensives
- Antipsychotics

- Benzodiazepines
- Diuretics
- Digoxin
- Opioids
- Diabetes medications (oral hypoglycaemics and insulin)

Clinical tool
How to perform a gait assessment

- Ask patient to stand from sitting position
  Look for: need for assistance; necessary use of upper limbs
- Ask patient to continue standing
  Ask about: light-headedness/sensation of spinning or movement
  Look for: ability to continue standing safely/ unsteadiness/stooped posture
- Ask patient to move feet together – ensure he/she is standing close by
  Look for: increasing unsteadiness
- Ask patient to close eyes (Romberg's test)
  Look for: increasing unsteadiness (be ready to catch patient)
- Ask patient to open eyes, walk 3 metres, then turn around and walk back, using an aid if required
  Look for: overall safety and stability; unilateral gait abnormality (stroke, peripheral nerve lesion, joint

disease, pain); short, shuffling steps (Parkinson's disease[1], diffuse cerebrovascular disease); high-stepping gait (foot-drop, sensory ataxia); broad-based/unsteady gait (cerebellar lesion, normal pressure hydrocephalus)
- Ask the patient to walk for a longer distance
  Ask about: chest pain, calf pain, breathlessness, fatigue
  Look for: ↑RR, laboured breathing, need to stop
- Repeat, if necessary, after correction of any reversible factors, e.g. treatment of acute illness, effective pain control, rehydration, removal of offending drug

[1] Other features of Parkinsonian gait include reduced arm-swing, stooped posture and, sometimes, difficulty in starting and stopping ('festinant' gait).

24

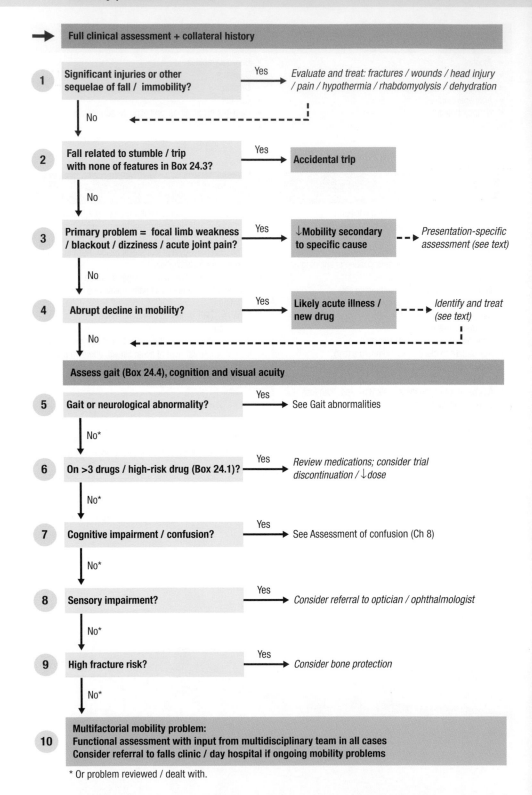

Full clinical assessment + collateral history

1 Significant injuries or other sequelae of fall / immobility? — Yes → *Evaluate and treat: fractures / wounds / head injury / pain / hypothermia / rhabdomyolysis / dehydration*

No

2 Fall related to stumble / trip with none of features in Box 24.3? — Yes → **Accidental trip**

No

3 Primary problem = focal limb weakness / blackout / dizziness / acute joint pain? — Yes → **↓Mobility secondary to specific cause** → *Presentation-specific assessment (see text)*

No

4 Abrupt decline in mobility? — Yes → **Likely acute illness / new drug** → *Identify and treat (see text)*

No

Assess gait (Box 24.4), cognition and visual acuity

5 Gait or neurological abnormality? — Yes → See Gait abnormalities

No*

6 On >3 drugs / high-risk drug (Box 24.1)? — Yes → *Review medications; consider trial discontinuation / ↓dose*

No*

7 Cognitive impairment / confusion? — Yes → See Assessment of confusion (Ch 8)

No*

8 Sensory impairment? — Yes → *Consider referral to optician / ophthalmologist*

No*

9 High fracture risk? — Yes → *Consider bone protection*

No*

10 Multifactorial mobility problem:
Functional assessment with input from multidisciplinary team in all cases
Consider referral to falls clinic / day hospital if ongoing mobility problems

* Or problem reviewed / dealt with.

1 Significant injuries or other sequelae of fall/immobility?

In all patients who have fallen (or who have been found on the floor), perform a rapid but thorough survey of the entire body for injuries. Fractures, lacerations or bruising may be not immediately apparent, and the cognitively impaired patient may not bring them to your attention. Assess the perfusion and function of any limb with bruising, deformity, pain or swelling and consider the need for X-rays. Pain will compound any existing mobility problems – ensure it is adequately treated. If there is a history of head injury, arrange neuroimaging if any of the features in Box 24.2 is present.

In patients with a prolonged period of immobility, e.g. lying on the floor or confined to bed, check temperature to exclude hypothermia, look for clinical/biochemical evidence of dehydration and examine the heels and sacrum for pressure sores. Consider aspiration/hypostatic pneumonia in patients with hypoxia, lung crackles or CXR changes. If there has been significant soft tissue pressure damage or any prolonged time on the floor, check CK and urinary myoglobin (suggested by haematuria on urinalysis with no red cells on microscopy) to exclude rhabdomyolysis and be vigilant for compartment syndrome (Box 21.3, p. 191).

2 Fall related to stumble/trip with none of features in Box 24.3?

Take care in making this diagnosis – a simple trip on a loose carpet tile at walking pace is usually

not 'normal' and the visual impairment that led to the trip or the poor balance that turned it into an injurious fall might be reversible. On the other hand, exhaustive assessment is inappropriate in patients with a genuinely accidental fall and no underlying mobility problems. Have a low threshold for further evaluation if any of the features in Box 24.3 is present or events leading up to the fall are unclear.

3 Primary problem = focal limb weakness/blackout/dizziness/acute joint pain?

If you identify new limb weakness on examination, assess as described in Chapter 22.

If mobility problems are consequent on dizziness, evaluate firstly for symptomatic postural hypotension: a fall of ≥20 mmHg in systolic BP or ≥10 mmHg in diastolic BP within 3 minutes of changing from a lying to standing position, accompanied by a feeling of light-headedness/pre-syncope. If this is detected, search for underlying causes, e.g. antihypertensives, dehydration, autonomic neuropathy. Otherwise, assess as in Chapter 10, but complete a full mobility assessment, especially if no specific disorder is identified.

Consider whether an apparent fall could have been a blackout. Beware of accepting rationalizations for the event ('I must have tripped') and make every attempt to obtain an eyewitness account of the current episode or previous ones. If patients cannot recall how they came to be lying on the ground, assess, in the first instance, as per transient loss of consciousness (see Ch. 31). Also suspect transient loss of consciousness if the patient was witnessed as having a period of unresponsiveness, sustained facial injuries during the fall (most conscious patients can protect the face) or experienced palpitation, chest pain, breathlessness or a pre-syncopal prodrome prior

24

Box 24.2 Indications for early neuroimaging in patients with head injury[1]

Immediate CT brain

- ↓GCS <12 or persistently <15
- Focal neurological signs
- Persistent headache or vomiting
- Features of basal skull fracture
- Coagulopathy or anticoagulation

CT brain within 8 hours

- Seizure
- >65 years + episode of loss of consciousness
- Retrograde amnesia
- Evidence of skull fracture

[1]Based on SIGN guideline 110.

Box 24.3 Features *not* consistent with a diagnosis of simple accidental trip

- Recurrent or multiple falls
- Recent decline in mobility or functional status
- Inability to get up from the ground
- Implausible mechanism for fall
- Witnessed period of unresponsiveness
- Inability to recall landing on ground
- Facial injuries

to 'falling'. Have a lower threshold for further evaluation of possible syncope in patients with ECG abnormalities (see Box 31.3, p. 273) or a history of major cardiac disease.

If mobility problems are secondary to an acutely painful joint, assess as in Chapter 20.

4 Abrupt decline in mobility?

An abrupt decline in mobility (acute fall, new onset of recurrent falls or being 'off legs') is one of the classical atypical presentations of acute illness in the elderly. Characteristic signs/symptoms of the specific precipitant may be absent and 'screening' investigations (Box 24.4) are often required to uncover the problem or identify a focus for further assessment.

Review all new drugs (including over-the-counter ones) started within the previous weeks and consider trial discontinuation of any high-risk agents (see Box 24.1). If significant loss of mobility was preceded by a fall, consider the possibility of fracture or head injury – ensure pain is adequately treated.

Weight loss, muscle wasting, hypoalbuminaemia and chronic anaemia may suggest a progressive disorder 'coming to a head'. Suspect significant acute illness in patients whose baseline mobility is relatively normal. Once this has been addressed, complete a full assessment to identify underlying mobility problems and reversible risk factors for falling.

In patients with a background of progressive mobility decline/deteriorating functional status/general frailty, the acute precipitant may be minor – do not over-emphasize it in comparison with the underlying contributory factors.

Box 24.4 Screening investigations to identify acute illness in elderly patients

- Capillary BG
- PR examination
- Urine dipstick and MSU/CSU (avoid diagnosing a urinary tract infection purely on the basis of abnormal dipstick results)
- Blood tests – FBC, U+E, LFTs, glucose, CRP (minimum)
- CXR

5 Gait or neurological abnormality?

Assessment of walking pattern is key to understanding mobility problems. It is a fundamental element of the neurological examination and can reveal abnormalities not elicited on gross testing of individual modalities. It may also unmask impaired effort tolerance due to cardiorespiratory or lower limb disease. Finally, the gait assessment is an opportunity to assess falls risk, even in the absence of specific findings. Check that patients are safe to mobilize, equip them with their normal walking aid and follow the steps in Clinical tool: Assessment of gait. Go to 'Gait abnormalities' (p. 220) if any abnormalities are detected.

6 On >3 drugs/high-risk drug (Box 24.1)?

Medications are one of the most readily modifiable of all factors influencing mobility problems but indiscriminate changes may do more harm than good. Individual medications that increase the risk of falling are listed in Box 24.1. Polypharmacy (≥5 regular medications) is a risk factor for falls. Review the indications for all drugs: are they still required? Look for opportunities to rationalize treatment, consider alternatives and consider decreasing the dose.

A gradual approach will allow the impact of individual changes to be assessed and is essential with psychotropic medication where abrupt withdrawal may be worse than the toxic syndrome. Explore a possible contribution from alcohol in all cases – in patients with underlying mobility/balance problems it may critically impair stability, even when consumed within recommended limits.

7 Cognitive impairment/confusion?

Acute delirium is a common cause of reduced mobility, and may not be readily apparent if it is hypoactive or superimposed on chronic impairment. Vigilance and collateral history are essential counterparts to objective measures of cognitive function; an Abbreviated Mental Test score of 6/10 is difficult to interpret without knowledge of baseline ability. Chronic cognitive impairment is also a risk factor for falls, but difficult to ameliorate. Consider silent precipitants of wandering/getting out of bed, such as urinary urgency or nicotine withdrawal. Further assessment of confusion is detailed in Chapter 8.

8 Sensory impairment?

Visual impairment increases the risk of falls and may be reversible, e.g. refractory errors, cataracts. Screen for ↓visual acuity. If detected, refer to an ophthalmologist (or an optician if a refractory error is suspected). Hearing loss may also contribute to instability and increased risk of falling, particularly in combination with some of the other risk factors.

9 High fracture risk?

Fractures, especially of the hip, are a devastating consequence of falls and selected patients may benefit from bone protection. This is a controversial area and specific indications change, but treatment, e.g. bisphosphonates, should be considered in patients with previous fragility fractures or a bone mineral density T-score of −2.5 or less and in those taking long-term or frequent courses of systemic steroids. In other cases, consider using the Q-fracture risk assessment tool, http://qfracture.org.

10 Multifactorial mobility problem: arrange multidisciplinary team assessment

All patients with recurrent falls or ↓mobility should be referred to physiotherapy/occupational therapy for assessment of functional ability, environmental contributors to the presentation, and scope for benefit from measures such as walking aids/strength and balance training/home alarms. In patients with ongoing problems, consider referral to day hospital or a specialist falls clinic for comprehensive assessment.

24

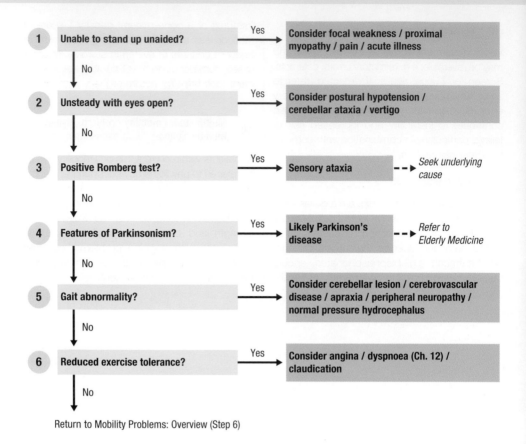

Return to Mobility Problems: Overview (Step 6)

1 Unable to stand up unaided?

Lower limb weakness may limit the ability to rise from a chair or necessitate use of the chair arms or pulling on nearby furniture. Systemic illness, toxic insults or metabolic derangement may cause mild generalized weakness. If weakness is persistent, asymmetrical or associated with wasting/neurological abnormalities, see Chapter 22.

2 Unsteady with eyes open?

Check lying/standing BP if the patient feels faint or light-headed. Consider vertigo if the patient has a sensation of spinning or movement. Observe standing posture, identify reduction in joint function, and evaluate pain. If patients can remain standing without assistance, ask them to move their feet close together – inability to do so indicates significant ataxia. Look for associated features of cerebellar disease, e.g. intention tremor, dysdiadochokinesis, dysmetria (past-pointing), dysarthria, nystagmus.

3 Positive Romberg test?

A marked increase in unsteadiness after eye closing is a positive test, suggesting a sensory (proprioceptive or vestibular) rather than cerebellar cause of ataxia. Reduction in sensation may be a normal part of ageing, e.g. reduced vibration sense in the feet is common and of limited significance in the older patient. Examine the patient during walking for an unsteady, ataxic or 'lead boot' gait. The list of possible causes of peripheral neuropathy is vast but screen routinely for diabetes mellitus, alcohol excess, liver disease, malnutrition (check vitamin B_{12}) or iatrogenic causes, e.g. anticonvulsants, chemotherapy.

4 Features of Parkinsonism?

Look for the typical features of Parkinson's disease:

- tremor: coarse, slow (5 Hz) and usually asymmetrical; present at rest, absent during sleep; decreased by voluntary movement; increased by emotion; adduction–abduction of the thumb with flexion–extension of the fingers ('pill-rolling')
- ↑tone: 'lead-pipe' rigidity or (in the presence of tremor) 'cog-wheel' with a jerky feel
- bradykinesia: slow initiation of movement, ↓speed of fine movements, expressionless face
- gait: delayed initiation, ↓arm swing, stooped posture, short, shuffling steps, difficulty turning.

The presence of these features makes idiopathic Parkinson's disease (PD) more likely, but Parkinsonism has other causes: most commonly, diffuse cerebrovascular disease. The classical description of vascular Parkinsonism is of signs of PD below the waist, with relative sparing of the arms.

New presentations or progression of PD are usually assessed in an outpatient setting. Mobility-related admissions in patients with PD are more likely to be connected with a superimposed acute illness or a medication problem. Make certain that hospitalized patients with PD receive their medication at the correct dose and time to ensure that their mobility does not deteriorate further.

5 Gait abnormality?

Gait screening is sensitive for neuromotor, sensory and musculoskeletal abnormalities in the lower limbs because walking is a complex task in comparison with the tests of neurological function used in the standard screening examination.

The gaits associated with Parkinsonism and sensory ataxia are described above. Suspect cerebellar ataxia if the gait is unsteady and broad-based with an inability to heel–toe walk (as if inebriated with alcohol). A hemiplegic gait is usually obvious and will be associated with focal neurological signs. Bilateral lower limb proximal muscle weakness may produce a 'waddling' gait.

Pain can limit exertion or alter gait, leading to a decrease in function or an increased risk of falling. The patient will typically place the foot of the affected side delicately on the floor for as little time as possible to avoid the pain of weight-bearing ('antalgic' gait). Osteoarthritis is frequently responsible but is usually chronic and slowly progressive, and thus unlikely to lead to hospital admission without additional factors. Acutely painful joints require careful assessment.

Consider gait apraxia if no specific neurological abnormality or gait pattern is noted but the gait is none the less abnormal. Apraxia, the inability to conduct learned, purposeful movements properly (in the absence of a focal insult), is a result of general or frontal cerebral insults such as dementia, cerebrovascular disease, normal pressure hydrocephalus, sedation or metabolic derangement.

Psychological causes of reduced mobility (especially the fear of falling) can also reduce mobility and increase the risk of falls, and may only be elicited by asking the patient to mobilize greater distances.

6 Reduced exercise tolerance?

Observe for/ask about exertional dyspnoea, chest discomfort and claudication. The latter may be due to peripheral vascular disease (diminished pulses, skin changes, vascular disease elsewhere) but consider neurogenic claudication secondary to spinal stenosis, especially if the discomfort responds to postural change, e.g. bending over, sitting down, more quickly than standing still.

24

Nausea is the unpleasant sensation of being about to vomit. Vomiting is the forceful expulsion of gastric contents, often preceded by nausea. Vomiting should be differentiated from regurgitation, where there is appearance of gastric contents without any effort. The assessment of acute (≤10 days) nausea and vomiting (N&V) differs from chronic presentations reflecting a different range of likely diagnoses.

This chapter focuses on N&V as a principal presenting complaint. Refer to the relevant chapter if a more specific clinical feature is present, e.g. jaundice, headache, chest pain. See Chapter 15 if the vomitus comprises fresh or altered blood.

Infection

Gastroenteritis is by far the most common cause of acute N&V. It may affect any age group but has a higher incidence in children, young adults and the elderly. The aetiology is usually viral, e.g. norovirus, rotavirus, adenovirus. Bacterial pathogens tend to come from poorly prepared/cooked foodstuffs, and can include *Bacillus cereus* and *Staphylococcus aureus*. There may be known contacts with similar symptoms, or a history of travel, eating out or eating unusual foods in recent days. Vomiting mediated by a bacterial toxin tends to develop within 1–6 hours. Accompanying features may include fever, abdominal cramping and diarrhoea.

Other infections, e.g. urinary tract infection, meningitis, hepatitis or otitis media may also cause N&V, particularly in more vulnerable groups such as children and the elderly. However, other clinical features usually predominate.

GI obstruction

Mechanical obstruction of the GI tract, e.g. due to tumour, adhesions or incarcerated hernia, may cause vomiting, usually accompanied by colicky abdominal pain (see Ch. 4) and absolute constipation +/− abdominal distension. The characteristics of the vomitus may suggest the location of obstruction: gastric juices – gastric outlet obstruction; bilious material – small bowel obstruction; feculent material – distal obstruction (or coloenteric/cologastric fistula).

Other GI tract disease

Peptic ulcer disease may present with N&V, typically associated with epigastric discomfort or a history of dyspeptic symptoms. Gastroparesis results in vomiting after food ingestion due to delayed gastric emptying; suspect this in patients with poorly controlled diabetes/multiple diabetes-related complications, scleroderma or previous gastric surgery. N&V may be a prominent feature of acute inflammatory abdominal pathology, e.g. acute pancreatitis/appendicitis/cholecystitis, but abdominal pain is almost always the principal complaint (Ch. 4). Severe constipation may lead to N&V, particularly in frail elderly patients.

Medications

Numerous medications or toxins can result in nausea or vomiting; some of the more common culprits are listed in Box 25.1. Alcohol misuse is a very frequent cause of both acute and chronic N&V. Heavy cannabis use can result in chronic vomiting, which may be cyclical, and tends to be alleviated by baths and showers.

Metabolic disturbance

Chronic renal failure with uraemia tends to present non-specifically and nausea +/− vomiting is often a prominent feature. Conversely, severe N&V is an important cause of acute kidney injury due to hypovolaemia. The assessment of renal failure is discussed on page 230.

Diabetic ketoacidosis (DKA) and, to a lesser extent, hyperosmolar hyperglycaemic state (HHS),

Box 25.1 Common toxic/therapeutic causes of nausea and vomiting	
Alcohol	Digoxin
Anti-arrhythmics	NSAIDs
Anticonvulsants	Oestrogen and progestogen-containing drugs
Antibiotics (esp. erythromycin)	Oestrogen and progestogen-containing drugs
Anti-Parkinsonian treatments	Opioids
Cannabinoids	Psychotropic meds
Chemotherapy agents	Theophylline

Box 25.2 Clinical / biochemical features often present in patients with adrenal insufficiency

Symptoms (often insidious)

- Lethargy, fatigue
- Anorexia, weight loss
- Nausea and vomiting
- Postural hypotension

Physical signs

- Pigmentation (skin, mucous membranes)
- Vitiligo
- Postural hypotension

Blood

- Hyponatraemia
- Hyperkalaemia
- Hypoglycaemia (fasting or spontaneous)
- Normal-anion gap metabolic acidosis (mild)

Other

- History of other autoimmune disorders

may present with N&V. Suggestive features include a history of polyuria and/or polydipsia and a background of diabetes (particularly type 1).

N&V may be the main presenting symptom in hypercalcaemia, especially since other features tend to be non-specific. Underlying causes are discussed on page 297.

GI upset, including N&V is also common in adrenal insufficiency, including acute adrenal crisis. Hypotension and illness severity are usually disproportionate to the degree of vomiting. Other suggestive features are shown in Box 25.2.

CNS causes

Raised intracranial pressure may produce vomiting, often without nausea. When chronic, e.g. space occupying lesion, vomiting classically occurs shortly after wakening and is associated with headache (worse on lying, bending or straining) and papilloedema. In acute causes, e.g. intracerebral haemorrhage, there may be sudden onset headache initially followed by a progressive decline in GCS. Nausea, with or without vomiting, occurs during episodes of migraine in ~80% of patients and is often severe; however headache +/− aura is usually the dominant symptom (Ch. 19).

N&V accompanied by vertigo suggests vestibular or brainstem pathology (Ch. 10). Vomiting may also occur in CNS infection, e.g. meningitis but usually not as the main presenting feature.

Other causes

Always consider pregnancy in women of child-bearing age with new-onset nausea +/− vomiting. Symptoms are not always confined to morning and may occur at any time of the day. In eating disorders, recurrent vomiting may be concealed by the patient and brought to light by a family member. There is frequently a history of psychiatric disorder, deliberate self harm, laxative abuse or evidence of altered body image.

Functional vomiting is a diagnosis of exclusion; symptoms are typically worse after eating with vomiting of undigested or chewed food. There may also be a history of early satiety and epigastric fullness.

25

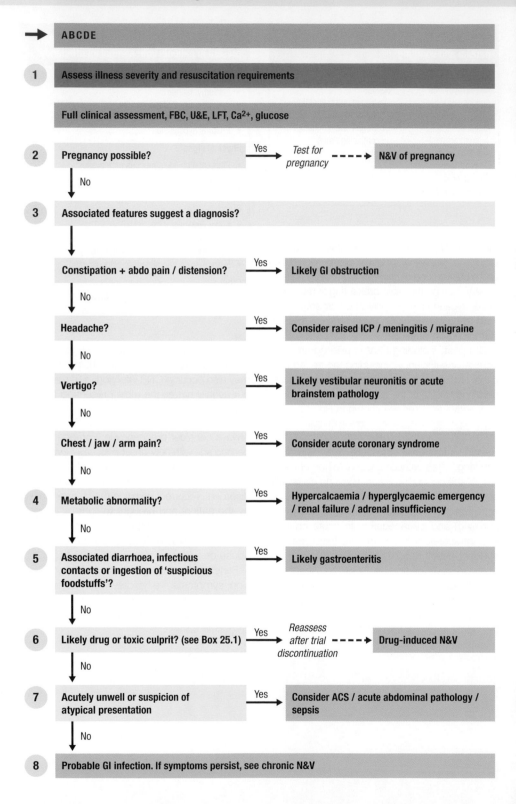

ABCDE

1 Assess illness severity and resuscitation requirements

Full clinical assessment, FBC, U&E, LFT, Ca^{2+}, glucose

2 Pregnancy possible? — Yes → *Test for pregnancy* - - - → N&V of pregnancy

No ↓

3 Associated features suggest a diagnosis?

↓

Constipation + abdo pain / distension? — Yes → Likely GI obstruction

No ↓

Headache? — Yes → Consider raised ICP / meningitis / migraine

No ↓

Vertigo? — Yes → Likely vestibular neuronitis or acute brainstem pathology

No ↓

Chest / jaw / arm pain? — Yes → Consider acute coronary syndrome

No ↓

4 Metabolic abnormality? — Yes → Hypercalcaemia / hyperglycaemic emergency / renal failure / adrenal insufficiency

No ↓

5 Associated diarrhoea, infectious contacts or ingestion of 'suspicious foodstuffs'? — Yes → Likely gastroenteritis

No ↓

6 Likely drug or toxic culprit? (see Box 25.1) — Yes → *Reassess after trial discontinuation* - - - → Drug-induced N&V

No ↓

7 Acutely unwell or suspicion of atypical presentation — Yes → Consider ACS / acute abdominal pathology / sepsis

No ↓

8 Probable GI infection. If symptoms persist, see chronic N&V

1 Assess illness severity and resuscitation requirements

Step 1 Are there features of shock?
Look for ↑HR, ↓BP (a late sign) or evidence of tissue hypoperfusion (see Box 30.1, p. 267). If present, reassess following aggressive IV fluid resuscitation and monitor urine output (consider urinary catheterization if necessary). Exclude diabetic ketoacidosis (see Clinical tool, p. 299) if ↑CBG, known type 1 diabetes or recent polydipsia/polyuria. Suspect adrenal insufficiency in patients with a history of Addison's disease (or other autoimmune disease), chronic corticosteroid use or suggestive clinical features (Box 25.2); also consider whenever the severity of shock appears disproportionate to fluid losses: take blood for random cortisol and treat immediately with intravenous hydrocortisone.

Step 2 Is there acute renal impairment?
Hypovolaemia may result in severe 'pre-renal' acute kidney injury (AKI), especially if compounded by antihypertensive or nephrotoxic medication such as diuretics, ACE inhibitors or NSAIDs. Patients with AKI due to volume depletion require IV rehydration with close monitoring of fluid balance, urine output and U+E. However, consider other potential drivers of both AKI and nausea/vomiting, (e.g. sepsis, drug toxicity) in patients without clinical evidence of hypovolaemia. Consider renal failure as the cause of N&V in patients with severe impairment. See page 230 for further assessment of renal failure.

Step 3 Does the patient otherwise require IV fluids/hospital admission?
Patients with clinical evidence of dehydration (thirst, dry mucous membranes, ↓skin turgor) and ongoing vomiting, require IV hydration.

Other features that may indicate a need for hospital admission include
- evidence of sepsis (Ch. 14)
- acute kidney injury
- frail, elderly or immunocompromised patient
- significant comorbidity, e.g. heart/renal/hepatic failure.

2 Pregnancy possible?

Ask about last menstrual period and formally test for pregnancy in any women of reproductive age presenting with N&V.

3 Associated features suggest a diagnosis?

Perform an AXR if N&V is accompanied by absent bowel movements and abdominal pain or distension. Consider acute gastritis, peptic ulcer disease or pancreatitis if there is severe upper abdominal pain. In either case, assess as per Chapter 4.

Headache may occur secondary to dehydration in acute vomiting but consider the possibility of serious CNS pathology. Assess as per Chapter 18 If headache is a prominent feature, especially if the onset is acute or there are any other concerning features, e.g. recent head injury, anticoagulant therapy, meningism, fever, reduced GCS, papilloedema or focal neurology.

Acute onset of N&V accompanied by vertigo (dizziness with an illusion of movement, e.g. spinning) is likely to represent either vestibular neuronitis or acute brainstem pathology such as infarction or haemorrhage; assess as per Chapter 10.

Suspect ACS and assess as per Chapter 6 if N&V occurs with chest, jaw, neck or arm pain.

25

4   Metabolic abnormality?

Test for diabetes and exclude ketoacidosis in any patient without a pre-existing diagnosis who has ↑CBG lab glucose (p. 299). Consider HHS in patients with known diabetes and markedly ↑BG (p. 299).

Assess patients with renal failure as described on page 230.

If ↑Ca^{2+} (corrected for albumin), assess further as described on page 297. Reassess symptoms after rehydration and other corrective treatment; remember that N&V may be due to the underlying cause, e.g. malignancy rather than ↑Ca^{2+} per se.

Consider adrenal insufficiency in patients with ↓Na^+/↑K^+ or ↓blood glucose, especially if there are suggestive clinical features (Box 25.2). If suspected, check a morning cortisol level +/– ACTH stimulation test ('Short Synacthen Test').

5   Associated diarrhoea, infectious contacts or ingestion of 'suspicious foodstuffs'?

Suspect acute gastroenteritis if any of these features are present. Most cases are self-limiting viral or toxin-mediated infections and do not require further investigation or antimicrobial treatment. However, consider AXR (to exclude colonic dilatation) and surgical review if there are concerning features such as bloody diarrhoea, abdominal pain or an excessive systemic inflammatory response. Re-evaluate if symptoms persist >10 days.

6   Likely drug or toxic culprit? (see Box 25.1)

Always ask about recent changes to drugs or dosages - including over-the-counter medicines – and check what the patient is actually taking. Enquire about recreational drug use and alcohol intake. In drugs with a narrow therapeutic window, e.g. digoxin or some anticonvulsants, check serum levels to exclude toxicity. Resolution of symptoms with drug discontinuation (where possible) confirms the diagnosis.

7 **Acutely unwell or suspicion of atypical presentation?**

Consider non-specific presentation of major pathology in patients who appear seriously unwell, (e.g. autonomic upset, physiological derangement). Be mindful of atypical presentations in frail elderly patients or those with cognitive impairment, immunocompromise (including chronic corticosteroid treatment) or longstanding diabetes. Perform an ECG to look for evidence of myocardial infarction/ischaemia (p. 51) and check blood chemistry (including CRP and amylase) and urinalysis. Undertake a septic screen (p. 142) if there is fever or ↑inflammatory markers. Have a low threshold for AXR +/− further abdominal imaging, e.g. CT or USS. Severe constipation may lead to N&V in immobile, frail or elderly patients so enquire about bowel movements and consider PR exam +/− AXR.

8 **Probable GI infection**

In the absence of alternative pathology, GI infection is the most likely cause; it is almost always self-limiting so further investigation is usually not required. Re-evaluate if the patient is unwell or deteriorating. Proceed to assessment of chronic N&V symptoms persist for >10 days.

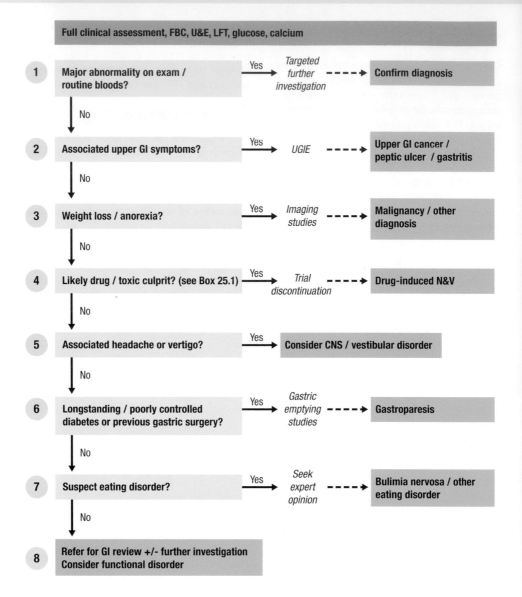

1 **Major abnormality on examination/ routine bloods?**

Screen patients with persistent or recurrent N&V for the following abnormalities to narrow the differential diagnosis.

Deranged LFTs +/– jaundice

If known chronic liver disease assess as per page 179. Otherwise, arrange urgent abdominal USS, review alcohol intake/all recent medications and assess further as described in Chapter 19 but continue to look for alternative causes of N&V if only minor LFT derangement without jaundice.

Palpable abdominal or pelvic mass

Arrange urgent imaging to exclude underlying malignancy. Consider USS initially, particularly for pelvic masses or hepatomegaly but arrange

CT abdomen/pelvis if no cause is found (or to further characterize/stage abnormalities).

Renal failure

Severe renal failure frequently presents non-specifically with nausea +/− vomiting, lethargy, anorexia. Distinguish this from 'pre-renal' renal impairment due to protracted vomiting and assess for an underlying aetiology (p. 230).

Anaemia

Arrange urgent upper GI endoscopy in any patient with persistent N&V and evidence of iron deficiency anaemia. In patients without iron-deficiency, continue anaemia work-up but consider other causes of N&V if no clear explanation identified.

Hypercalcaemia

Assess as described on page 297. If mildly $\uparrow Ca^{2+}$ continue to evaluate for other causes of N&V.

2 Associated upper GI symptoms?

Associated symptoms of dysphagia, early satiety, epigastric discomfort or dyspepsia suggest upper GI tract pathology such as oesophageal/gastric cancer; peptic ulcer disease or gastritis. Ask about NSAID use/alcohol intake and arrange upper GI endoscopy if any of these are present or if vomiting persists for >4 weeks (urgently if weight loss, dysphagia or new onset symptoms in patient aged ≥50 years). Refer for formal GI review if persistent symptoms with no cause identified on endoscopy.

3 Weight loss/anorexia?

Investigate for underlying malignancy if N&V is accompanied by significant weight loss, (e.g. ≥5% of body weight in ≤12 months) +/− anorexia, especially in patients with relatively recent onset of symptoms. Arrange upper GI endoscopy if not already performed and, if normal, request CT abdomen/pelvis. If no cause identified, continue to assess as below. Consider chronic presentation of adrenal insufficiency if there are other suggestive clinical features (Box 25.2).

4 Likely drug/toxic culprit?

Ask about all medications (including over the counter), particularly those in Box 25.2;

suspect a toxic aetiology if there is a clear temporal relationship between starting the drug and symptom onset. Reassess after trial discontinuation (if safe to do so) and look for alternative causes if symptoms persist. Check serum levels to exclude toxicity in drugs with a narrow therapeutic window, e.g. digoxin, lithium, theophylline. Establish alcohol intake and ask specifically about cannabis use.

5 Associated headache or vertigo?

Consider $\uparrow$intracranial pressure if vomiting is associated with recurrent headache that is: most prominent on waking from sleep; aggravated by bending, straining or lying; or accompanied by papilloedema – arrange urgent CT brain. See Chapter 10 for assessment of patients with vertigo.

6 Longstanding/poorly controlled diabetes or previous gastric surgery?

Suspect gastroparesis in diabetic patients with longstanding poor control and/or significant microvascular complications or in patients with previous gastric surgery (including weight reduction surgery). Delayed gastric emptying on a nuclear scintigraphy scan confirms the diagnosis.

7 Suspect eating disorder?

Consider this in patients with persistent/recurrent vomiting despite reassuring GI investigation who have evidence of low mood or self-esteem, a history of psychiatric disorder or where family members raise concern. Typically, vomiting occurs after eating and is not directly witnessed. Explore the issue sensitively and, if suspected, seek expert input at an early stage.

8 Refer for GI review/further investigation

Arrange UGIE (if not already performed) and refer for GI evaluation if symptoms persist without a clear cause. Investigate for chronic pancreatitis if there is associated epigastric discomfort, a history of chronic alcohol excess and/or steatorrhoea; check faecal elastase and arrange abdominal CT. Consider functional vomiting if investigations are consistently reassuring but be vigilant for underlying eating disorder.

25

Further assessment of renal failure

Step 1 Recognize renal impairment

Diagnostic criteria for AKI and CKD are shown in Box 25.3 and Table 25.1.

Step 2 Identify and treat hyperkalaemia

$\uparrow$K$^+$ may cause life-threatening arrhythmias and cardiac arrest. Perform an ECG if ≥5.5 mmol/L to look for:

- early changes: tall, peaked T waves
- advanced changes: flattened P waves, $\uparrow$PR interval, $\uparrow$QRS duration.

Treat as follows:

- give IV calcium, e.g. 10% calcium gluconate, with continuous ECG monitoring

---

Box 25.3 Diagnostic criteria for acute kidney injury

1. Increase in serum creatinine by ≥26 µmol/L from baseline within 48 hours
2. Increase in serum creatinine ≥1.5-fold from baseline within 1 week
3. Urine output <0.5 mL/kg/hr for >6 consecutive hours

Source: Kidney Disease: Improving Global Outcomes. 2010. Clinical practice guideline on acute kidney injury. Available online at http://www.kdigo.org

---

Table 25.1 Classification of chronic kidney disease

Stage	Category	GFR (mL/min/1.73 m²)
1	Evidence of chronic kidney damage[1] with normal GFR	≥90
2	Evidence of chronic kidney damage[1] with mild impairment of GFR	60–89
3	Moderate impairment of GFR	30–59
4	Severe impairment of GFR	15–29
5	End-stage renal failure	<15

[1]Evidence of chronic kidney damage includes:
- *persistent microalbuminuria/proteinuria/haematuria*
- *structural kidney abnormalities on imaging*
- *features of chronic glomerulonephritis on renal biopsy.*
Source: Kidney Disease Outcome Quality Initiative 2002. K/DOQI clinical practice guidelines for chronic kidney disease: evaluation, classification, and stratification. Am J Kidney Dis. 39(2 Suppl 2):S1–246.

---

if there are ECG changes – titrate up to 10 mL until changes resolve

- give treatment to lower K$^+$, e.g. IV dextrose and insulin, especially if K$^+$ >6.0 mmol/L or ECG changes. Repeat U+E and ECG following treatment
- consider the need for urgent renal review (Box 25.4).

Step 3 Distinguish CKD from AKI

Previous U+E results are the best guide to the chronicity of renal impairment. If unavailable, possible clues to CKD include:

- evidence of metabolic bone disease (especially $\uparrow$parathyroid hormone)
- bilateral small kidneys on USS
- gradual onset of oedema over weeks to months.

Assume AKI, at least initially, if none of these features is present and there are no previous U+E results for comparison.

Step 4 If de novo presentation, perform a full diagnostic work-up

- Assess volume status: renal hypoperfusion ('pre-renal' failure) is the most common cause of AKI. Look for:
  - predisposing factors (diarrhoea, vomiting, blood loss, $\downarrow$oral intake, diuretics),
  - features of dehydration ($\downarrow$skin turgor, dry mucous membranes, thirst) and
  - signs of shock (see Box 30.1, p. 267).

If you suspect hypovolaemia, assess the response of urine output and U+E to fluid resuscitation and correction of underlying causes.

- Exclude obstruction: bladder outflow obstruction occurs most frequently in males

---

Box 25.4 Reasons for urgent renal referral

- Indication for urgent renal replacement therapy
  - $\uparrow$K$^+$ or pulmonary oedema refractory to medical management
  - Severe metabolic acidosis
  - Uraemic pericarditis
  - Uraemic encephalopathy
- Progressive increase in serum creatinine despite fluid resuscitation/withholding of nephrotoxins
- Persistently oliguric or anuric patients
- Suspected glomerular disease
- CKD patients with increasing symptoms of uraemia or likely progression to stage 5 CKD

with prostatic enlargement. Insert a urinary catheter if there is a palpable bladder or ↑post-void residual urine on bladder scanning. Request a renal USS to exclude upper renal tract obstruction.

- Review all recent prescriptions and ask about non-prescribed drugs. Common culprits include radiographic contrast media, NSAIDs, ACE inhibitors/angiotensin receptor blockers, antimicrobials (gentamicin, vancomycin, penicillins, amphotericin B) and ciclosporin.
- Seek evidence of sepsis (Box 14.1, p. 141), and, if present, perform a full septic screen as per Chapter 14.
- Consider other causes: suspect *glomerulonephritis* in any patient with heavy, e.g. ≥3+, haematuria/proteinuria on dipstick. Evaluate for multisystem disease (rash, joint disease, haemoptysis), perform serological investigations (Table 25.2) and discuss urgently with the renal team.
- Consider *haemolytic uraemic syndrome/ thrombotic thrombocytopenic purpura* if AKI is accompanied by an acute diarrhoeal illness or neurological features. Review the FBC/blood film for: ↓Hb, ↓platelets, ↑reticulocytes and red cell fragments. Seek immediate expert advice if suspected.
- Consider *rhabdomyolysis* in patients with a history of trauma, a long period lying on the floor or recreational drug use, e.g. cocaine. Check CK (>×5 upper limit of normal) and perform urinalysis +/– urine microscopy

(dipstick haematuria with no red cells on microscopy suggests myoglobinuria).

- Send plasma for protein electrophoresis and urine for Bence Jones protein if you suspect *multiple myeloma*, e.g. hypercalcaemia, bone pain pathological fractures, or if the cause of renal dysfunction remains unclear.

Step 5 If acute-on-chronic impairment, consider reasons for deterioration

Acute deterioration is often due to

- dehydration
- infection
- hypotension
- nephrotoxic agent (see above).

Identify and reverse these causes, monitor renal function and discuss with the renal team if there is any further decline in GFR.

Step 6 If stable CKD, seek evidence of complications

Sequelae of CKD should be sought and corrected, if possible.

- *Renal anaemia*: this may result from inadequate renal production of erythropoietin. Measure ferritin and transferrin saturation to ensure that the patient is iron-replete (ferritin >100 ng/mL; transferrin saturation >20%), exclude other causes of anaemia (p. 136) and refer to a nephrologist for consideration of erythropoiesis-stimulating agents.
- *Metabolic acidosis*: this is indicated by a low venous bicarbonate and can be corrected by oral sodium bicarbonate.
- *Metabolic bone disease*: ↓phosphate excretion and ↓renal activation of vitamin D result in ↑PO_4^{3-}, ↓Ca^{2+} and ↑parathyroid hormone (secondary hyperparathyroidism). Treat with phosphate binders and vitamin D analogues, aiming to maintain plasma Ca^{2+} and PO_4^{3-} within normal limits.
- *Volume overload*: in advanced CKD, oliguria may result in significant fluid overload, with peripheral ± pulmonary oedema. Liaise with a nephrologist if this is refractory to diuretic therapy and salt restriction.
- *Hypertension*: ↑BP is common in CKD, accelerates the decline in renal function and increases cardiovascular risk. Monitor BP and aim for strict targets, e.g. <130/80 mmHg.

25

Table 25.2 Serological investigations in suspected glomerulonephritis

Test	Underlying diagnosis
ANA	Connective tissue disease, e.g. SLE
Anti ds-DNA	
Extractable nuclear antigens	
Anti GBM antibodies	Goodpasture's disease
ANCA	Vasculitis, e.g. granulomatosis with polyangiitis
Antistreptolysin O titre	Post-streptococcal glomerulonephritis
Cryoglobulins	Cryoglobulinaemia

Palpitation is an unpleasant awareness of the heartbeat. Patients may describe the sensation as skipping, fluttering, racing, pounding, thudding or jumping. Episodes can be unpleasant and frightening but most are benign and less than half are due to a heart rhythm abnormality. In most cases, the key to diagnosis lies in documenting the cardiac rhythm during symptoms. Establish the frequency, intensity and impact of symptoms as this is essential to guide treatment.

Heightened awareness of normal heartbeat

Awareness of the normal heartbeat is common but may produce anxiety in patients with psychosocial stress or health concerns, e.g. recent heart 'scare', death of family member. It is most commonly noted when lying awake in bed or sitting at rest.

Sinus tachycardia/↑stroke volume

Causes of sinus tachycardia are shown in Box 26.1; anxiety is the most frequent aetiology, with patients typically reporting episodes of a fast, regular, pounding heartbeat that builds up and resolves over minutes. Increased stroke volume due to aortic regurgitation or vasodilator drugs may produce a forceful heartbeat without tachycardia.

Extrasystoles

Atrial or ventricular extrasystoles (ectopics or premature beats) do not usually cause symptoms but, in some patients, produce a sensation of dropped beats (due to ↓stroke volume of the ectopic beat), 'jolts' or 'thumps' (due to ↑stroke volume of the post-ectopic sinus beat), or, if frequent, an irregular heartbeat. Extrasystoles are common in healthy individuals and usually benign, but frequent ventricular extrasystoles, particularly in older patients may indicate underlying structural or coronary heart disease.

Paroxysmal supraventricular tachycardia

'Supraventricular tachycardia' (SVT) refers to atrioventricular nodal re-entry tachycardia (AVNRT) and AV re-entry tachycardia (AVRT). AVNRT is due to right atrial and AV node re-entry, usually in structurally normal hearts; AVRT (known as *Wolff–Parkinson–White syndrome*) is caused by a re-entry circuit formed from the AV node and an 'accessory pathway' – an abnormal band of conducting tissue connecting atria and ventricles.

Both produce episodes of regular tachycardia (± light-headedness and breathlessness) with an abrupt onset and offset. The ECG shows a regular narrow-complex tachycardia at 140–220/min (Fig. 26.1).

In 50% of patients with an accessory pathway, the ECG in sinus rhythm shows a short PR interval and slurring of the QRS upstroke ('delta wave') due to premature activation of ventricular tissue by the pathway – 'pre-excitation' (Fig. 26.2).

Most cases of AVNRT and AVRT are curable with radiofrequency catheter ablation.

Atrial arrhythmias (atrial tachycardia, flutter and fibrillation)

Atrial tachycardia produces symptoms similar to SVT; the ECG shows a regular narrow-complex tachycardia with abnormal P waves.

Atrial flutter is caused by a large re-entry circuit within the right atrium that generates an atrial rate of 300/min. This is usually associated with AV block, resulting in a ventricular rate of 150/min (2:1 block) or 100/min (3:1). Symptoms are similar to SVT. The ECG shows a regular narrow-complex tachycardia with 'saw-toothed' flutter waves (Fig. 26.3). With 2:1 block these may be obscured, so suspect atrial flutter in any patient with a regular narrow-complex tachycardia of 150/min.

Atrial fibrillation is common. Underlying causes are shown in Box 26.2. Atrial activity is chaotic and the ventricles are activated rapidly and

Box 26.1 Causes of sinus tachycardia

- Anxiety or panic disorder
- Stress or strong emotion
- Drugs: beta$_2$ agonists, anticholinergics, cocaine, amphetamines
- Anaemia
- Thyrotoxicosis
- Fever
- Pregnancy
- Phaeochromocytoma

irregularly. Patients with paroxysmal atrial fibrillation experience an erratic or irregular heartbeat that is usually fast and may be associated with breathlessness, light-headedness or ↓effort tolerance. The ECG shows an irregular narrow-complex tachycardia with no P waves (Fig. 26.4). Patients with atrial fibrillation or flutter are at greater risk of thromboembolic complications, including stroke.

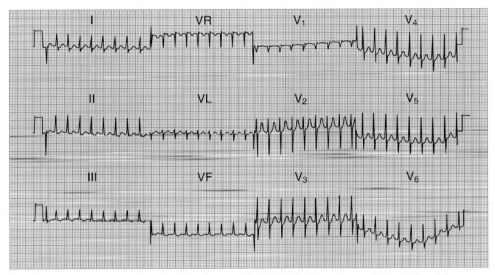

Fig. 26.1 Supraventricular tachycardia. (From Hampton JR. 150 ECG Problems, 3rd edn. Edinburgh: Churchill Livingstone, 2008.)

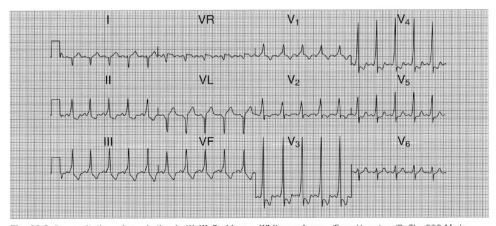

26

Fig. 26.2 Pre-excitation: sinus rhythm in Wolff–Parkinson–White syndrome. (From Hampton JR. The ECG Made Easy, 7th edn. Edinburgh: Churchill Livingstone, 2008.)

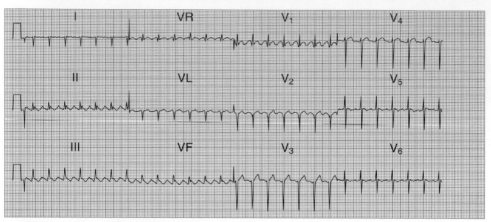

Fig. 26.3 Atrial flutter with 2 : 1 AV block. (From Hampton JR. The ECG in Practice, 5th edn. Edinburgh: Churchill Livingstone, 2008.)

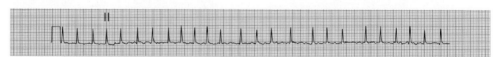

Fig. 26.4 Atrial fibrillation with a rapid ventricular response. (From Hampton JR. The ECG in Practice, 5th edn. Edinburgh: Churchill Livingstone, 2008.)

Box 26.2 Common causes of atrial fibrillation

- Hypertension
- Ischaemic heart disease
- Valvular heart disease (especially mitral stenosis)
- Alcohol
- Cardiomyopathy
- Sick sinus syndrome
- Congenital heart disease
- Constrictive pericarditis
- Hyperthyroidism
- Idiopathic ('lone' atrial fibrillation)

Ventricular tachycardia

Ventricular tachycardia (VT) is a potentially life-threatening arrhythmia that most frequently occurs in patients with previous MI or cardiomyopathy but can arise in structurally normal hearts. Rapid palpitation is often accompanied by pre-syncope (a feeling of faintness and near-collapse), syncope, breathlessness or chest pain. In patients with significant underlying left ventricular impairment, palpitation is frequently absent. The ECG shows a regular broad-complex tachycardia (Fig. 26.5). A variant, torsades de pointes, with a characteristic ECG appearance (Fig. 26.6), may occur in patients with a prolonged QT interval.

Bradyarrhythmia, e.g. sick sinus syndrome, intermittent AV block

Bradyarrhythmias more commonly present with light-headedness or syncope but the patient may report intermittent episodes of a slow but forceful heartbeat. Associated ECG findings include sinus pauses, junctional bradycardia and intermittent second- or third-degree AV block (Figs 31.1 and 31.2, p. 279).

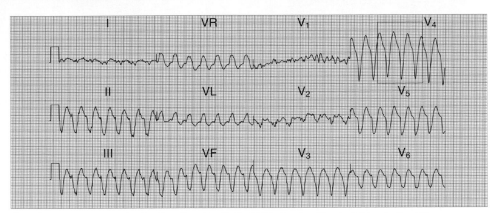

Fig. 26.5 Ventricular tachycardia. (From Hampton JR. The ECG in Practice, 5th edn. Edinburgh: Churchill Livingstone, 2008.)

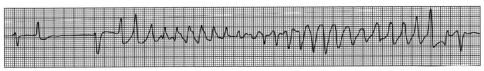

Fig. 26.6 Torsades de pointes. (From Boon NA, Colledge NR, Walker BR. Davidson's Principles & Practice of Medicine, 20th edn. Edinburgh: Churchill Livingstone, 2006.)

26

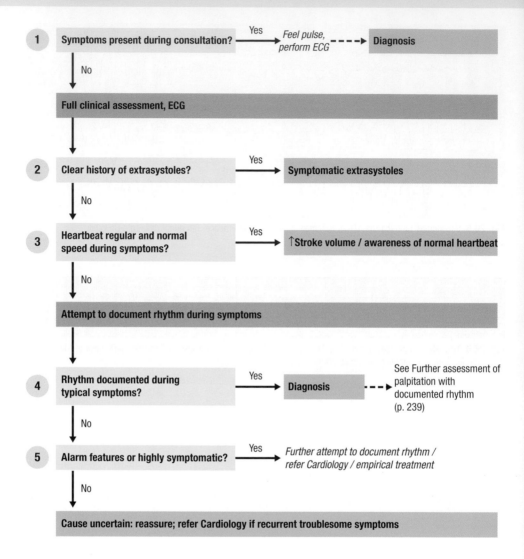

1 Symptoms present during consultation? —Yes→ *Feel pulse, perform ECG* - - - -▶ Diagnosis

No ↓

Full clinical assessment, ECG

2 Clear history of extrasystoles? —Yes→ Symptomatic extrasystoles

No ↓

3 Heartbeat regular and normal speed during symptoms? —Yes→ ↑Stroke volume / awareness of normal heartbeat

No ↓

Attempt to document rhythm during symptoms

4 Rhythm documented during typical symptoms? —Yes→ Diagnosis - - -▶ See Further assessment of palpitation with documented rhythm (p. 239)

No ↓

5 Alarm features or highly symptomatic? —Yes→ *Further attempt to document rhythm / refer Cardiology / empirical treatment*

No ↓

Cause uncertain: reassure; refer Cardiology if recurrent troublesome symptoms

1 Symptoms present during consultation?

If the patient has symptoms during the consultation, feel the pulse straight away and perform an ECG as soon as possible. This may sound overly simple but much of the difficulty in diagnosing palpitation lies in trying to document the rhythm during a typical episode of symptoms. Do not miss the opportunity!

2 Clear history of extrasystoles?

It is not always possible to distinguish frequent extrasystoles from sustained arrhythmias such as atrial fibrillation on the history alone. However, a clear history of an occasional 'jolt' or 'jump' in the chest or isolated 'dropped' or 'skipped' beats is highly suggestive – such patients can usually be reassured without further investigation.

3 Heartbeat regular and normal speed during symptoms?

Many patients with palpitation describe the heartbeat as 'forceful' or 'strong' rather than fast, slow or irregular. This may reflect ↑stroke volume, e.g. aortic regurgitation, anaemia, vasodilators, or simply awareness of the normal heartbeat but, in either case, it argues strongly against an arrhythmic cause. Look for underlying physical and psychosocial factors, but further investigation is usually unnecessary unless there is a specific additional concern.

Attempt to document rhythm during symptoms

This is a key diagnostic step. The chosen method will be dictated predominantly by the frequency of symptoms.

- Consider inpatient telemetry if the patient has experienced a recent episode, e.g. in the last 72 hours, with syncope or pre-syncope, or has other high-risk features (p. 280).
- Use Holter monitoring if symptoms are occurring frequently. A 24-hour Holter monitor is useful only in patients who have at least daily symptoms, a 48-hour Holter monitor can be used in those with symptoms on most days, and a 7-day monitor is useful for those with weekly symptoms,
- If symptoms are occurring less than weekly, consider more prolonged ambulatory monitoring through a wireless ECG patch recorder or an external patient-activated recorder. Ambulatory smart phone monitors are now available that are patient activated and allow an ECG to be recorded and sent to the clinician.
- If symptoms are very infrequent, ask the patient to phone for an ambulance or report to their family doctor or to an emergency department during an episode (advise not to drive) or, depending on symptom severity, consider referral for insertion of an implantable loop recorder.
- If symptoms are induced by physical exertion, refer for a supervised exercise ECG.

4 Rhythm documented during typical symptoms?

Diagnose arrhythmia as the cause of palpitation if you obtain an ECG recording of rhythm disturbance that corresponds with symptoms – proceed to 'Further assessment of palpitation with documented rhythm'.

Clear documentation of sinus rhythm during a typical attack excludes an arrhythmic cause for symptoms.

Asymptomatic rhythm disturbances may occur during prolonged ECG monitoring. The patient may need further assessment for the specific arrhythmia but symptoms should not automatically be attributed to it – especially if typical symptoms occur during periods of sinus

26

rhythm. Consult a cardiologist if there is any doubt as to the significance of an ECG recording.

Continue to step 5 if the patient did not experience a typical episode of palpitation during the period of rhythm monitoring.

5 Alarm features or highly symptomatic?

The lengths to which you should go to document the ECG during symptoms depends on both the severity of symptoms and the estimated risk of a life-threatening arrhythmia, e.g. VT or complete heart block.

Consider reassurance without further investigation for patients with mild, infrequent symptoms and no high-risk features; reassess if symptoms subsequently become more frequent or intrusive. Persist with attempts to document the rhythm in patients with symptoms that are frequent, unpleasant or which interfere with occupation or lifestyle.

Irrespective of symptom frequency and intensity, refer patients with any of the following features to cardiology for further investigation:

- palpitation associated with syncope or pre-syncope
- family history of sudden cardiac death or inheritable cardiac conditions
- significant abnormality on resting ECG
- risk factors for VT, e.g. previous MI, ventricular surgery, cardiomyopathy.

Table 26.1 CHA$_2$DS$_2$-VASc thromboembolic risk score	
Thromboembolic risk factor	Points
Congestive heart failure: clinical evidence of heart failure or reduced LV ejection fraction	1
Hypertension	1
Age: ≥75 years	2
Diabetes mellitus	1
Stroke: previous stroke, TIA or systemic embolism	2
Vascular disease: history of MI, peripheral arterial disease or aortic atheroma	1
Age: 64–75 years	1
Sex: female sex	1
Risk of thromboembolic events (event rate/100 person years) according to score Score 0 = low risk (0.78) Score 1 = intermediate risk (2.01) Score ≥2 = high risk (8.82)	

Modified from Kirchhof P et al. 2016. 2016 ESC Guidelines for the management of atrial fibrillation developed in collaboration with EACTS. Eur Heart J. 37(38):2893–2962 and Olesen JB et al. 2011. Validation of risk stratification schemes for predicting stroke and thromboembolism in patients with atrial fibrillation: nationwide cohort study. Br Med J. 342:d124.

Table 26.2 HAS-BLED bleeding risk score	
Bleeding risk factor	Points
Hypertension: uncontrolled hypertension (systolic BP >160 mmHg)	1
Abnormal renal/liver function: Dialysis or serum creatinine >200 micromol/L	1
Cirrhosis or bilirubin >2× normal or ALT >3× normal	1
Stroke: previous stroke	1
Bleeding: previous major bleed or predisposition to bleeding	1
Labile INR: time in therapeutic range <60%	1
Elderly: age >65 years	1
Drugs/alcohol: Concomitant use of antiplatelet or non-steroidal anti-inflammatory drugs	1
≥8 alcoholic drinks per week	1
Score ≥3 indicates higher risk of major bleeding.	

Modified from Pisters R et al. 2010. A novel user-friendly score (HAS-BLED) to assess 1-year risk of major bleeding in patients with atrial fibrillation: the Euro Heart Survey. Chest. 138(5):1093–1100.

Further assessment of palpitation with documented rhythm

Assess the frequency and intensity of symptoms and the impact on occupation and lifestyle. Establish the efficacy and side-effects of previous treatments.

Sinus tachycardia

- Review all prescribed and 'recreational' drugs, screen for anaemia and hyperthyroidism with FBC/TFTs and, where appropriate, perform a pregnancy test.
- If ↑BP or if episodes are associated with headache, flushing or GI upset, measure 24-hour urinary metanephrines to exclude phaeochromocytoma.
- Request an echocardiogram if there are any features to suggest structural heart disease, e.g. unexplained murmur, signs of heart failure.
- Look for evidence of an anxiety or panic disorder.

Extrasystoles

- Seek potential exacerbating factors including ↓K^+, ↓Mg^{2+}, drugs, e.g. tricyclic antidepressants, digoxin, alcohol, tobacco or (possibly) caffeine consumption.
- Consider further investigation, e.g. echocardiography, exercise ECG if frequent or associated with other signs/symptoms of CVS disease.

Supraventricular tachycardia

- Look for pre-excitation on resting ECG (see Fig. 26.2) to suggest an accessory pathway-mediated tachycardia.
- Refer to cardiology for electrophysiology study ± radiofrequency ablation if symptoms are frequent, disabling or unpleasant or if there are side-effects on medical therapy.

Atrial flutter/fibrillation

- Perform echocardiography to exclude structural heart disease, e.g. cardiomyopathy, left ventricular hypertrophy, valvular disease.
- Seek causative or exacerbating factors: measure BP, electrolytes and TFT; enquire about alcohol intake and symptoms of angina.
- Use the CHA_2DS_2-VASc score (Table 26.1) to assess thromboembolic risk in patients with non-valvular atrial fibrillation (all patients with mitral stenosis are at high risk) and the HAS-BLED score (Table 26.2) to assess the risk of major bleeding.
- Refer to Cardiology if symptoms are frequent, distressing or disabling despite first-line medical therapy, e.g. beta-blockers.

Ventricular tachycardia

- Perform an ECG to look for evidence of underlying structural heart disease, e.g. cardiomyopathy.
- Enquire about previous MI and symptoms of/risk factors for ischaemic heart disease.
- Measure the QT interval on the ECG in sinus rhythm.
- Measure electrolytes – especially K^+, Mg^{2+} and Ca^{2+}.
- Refer all patients to Cardiology for further investigation, risk stratification and treatment.

Bradyarrhythmia

- Seek an underlying cause: check TFTs and review drugs for rate-limiting agents, e.g. digoxin, beta-blockers, verapamil.
- Refer symptomatic bradyarrhythmia or asymptomatic second-degree AV block (Mobitz type 2), complete heart block or sinus pauses >3 seconds to Cardiology.

26

The accurate diagnosis of skin disease is usually based on visual pattern recognition developed through experience rather than analytical rule-based approaches. This is a step-by-step approach to assist identification of important acute generalized eruptions that require urgent advice and treatment.

Erythroderma

Erythroderma (red skin) describes inflammatory skin disease manifesting predominantly as erythema and involving >90% of the body surface area (BSA; Fig. 27.1). The term 'sub-erythrodermic' is sometimes used to describe extensive erythema covering <90% BSA. Acute erythroderma can be life-threatening and most cases need hospitalization and urgent dermatology review. The major causes are eczema (40%), psoriasis (25%), cutaneous lymphoma (15%) and drug eruptions (10%).

Eczema

'Eczema' and 'dermatitis' are interchangeable terms. Dermatitis is used to denote a group of non-infective inflammatory skin diseases that represent a reaction pattern to various stimuli. Dermatitis may be classified by aetiology (atopic, irritant, allergic/contact, venous/stasis), morphology (seborrhoeic, discoid) or site (palmar, plantar, pompholyx). All produce the same key clinical feature: pruritic, erythematous lesions with typically indistinct margins. The lesions can progress through a number of phases: acute (with vesicles and bullae – Fig. 27.2), subacute (with scaling and crusting) and chronic (with acanthosis, lichenification and fissuring). Lesions may become secondarily infected by bacteria forming a crusted yellow exudate ('impetigo') (Fig. 27.3), or by viruses, e.g. herpes simplex, producing a vesicular pattern ('eczema herpeticum').

Psoriasis

Psoriasis, a very common papulosquamous eruption, is characterized by well-demarcated erythematous or purple papules and plaques, topped with silvery scale. There are three forms of acute eruption: erythroderma (see above), pustular psoriasis (Fig. 27.4) – a form that can deteriorate rapidly and guttate psoriasis (Fig. 27.5) – with characteristic widespread multiple 'drop-like' lesions, most commonly seen in young adults in association with streptococcal pharyngitis. Pityriasis rosea is often confused with psoriasis. It may be a reaction to a viral infection and initially presents with a single 'herald patch' followed by the subsequent development of multiple lesions on the torso (Fig. 27.6).

Toxic epidermal necrolysis, Stevens–Johnson syndrome and erythema multiforme

Toxic epidermal necrolysis (TEN) is the severe end of a spectrum of acute eruptions caused by a cell-mediated cytotoxic reaction against epidermal cells (Fig. 27.7). It is characterized by fever (>38° C), widespread tender erythema affecting >30% of the skin surface, and mucosal involvement (see below). Erythema is followed by extensive, full-thickness, cutaneous and mucosal necrosis and denudation within a couple of days. Similar features involving <10% of the body surface are termed Stevens–Johnson syndrome (SJS), also known as 'erythema multiforme major'; if 10–30% of body surface area is affected, this is often classified as TEN/SJS overlap. Drugs, e.g. allopurinol, anticonvulsants, NSAIDs, cause >80% of cases and have usually been commenced 1–3 weeks prior to presentation.

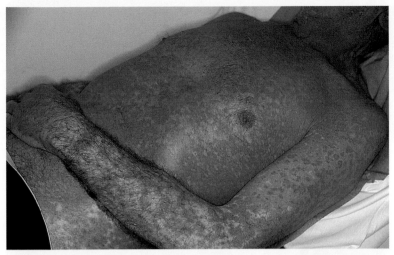

Fig. 27.1 Erythroderma. (From Gawkrodger DJ. Dermatology ICT, 4th edn. Edinburgh: Churchill Livingstone, 2008.)

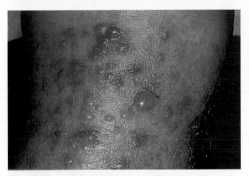

Fig. 27.2 Acute dermatitis. (From Gawkrodger DJ. Dermatology ICT, 4th edn. Edinburgh: Churchill Livingstone, 2008.)

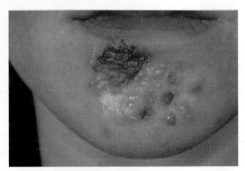

Fig. 27.3 Impetigo. (From Kumar P, Clark M. Kumar & Clark's Clinical Medicine, 7th edn. Edinburgh: Churchill Livingstone, 2009.)

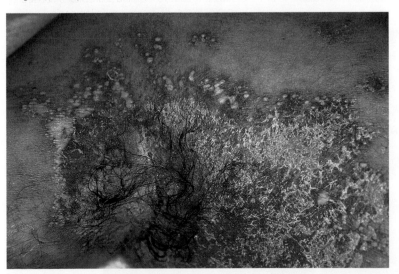

Fig. 27.4 Pustular psoriasis. (From Gawkrodger DJ. Dermatology ICT, 4th edn. Edinburgh: Churchill Livingstone, 2008.)

27

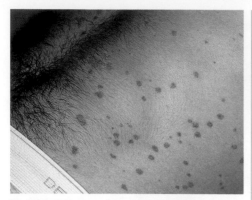

Fig. 27.5 Guttate psoriasis. (From Bolognia J, Jorizzo J, Rapini R. Dermatology, 1st edn. London: Mosby, 2003.)

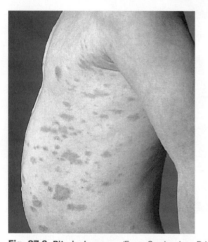

Fig. 27.6 Pityriasis rosea. (From Gawkrodger DJ. Dermatology ICT, 4th edn. Edinburgh: Churchill Livingstone, 2008.)

Erythema multiforme (minor) represents a similar but milder type of cytotoxic reaction. Classically, it presents with 'target' lesions, consisting of three zones: a dark or blistered centre (bull's-eye) surrounded by a pale zone and an outer rim of erythema (Fig. 27.8). The lesions predominantly occur on the hands/feet and affect <10% of the BSA without mucous membrane involvement. The underlying cause is more often viral (especially herpes simplex) than drug-induced.

Pemphigus/pemphigoid/dermatitis herpetiformis

Separation of keratinocytes from each other, or from the underlying dermis, produces blistering. The three most common blistering disorders are pemphigus (Fig. 27.9), pemphigoid (Fig. 27.10)

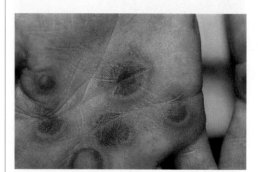

Fig. 27.8 Erythema multiforme-target lesions. (From Bolognia J, Jorizzo J, Rapini R. Dermatology, 1st edn. London: Mosby, 2003.)

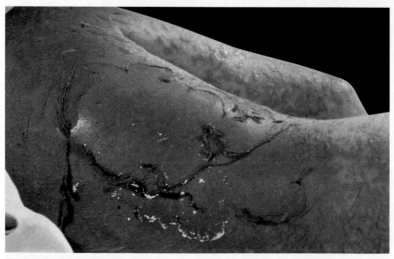

Fig. 27.7 Toxic epidermal necrolysis. (From Gawkrodger DJ. Dermatology ICT, 4th edn. Edinburgh: Churchill Livingstone, 2008.)

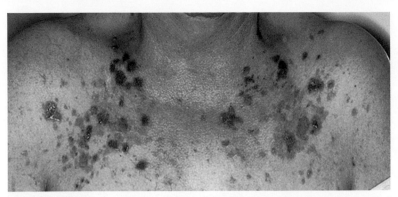

Fig. 27.9 Pemphigus. (From Bolognia J, Jorizzo J, Rapini R. Dermatology, 1st edn. London: Mosby, 2003.)

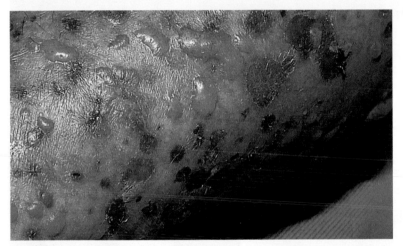

Fig. 27.10 Pemphigoid. (From Bolognia J, Jorizzo J, Rapini R. Dermatology, 1st edn. London: Mosby, 2003.)

and dermatitis herpetiformis (Fig. 27.11) which is commonly associated with coeliac disease.

Urticaria/angioedema

Urticaria (Fig. 27.12) is oedema within the dermis secondary to mast cell degranulation, and is a common skin reaction. Angioedema results from oedema deeper within the dermis and subcutaneous tissues, and may occur in up to 40% of cases. Although commonly thought to be allergic, most cases of acute urticaria are not mediated by immunoglobulin E (IgE). Those that are, arise in response to drugs (especially antibiotics), foods (peanuts, eggs, shellfish) and skin contact (latex, plants, bee/wasp stings), and may progress to anaphylaxis. Non-IgE causes include concurrent

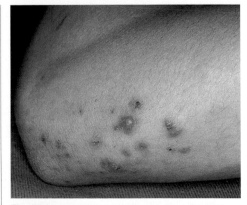

Fig. 27.11 Dermatitis herpetiformis. (From Gawkrodger DJ. Dermatology ICT, 4th edn. Edinburgh: Churchill Livingstone, 2008.)

27

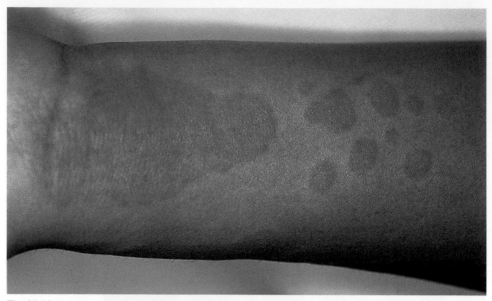

Fig. 27.12 Urticaria. (From Gawkrodger DJ. Dermatology ICT, 4th edn. Edinburgh: Churchill Livingstone, 2008.)

infection (especially upper respiratory tract infections), drugs that promote mast cell degranulation (opiates, aspirin, NSAIDs, ACE inhibitors) and foods that contain salicylates and additives.

Purpura (including vasculitis)

Purpura (Fig. 27.13) is fixed staining of the skin by leakage of blood from the intravascular space and needs to be distinguished from simple bruising. Causes include:

* septic emboli from systemic infectious diseases
* haematological disorders
* thrombosis involving microcirculation
* vasculitis (inflammation in vessel walls).

Acute exanthems

'Exanthem' simply means 'breakout' and, although the term is mostly used for rashes with an infectious aetiology, it may be regarded as a pseudonym for any acute eruption or rash.

Drug eruptions are common and do not necessarily indicate allergy; ~3% of all patients admitted to hospital have an eruption due to adverse drug reactions. Those most commonly

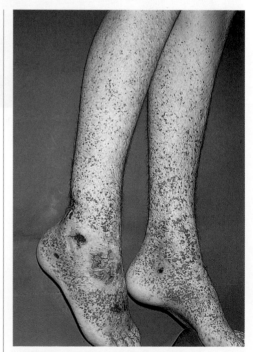

Fig. 27.13 Vasculitis/purpura. (From Gawkrodger DJ. Dermatology ICT, 4th edn. Edinburgh: Churchill Livingstone, 2008.)

Box 27.1 Drugs that cause rashes in >1% of the population

- Penicillins
- Carbamazepine
- Allopurinol
- Gold
- Sulphonamides
- NSAIDs
- Phenytoin
- Isoniazid
- Chloramphenicol
- Erythromycin
- Streptomycin

implicated are listed in Box 27.1. In hospital, rashes are commonly attributed to and often caused by medications, but similar cutaneous signs can be due to underlying or intercurrent illness, e.g. viral or bacterial exanthems or internal disease, non-specific reactions to treatment, e.g. sweat rash due to prolonged bed-rest or previously unidentified independent skin disease.

Infective exanthems are largely viral. Many of the conditions described above could be considered specific examples of infective exanthems, e.g. erythema multiforme post-herpes simplex, guttate psoriasis post-pharyngitis and pityriasis rosea.

27

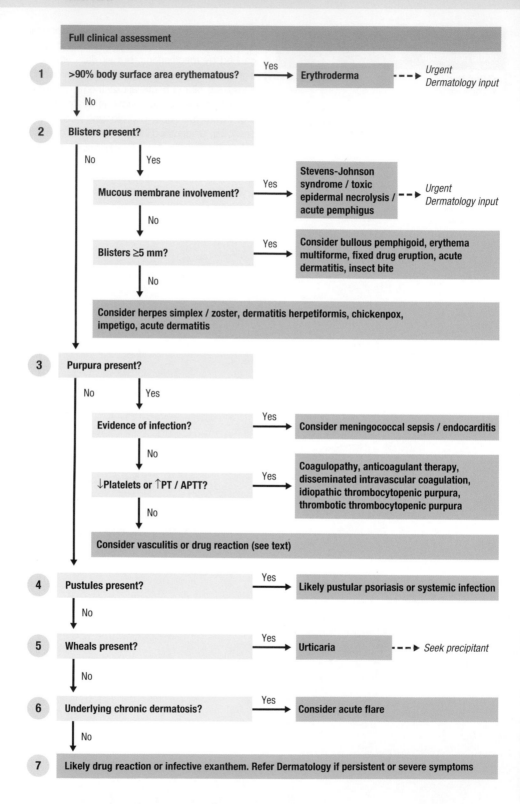

Full clinical assessment

1 >90% body surface area erythematous? — **Yes** → **Erythroderma** ----→ *Urgent Dermatology input*

No ↓

2 Blisters present?

No / Yes

Mucous membrane involvement? — **Yes** → **Stevens-Johnson syndrome / toxic epidermal necrolysis / acute pemphigus** ----→ *Urgent Dermatology input*

No ↓

Blisters ≥5 mm? — **Yes** → **Consider bullous pemphigoid, erythema multiforme, fixed drug eruption, acute dermatitis, insect bite**

No ↓

Consider herpes simplex / zoster, dermatitis herpetiformis, chickenpox, impetigo, acute dermatitis

3 Purpura present?

No / Yes

Evidence of infection? — **Yes** → **Consider meningococcal sepsis / endocarditis**

No ↓

↓Platelets or ↑PT / APTT? — **Yes** → **Coagulopathy, anticoagulant therapy, disseminated intravascular coagulation, idiopathic thrombocytopenic purpura, thrombotic thrombocytopenic purpura**

No ↓

Consider vasculitis or drug reaction (see text)

4 Pustules present? — **Yes** → **Likely pustular psoriasis or systemic infection**

No ↓

5 Wheals present? — **Yes** → **Urticaria** ----→ *Seek precipitant*

No ↓

6 Underlying chronic dermatosis? — **Yes** → **Consider acute flare**

No ↓

7 Likely drug reaction or infective exanthem. Refer Dermatology if persistent or severe symptoms

1 >90% body surface area erythematous?

Estimate the proportion of skin that is erythematous using the guide in Box 27.2; >90% of BSA indicates erythroderma. Admit any patient with acute erythroderma to hospital, assess and stabilize as described in Box 27.3 and arrange urgent dermatology review. Subsequent treatment is based on the exact diagnosis and guided by expert dermatological assessment.

2 Blisters present?

Blisters form when fluid separates the layers of the skin; blisters <5 mm diameter are termed 'vesicles', those >5 mm are called 'bullae'. Mucous membranes are involved (Fig. 27.14)

Box 27.2 Calculating body surface area

Originally developed for calculating surface area for burn victims, in adults a simple way of calculating the BSA affected by a cutaneous disorder is the 'Wallace rule of nines'. This system allocates to different body parts 9% (or half thereof) of the total BSA. In extensive skin disease it is sometimes easier to identify unaffected skin, and assessment is aided by remembering that the patient's hand is approximately 1% of BSA.

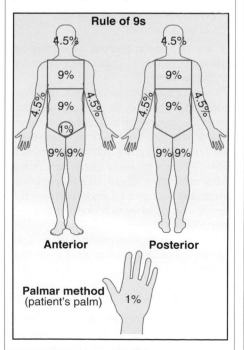

Rule of 9s

Anterior   Posterior

Palmar method (patient's palm) 1%

---

when erosions and ulceration (with subsequent crusting) occur on oral, genital and ocular epithelium; examine these sites in any acute severe skin eruption.

Suspect TEN if there is extensive blistering with peeling of the skin to reveal bright red oozing dermis (see Fig. 27.6), along with mucous membrane involvement; seek immediate Dermatology review and manage in a burns or critical care unit. If bullae and mucosal lesions are present but blistering is less extensive, consider SJS and pemphigus (see Fig. 27.9) – arrange prompt dermatological review in all cases.

In the absence of mucous membrane involvement, look for target lesions (see Fig. 27.8) on the hands and feet suggestive of erythema multiforme; otherwise, consider bullous pemphigoid (see Fig. 27.10), fixed drug eruption or, if lesions are well localized, an insect bite or contact dermatitis.

If the patient has a painful eruption of vesicles, suspect infection with herpes simplex if it is confined to the face, lip or finger (herpetic whitlow) and herpes zoster (shingles; Fig. 27.15) if it follows a dermatomal distribution. In febrile patients with widespread vesicles consider

---

Box 27.3 Assessment and immediate management of skin dysfunction

The mainstay of emergency dermatology treatment is to provide surrogate skin function until the underlying condition has resolved or is suppressed with suitable medication. Look for evidence of shock (see Box 30.1, p. 267) and dehydration, and monitor U+E regularly. Replenish fluid lost through defective skin barrier function with IV fluids and supplementary electrolytes. Take swabs of all areas of suspected infection and, if the patient is pyrexial, take blood cultures before commencing antibiotic therapy. Use strict aseptic technique for blood cultures, ideally through non-affected skin, to try to avoid contaminants (more likely in dermatological patients due to ↑skin flora load). Remember that many acute cutaneous eruptions are associated with pyrexia, due not to systemic infection but to loss of temperature homeostasis through vasodilatation. Maintain body temperature with a warm room and regular antipyretics. Assess the extent of skin compromise as detailed above and restore its barrier function with regular application of thick emollients (liquid paraffin : white soft paraffin, 50:50). Remove any potential exacerbates by discontinuing all unnecessary medication.

27

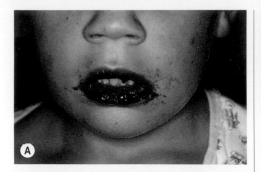

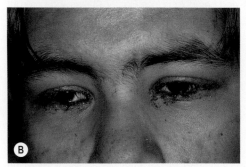

Fig. 27.14 Mucous membrane involvement in Stevens–Johnson syndrome. [A] Oral. [B] Ocular. (From Gawkrodger DJ. Dermatology ICT, 4th edn. Edinburgh: Churchill Livingstone, 2008.)

chickenpox or, if there is known eczema, eczema herpeticum. Suspect dermatitis herpetiformis if the vesicles are intensely itchy and occur on the extensor surfaces (see Fig. 27.11).

3 Purpura present?

Classify the rash as purpuric if there are dark red or purple macules/patches that do not blanch with pressure (see Fig. 27.13).

Take urgent blood cultures and treat empirically for meningococcal sepsis pending further investigation if the patient has fever, shock, drowsiness or meningism (see Box 18.2, p. 169). Consider septic emboli from endocarditis if the patient is febrile and has a predisposing cardiac lesion or a new murmur.

Look for evidence of an underlying bleeding tendency – ask about/examine for ecchymoses, epistaxis, GI bleeding, menorrhagia, haemarthrosis and mucosal haemorrhage, and check FBC, PT and APTT. Unless the cause is obvious, e.g. excessive anticoagulation, chronic

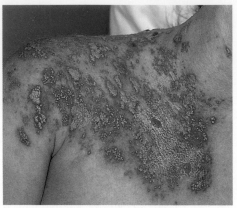

Fig. 27.15 Herpes zoster. (From Gawkrodger DJ. Dermatology ICT, 4th edn. Edinburgh: Churchill Livingstone, 2008.)

liver disease, discuss with Haematology if there is coagulopathy or ↓platelets.

If ↓platelets are present with normal coagulation, look for associated features of thrombotic thrombocytopenic purpura:

- ↓Hb without an obvious alternative cause
- red cell fragmentation on blood film
- ↑↑LDH
- neurological abnormalities (↓GCS, headache, seizures).

If any of these is present, seek immediate Haematology input, as urgent plasma exchange may be life-saving.

Suspect a systemic vasculitis, e.g. polyarteritis nodosa, Henoch–Schönlein purpura, microscopic polyangiitis, cryoglobulinaemia, rheumatoid vasculitis or other systemic inflammatory disorder – if there is palpable purpura accompanied by fever, ↑ESR/CRP, constitutional upset, joint disease and/or renal involvement (↓GFR, proteinuria, haematuria). Perform a full vasculitis/autoimmune 'screen' and consider skin biopsy ± biopsy of other affected organs.

Also consider cholesterol embolization or drug reaction – seek Dermatology input if the cause remains unclear.

4 Pustules present?

Pustules are best thought of as small blisters filled with pus (see Fig. 27.3). The key diagnostic conundrum is whether they are infective or sterile.

In both cases, the patient may be unwell, with significant constitutional upset.

Assume an infective pustulosis, at least initially, if the patient has a fever and the lesions have a follicular appearance (individual, palpably raised lesions, following the distribution of hair follicles). Suspect sterile pustulosis due to either pustular psoriasis or drug reaction if the pustules have a subcorneal appearance (more superficial, often confluent lesions). In either case, admit the patient and seek an urgent dermatological opinion.

5 Wheals present?

Classify the rash as urticaria if there are wheals: transient (<24 hours), erythematous, intensely pruritic raised skin lesions (see Fig. 27.12). Look for swelling of the lips, face and throat, suggesting associated angioedema; patients may describe the skin sensation as burning rather than itchy. Take a careful food and drug history to identify possible precipitants, although in many cases a cause cannot be identified (idiopathic urticaria). Other than avoidance of any identified precipitant, the mainstay of treatment is regular antihistamines; most cases subside quickly with avoidance of the precipitant and/or antihistamine treatment. Refer patients with persistent (>24 hours) or chronic (>6 weeks) lesions for outpatient dermatological assessment.

6 Underlying chronic dermatosis?

Ask about previous skin disease, recent changes to dermatological or other medications and specifically whether the present eruption resembles previous rashes. It is very common for hospital patients to miss their dermatological medications due to lack of prescription or interruption of their regular topical application routine; if this is the case, suspect an acute flare and look for resolution of the rash after reinstating routine treatment.

7 Likely drug reaction or infective exanthem. Refer to Dermatology if persistent or severe symptoms

Occasionally, serious acute drug eruptions lack the specific features detailed above; seek prompt dermatological advice in any patient with signs of significant systemic upset, mucous membrane involvement or associated lymphadenopathy, or if symptoms are persistent and troublesome.

Consider guttate psoriasis and pityriasis rosea if there is an acute papulosquamous eruption (see above) over the trunk. Suspect the former if the lesions are 'drop-like' (see Fig. 27.5) and there is a history of upper respiratory tract infection within the past 2–3 weeks; suspect the latter if the lesions form a 'Christmas tree' pattern on the back (see Fig. 27.6) and follow a 'herald patch'.

Precise identification of infective exanthems is seldom required as most do not need specific treatment and will settle conservatively, but seek specialist advice if the patient is a returning traveller with fever or an unusual rash.

Review all recent medications, both prescribed and over-the-counter drugs. There is significant variation in the morphology and exposure-to-onset time (minutes to years) of cutaneous drug eruptions. If a drug reaction is suspected, e.g. a drug from Box 27.1 is involved or there is a clear temporal association, attempt to confirm by trial discontinuation wherever feasible.

27

28 Red eye

The acute red eye (or eyes) is a common presentation. Check visual acuity (VA) in all cases. Patients with associated reduced ↓VA, severe pain or photophobia require urgent specialist ophthalmology referral.

Conjunctivitis

Inflammation of the conjunctiva is common. It can be infective: viral – commonly adenoviruses and *Herpes simplex*; bacterial (*Streptococcus pneumoniae, Staphylococcus aureus, Haemophilus influenzae, Chlamydia trachomatis, Neisseria gonorrhoeae*; or fungal; allergic or chemical. It can affect one or both eyes and commonly presents with eye redness, eyelid swelling (usually mild), gritty discomfort and discharge (Fig. 28.2). Bacterial and viral conjunctivitis usually produce a mucopurulent discharge and are highly contagious. Patients may have difficulty opening the eye after sleep because the discharge 'glues' the eyelid margins together. Photophobia and ↓VA are unlikely.

Foreign body

The patient often reports a sensation of something going into the eye – often wind-blown. There is redness and often copious watering. On examination a small foreign body will be seen, superficially adherent to, or embedded in, the cornea, or under the upper or lower eyelid (Fig. 28.3). Photophobia and discomfort may occur, aggravated by blinking if the foreign body is

---

Clinical tool
Acute red eye examination

- Ask about subjective VA in both eyes, unilateral versus bilateral symptoms, pain, itchiness, burning and grittiness, eye discharge and its character (mucopurulent, watery), abnormality of eyelashes, eyelid or eye closure, photophobia and a history of a foreign body going into the eye (and the mechanism, e.g. hammering, grinding, blowing in with wind).
- If the patient is uncomfortable, put topical anaesthetic drops (e.g. oxybuprocaine 0.4%) into the eye. Warn the patient that this stings for a few seconds before it works.
- Examine eye movements and if appropriate visual fields. Pain on eye movement is suggestive of scleritis or orbital cellulitis. Look at the fundus with an ophthalmoscope.
- Always check and document objective **VA in BOTH eyes** with their spectacles or a pinhole using a Snellen chart.
- Check the position of the lid margins and the position of the lashes.
- Assess pupil size, shape, symmetry and reactivity. Assess the clarity of the iris. A hazy iris suggests corneal oedema (such as in acute angle glaucoma) or inflammatory cells in the anterior chamber (such as in iritis). A fluid level may be seen in iritis (collection of pus cells; hypopyon) or trauma (collection of blood; hyphaema)
- Assess the pattern of redness. Diffuse redness involving inner eyelid suggests conjunctivitis. Segmental redness may indicate episcleritis or scleritis (although this may be generalized with deeper scleral vessel engorgement). Ciliary injection occurs in iritis and corneal conditions. Well-demarcated red eye with quiet adjacent conjunctiva is seen with subconjunctival haemorrhage.
- With the slit lamp, carefully inspect the ocular and corneal surfaces for ulceration, foreign bodies, abrasions and trauma. Examine the anterior chamber for pus cells.
- In addition to carefully examining the cornea and globe for foreign bodies, look in the lower lid by gently pulling it down and also evert the upper lid with a cotton wool bud (Fig. 28.1).
- Instil fluorescein and with the slit lamp and with the blue light, carefully re-inspect the ocular and corneal surfaces for uptake suggesting ulceration, abrasions and trauma.
- Irrespective of the suspected diagnosis, if ↓VA ± severe pain ± photophobia, get emergency Ophthalmology review.

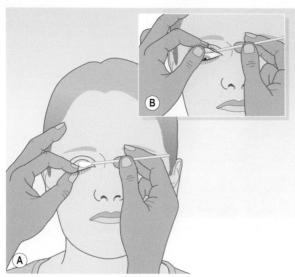

Fig. 28.1 Everting the upper eyelid to look at the conjunctiva. (From Douglas G, Nicol F, Robertson C. Macleod's Clinical Examination, 13th edn. Edinburgh: Churchill Livingstone, 2013.)

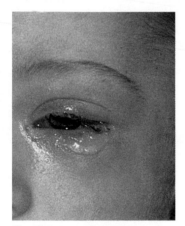

Fig. 28.2 Conjunctivitis. (From Batterbury M, Bowling B, Murphy C. Ophthalmology, 3rd edn. Edinburgh: Churchill Livingstone, 2009.)

lodged under the tarsal plate, but ↓VA is unlikely unless the foreign body is in the centre of the cornea. Fluorescein staining will aid identification.

Suspect an intraocular foreign body (i.e. one which has penetrated the anterior chamber or globe) with trauma from mechanical saws, grinding or hammering which can produce high-velocity foreign bodies, or if ↓VA, a hyphaema (blood in the anterior chamber) or an abnormal pupil is present.

Subconjunctival haemorrhage

This is benign self-limiting bleeding from underneath the conjunctiva (Fig. 28.4). It is most often idiopathic, but is associated with hypertension, straining (coughing, sneezing, Valsalva manoeuvre), NSAIDs, anticoagulants and bleeding disorders, and febrile illnesses, e.g. meningococcaemia, typhoid, malaria. The appearance may be dramatic, but is usually asymptomatic, painless, and with normal VA. If covering the entire conjunctiva there can be associated oedema (chemosis).

Ectropion/entropion/trichiasis/blepharitis

Ectropion occurs when the eyelid turns outward. With entropion the eyelid turns in (Fig. 28.5). Both more commonly affect the lower lid and cause redness, irritation, and watering and increased vulnerability to infections such as conjunctivitis. Trichiasis is due to eyelashes that grow back towards the eye causing pain and eye redness. Blepharitis is an inflammation (usually chronic) of the eyelids.

Keratitis

Keratitis is an inflammation/ulceration of the cornea causing an intensely painful red eye with photophobia and watering. VA may be ↓ and the eyelids swollen. Keratitis can be infective,

28

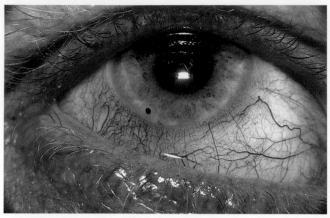

Fig. 28.3 Foreign body. (From Atkinson P, Kendall R, Rensburg LV. Emergency Medicine, 1st edn. Edinburgh: Churchill Livingstone, 2010.)

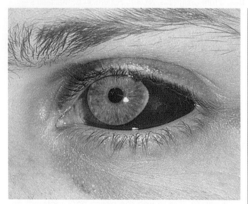

Fig. 28.4 Subconjunctival haemorrhage. (From Scully C. Medical Problems in Dentistry, 6th edn. Edinburgh: Churchill Livingstone, 2010.)

e.g. viral (herpes simplex infection can produce corneal ulcers with a characteristic dendritic branching pattern), bacterial, fungal, amoebic or parasitic; environmental, e.g. exposure, ultraviolet (as in snow blindness or welder's arc); chemical; traumatic or due to contact lens wearing; the main risk factor for keratitis is contact lens use. Keratitis, if untreated or severe, can lead to sight-threatening complications.

Acute iritis (anterior uveitis)

Inflammation of the iris, which is often recurrent (Fig. 28.6), occurs in young and middle-aged patients and may be associated with systemic diseases including seronegative spondyloarthropathies, inflammatory bowel disease, rheumatoid disease, SLE, sarcoid, HIV, etc. Presents with (usually unilateral) eye redness, typically ciliary or limbal (at the junction of the cornea and sclera), blurred vision/↓VA, watering, photophobia (experienced when a light is shone into the affected eye and also the normal eye) and pain. Pain may be aggravated by reading or close work. The pupil is commonly small and irregular.

Episcleritis/scleritis

In episcleritis there is localized inflammation of the episclera (which lies between the conjunctiva and the sclera) (Fig. 28.7). Pain is usually mild and there is redness and watering and a nodule may be seen or felt by the patient. Scleritis is a more serious localized inflammation of the sclera (Fig. 28.8). Pain is a dominant feature and is more severe than with episcleritis and it is often recurrent. It responds poorly to analgesics, is worse with eye movements and can radiate to the periorbital region, forehead, temple and jaw. Both conditions are associated with autoimmune diseases and rheumatoid arthritis. ↓VA is unlikely in episcleritis but present in up to 20% with scleritis.

Acute angle-closure glaucoma

A sight-threatening ophthalmic emergency caused by sudden blockage of aqueous humour leading to ↑↑↑intraocular pressure (Fig. 28.9).

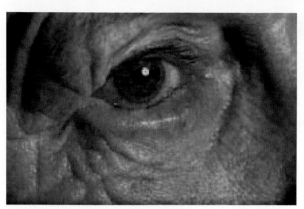

Fig. 28.5 Senile entropion of the lower lid. (From Douglas G, Nicol F, Robertson C. Macleod's Clinical Examination, 13th edn. Edinburgh: Churchill Livingstone, 2013.)

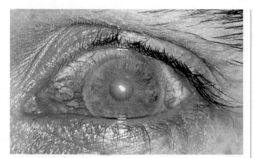

Fig. 28.6 Iritis (anterior uveitis). (From Swartz MH. Textbook of Physical Diagnosis: History and Examination, 6th edn. Philadelphia: Saunders, 2009.)

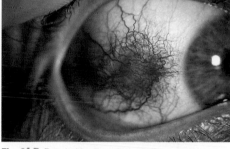

Fig. 28.7 Episcleritis. (From Rutter P. Community Pharmacy, 2nd edn. Edinburgh: Churchill Livingstone, 2009.)

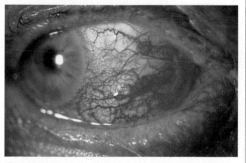

Fig. 28.8 Scleritis. (From Kanski JJ. Clinical Diagnosis in Ophthalmology, 1st edn. St Louis: Mosby, 2006.)

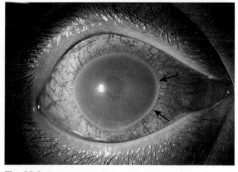

Fig. 28.9 Acute angle-closure glaucoma. Arrows show dilated conjunctival vessels at corneal edge. Note hazy cornea. (From Roberts JR, Hedges JR. Clinical Procedures in Emergency Medicine, 5th edn. Philadelphia: Saunders, 2010.)

28

Middle-aged/elderly, long-sighted patients with shallow anterior chambers are at particular risk. Pupil dilation can precipitate the condition so the onset may be more common in the evening and be precipitated by sympathomimetic, anticholinergic and other drugs.

Presentation is with acute, usually unilateral, severe eye pain with redness, ↓VA, seeing halos around lights, nausea and vomiting, a cloudy cornea and a fixed, mid-dilated non-reactive, often oval-shaped, pupil. The globe feels 'hard' on (gentle) palpation through the eyelid.

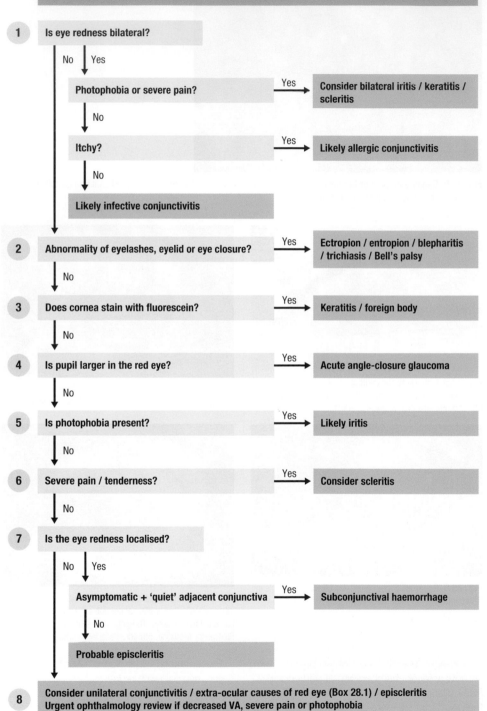

Eye examination (see clinical tool)

1 Is eye redness bilateral?

No | Yes

Photophobia or severe pain? — Yes → Consider bilateral iritis / keratitis / scleritis

No ↓

Itchy? — Yes → Likely allergic conjunctivitis

No ↓

Likely infective conjunctivitis

2 Abnormality of eyelashes, eyelid or eye closure? — Yes → Ectropion / entropion / blepharitis / trichiasis / Bell's palsy

No ↓

3 Does cornea stain with fluorescein? — Yes → Keratitis / foreign body

No ↓

4 Is pupil larger in the red eye? — Yes → Acute angle-closure glaucoma

No ↓

5 Is photophobia present? — Yes → Likely iritis

No ↓

6 Severe pain / tenderness? — Yes → Consider scleritis

No ↓

7 Is the eye redness localised?

No | Yes

Asymptomatic + 'quiet' adjacent conjunctiva — Yes → Subconjunctival haemorrhage

No ↓

Probable episcleritis

8 Consider unilateral conjunctivitis / extra-ocular causes of red eye (Box 28.1) / episcleritis
Urgent ophthalmology review if decreased VA, severe pain or photophobia

1 Is the eye redness bilateral?

A foreign body or trauma and acute glaucoma are usually unilateral. Conjunctivitis often starts unilaterally and then becomes bilateral. Iritis and keratitis can be bilateral although are more commonly unilateral.

Allergic conjunctivitis is almost always bilateral; it is often seasonal, worse in the morning, itchy and there may be a history of atopy.

Viral and bacterial conjunctivitis cannot be reliably differentiated based on clinical features; however, a watery discharge is more commonly seen with viral infection and a mucopurulent discharge with bacterial infection. Severe purulent discharge is common in gonococcal infection. Take conjunctival swabs for culture and sensitivity and to guide antibiotic/antiviral therapy.

2 Abnormality of eyelashes, eyelid or eye closure?

Check the position of the lid margins and the position of the lashes. The appearances of ectropion, entropion and trichiasis are usually obvious. Fluorescein staining may be present if the lashes have rubbed on the cornea.

Bell's palsy commonly presents with unilateral mouth droop and an inability to close the eye on the affected side. Differentiate from acute stroke as the forehead is not spared (patient is unable to wrinkle forehead). Bell's palsy can cause eye redness because of drying and/or corneal abrasion/ulceration and temporary taping at night can help prevent exposure keratitis and corneal ulceration. In blepharitis the lid margins/lashes are inflamed and crusty.

3 Does the cornea stain with fluorescein?

Examine carefully for fluorescein staining and foreign bodies as described (see Clinical tool). Infective causes of keratitis and corneal ulceration can be rapidly sight-threatening and may be caused by viral, bacterial, fungal or amoebic infection. Herpes simplex virus infection may produce characteristic dendritic staining of the cornea (Fig. 28.10). In addition to examining the cornea with fluorescein staining for ulceration, look for cloudiness or frank pus (hypopyon) in the anterior chamber; seek urgent specialist ophthalmological review regarding confirmation of

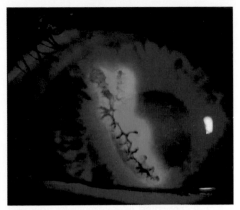

Fig. 28.10 Dendritic conjunctival ulcer. Fluorescein staining showing branching dendritic ulcer. (From Douglas G, Nicol F, Robertson C. Macleod's Clinical Examination, 13th edn. Edinburgh: Churchill Livingstone, 2013.)

the diagnosis and antimicrobial/antiviral therapy. Many foreign bodies can be simply removed with a cotton bud. Embedded metallic corneal foreign bodies require specialist review for removal and treatment of associated 'rust-rings'. A history consistent with penetrating injury or of hammering/grinding mandates specialist review and imaging.

4 Is the pupil larger in the red eye?

Suspect acute angle-closure glaucoma in any patient with periorbital pain, blurred vision/visual defect and a mid-dilated non-reactive pupil. The pain is usually severe and may be mistaken for other causes of severe headache, e.g. migraine or subarachnoid haemorrhage. Similarly, the associated nausea/vomiting/abdominal pain may lead to a misdiagnosis of gastroenteritis. The decreased VA may be profound, e.g. detection of hand movements only. The cornea is usually cloudy and the pupil irregular and unreactive.

Acute angle-closure is a medical emergency, any time delay in diagnosis and treatment may compromise sight drastically. Get emergency ophthalmological advice and review. Keep the patient supine if possible and do not cover the eye. Analgesics and anti-emetics may be indicated.

5 Is photophobia present?

Photophobia indicates iritis or corneal epithelial disturbance. Ask about previous similar episodes

28

(common in iritis) and underlying systemic conditions (e.g. ankylosing spondylitis, reactive arthritis, inflammatory bowel disease, connective tissue disorders) known to be associated with iritis or scleritis. Cloudiness or hypopyon of the anterior chamber may be present. Get emergency ophthalmological review.

6 Severe pain/tenderness?

Consider scleritis if the red eye is associated with severe pain (present in ≥80% of cases) or is very tender. Typically the redness will be localized but in severe cases it can involve most of the sclera. If suspected refer urgently for specialist assessment.

7 Is the eye redness localized?

Diagnose subconjunctival haemorrhage if there is a localized region of redness with no associated symptoms (except possibly mild dryness) and normal appearances of the surrounding conjunctiva. Suspect episcleritis if there is segmental redness associated with mild pain, eye watering or injection of the adjacent vessels. Consider scleritis if there is localized redness associated with reduced VA or pain that radiates to the periorbital region, forehead, temple or jaw.

8 Consider other causes (Box 28.1)

Infective conjunctivitis may be unilateral, particularly in the early stages; consider the diagnosis if there is associated discharge and no other

---

Box 28.1 Extraocular causes for a red eye

- Orbital cellulitis
- Cavernous sinus thrombosis
- Carotid-cavernous fistula
- Cluster headache

Box 28.2 Features suggestive of a benign cause for a red eye

- Pupils exhibit normal size and reactivity
- Normal VA (NB: occasionally a central corneal abrasion can reduce visual acuity)
- Clear cornea
- Clear anterior chamber
- No proptosis
- Eyeball not tender on palpation
- Normal extraocular eye movements

---

concerning features, e.g. photophobia or reduced VA. Though usually localized, both scleritis and episcleritis may cause diffuse eye redness. Reconsider the possibility of acute angle closure glaucoma if there are any suggestive features, e.g. cloudy cornea, severe orbital/periorbital pain or reports of seeing halos around objects. In the absence of a definite diagnosis, Box 28.2 lists features that would point to a benign underlying cause. Irrespective of the suspected diagnosis, get emergency Ophthalmology review if there is decreased VA, severe pain or photophobia.

Most causes of scrotal swelling are benign, but germ cell tumours are a leading cause of malignancy in young men whilst testicular torsion and strangulated herniae are surgical emergencies. It is important to ascertain whether the scrotal swelling arises from within the scrotum or from outside (inguinal hernia).

Indirect inguinal hernia

Inguinal hernia (Fig. 29.1) may occur at any age but is increasingly common from middle age and is the most frequent cause of scrotal swelling. Herniated bowel passes through the inguinal ring and may descend into the scrotal sac. Left-sided hernias may contain the sigmoid colon. As the swelling arises from the abdominal cavity, it is not possible to 'get above' it. Typically, the swelling is more prominent on standing, associated with a cough impulse and can be pushed back into the abdomen ('reduced'). A non-reducible or 'incarcerated' hernia may lead to bowel obstruction or strangulation with ischaemia.

Scrotal swellings

Scrotal swellings may arise from either the contents of the scrotum or the skin of the scrotum. Abnormalities of the contents should be divided into spermatic cord, epididymis and testicular pathologies.

Testicular abnormalities

Hydrocoele

Hydrocoele (see Fig. 29.1) is the most common cause of scrotal swelling, especially in older men. Fluid accumulates within the tunica vaginalis (analogous to the peritoneal space in the abdomen), producing a painless, cystic swelling that typically transilluminates. With substantial swelling, the underlying testes may be impalpable. Most cases are idiopathic, but some have an underlying inflammatory or, rarely, malignant process.

Orchitis

This may arise as a complication of epididymitis (epididymo-orchitis) or, with mumps (now rare due to vaccination). It presents with acute scrotal pain and swelling, over days rather than hours, often accompanied by fever, urinary symptoms and/or urethral discharge. There may be a tender, swollen (soft) epididymis/testis or a reactive hydrocoele.

Testicular tumour

These typically present as painless, irregular, firm testicular lumps. Non-seminomatous germ cell tumours (NSGCT) (see Fig. 29.1) are the most common malignancy amongst men aged 20–30 years. These comprise yolk sac tumours, choriocarcinoma, mixed type or embryonal tumours. Seminomatous tumours present later in life and have a slightly less aggressive course. Scrotal USS confirms the diagnosis and CT thorax/abdomen/pelvis is used in staging. Tumours are very chemosensitive (platinum-based chemotherapy) and 5-year survival is greater than 90% even if metastasis has occurred. The tumour markers alpha-fetoprotein (yolk sac tumours), beta-human chorionic gonadotropin (choriocarcinomas) and LDH (tumour burden) should be tested. Suspected testicular cancer requires urgent inpatient management due to the very rapid progression of these tumour types.

Torsion of the testis

Twisting of the testis may compromise its own blood supply; initially impeding venous outflow until the pressure in the testis reached mean arterial pressure and arterial inflow is then occluded. Acute, severe, unilateral testicular

Normal

Hydrocoele

Fig. 29.1 Common causes of scrotal swelling.

Spermatic cord

Epididymis

Testis

Indirect inguinal hernia

Epididymitis

Varicocoele

Tumour of testicle

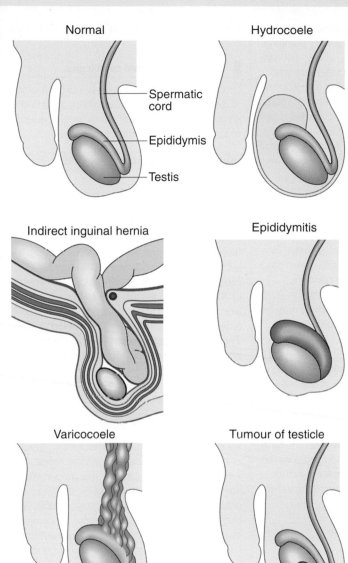

pain is the dominant presenting symptom, often accompanied by nausea and vomiting. On examination there may be a red, swollen, exquisitely tender hemiscrotum (often too tender to palpate), with the testis lying in a high position due to shortening of the spermatic cord. Patients are typically young adolescent males but consider torsion in all acute scrotal presentations. Suspected torsion mandates immediate surgical correction (de-torsion and pexy), as any delay threatens testicular viability.

Epididymis abnormalities

Epididymo-orchitis

Inflammation of the epididymis ± testis (see Fig. 29.1) is usually due to sexually transmitted infection (mainly chlamydia and gonorrhoea) in younger men, and urinary tract infection (UTI) in older men. Acute epididymo-orchitis may be difficult to distinguish clinically from torsion.

Epididymal cyst

These are common, benign, simple cysts arising from the head of the epididymis. They may be multiple or bilateral. They are palpable separately from the testis. Differential diagnosis includes hydrocele, spermatocoele (which is similar to an epididymal cyst but contains sperm) and haematocoele (collection of blood in the tunica vaginalis following trauma). Symptoms include a dragging or painful sensation due to the weight of the cyst.

Spermatic cord abnormalities

Varicocoele

Varicocoeles, varicosities of the gonadal vessels and their tributaries (see Fig. 29.1), are the commonest abnormalities of the spermatic cord. They typically present with a dragging sensation of the testis and feel like a 'bag of worms' on palpation. Left-sided varicocoeles may be caused by outflow obstruction of the left renal vein due to

renal tumours (e.g. tumour thrombus of renal cell carcinoma).

Other spermatic cord pathologies

Other abnormalities uncommonly include lipomas of the cord (usually identified whilst undertaking an inguinal hernia repair) and, rarely, adenomyoma and liposarcoma of the cord.

Abnormalities of the scrotal skin

Scrotal wall oedema

This is the most common abnormality of the scrotal skin, presenting as thickened, indurated skin, usually as a result of congestive cardiac failure or other causes of peripheral oedema. Lymphatic filariasis (*Wuchereria bancrofti* [90%], *Brugia malayi*, and *Brugia timori*) causes oedema of the legs and genitals due to parasitic invasion of the pelvic lymphatics. Treatment is with anti-parasitic agents such as mebendazole. The scrotum may rarely become enormously enlarged, for example necessitating carriage of the scrotum in a wheelbarrow. In instances such as these, debulking scrotal surgery is required.

Cellulitis/Fournier's gangrene

Fournier's gangrene refers to necrotizing fasciitis of the genitalia, perineum or perianal region; it is a life-threatening emergency requiring immediate surgical debridement and broad spectrum antibiotics. Infection is typically polymicrobial with both aerobic and anaerobic bacteria, including streptococcus, staphylococcus, enterobacteriacea and clostridium species. The condition tends to arise in older patients, with diabetes as the main risk factor. Intense genital pain and tenderness is the clinical hallmark and, importantly, the overlying inflammatory skin changes (erythema, oedema) may be relatively mild or even absent in the early stages. In advanced disease there may be subcutaneous crepitation or frank gangrene.

Clinical tool
Examination of the scrotum

Testicular examination

- Obtain consent and offer a chaperone.
- With the patient standing, then supine, inspect the scrotum for redness, swelling and position of the testes.
- Wearing gloves, palpate each testis in turn between forefinger and thumb; identify the spermatic cord and epididymis and assess any irregularity, swelling or tenderness.
- Use your fingers to see whether you can feel above the swelling (Fig. 29.2); if so, it originates in the scrotum.

- If you cannot 'get above' the swelling, check for a cough impulse and attempt to reduce the swelling by very gently 'massaging' it back into the abdomen.
- Determine whether the swelling transilluminates using a pen-torch.
- In patients with an acutely painful scrotum or tender/ inflamed scrotal swelling, check the cremasteric reflex. With the patient's thigh abducted and externally rotated, stroke the upper medial aspect – normally, the testis on that side will rise briskly.

Fingers can 'get above' mass   Fingers cannot 'get above' mass

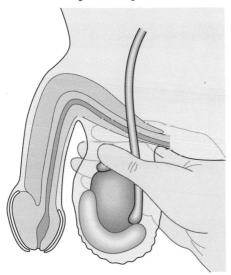

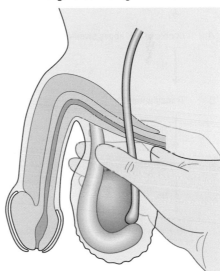

Fig. 29.2 Assessing the origin of a scrotal swelling. (From Douglas G, Nicol F, Robertson C. Macleod's Clinical Examination, 12th edn. Edinburgh: Churchill Livingstone, 2009.)

29

Full clinical assessment + testicular examination

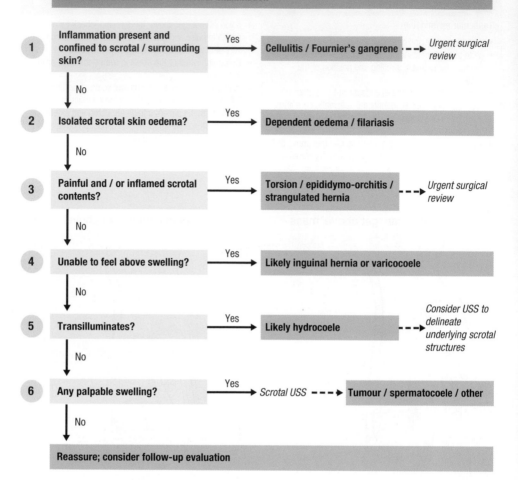

1 Inflammation present and confined to scrotal / surrounding skin? — Yes → Cellulitis / Fournier's gangrene ⤑ *Urgent surgical review*

No ↓

2 Isolated scrotal skin oedema? — Yes → Dependent oedema / filariasis

No ↓

3 Painful and / or inflamed scrotal contents? — Yes → Torsion / epididymo-orchitis / strangulated hernia ⤑ *Urgent surgical review*

No ↓

4 Unable to feel above swelling? — Yes → Likely inguinal hernia or varicocoele

No ↓

5 Transilluminates? — Yes → Likely hydrocoele ⤑ *Consider USS to delineate underlying scrotal structures*

No ↓

6 Any palpable swelling? — Yes → *Scrotal USS* ⤑ Tumour / spermatocoele / other

No ↓

Reassure; consider follow-up evaluation

1 Inflammation present and confined to scrotal/surrounding skin?

Consider Fournier's gangrene in any patient with inflammatory skin changes affecting the scrotal skin (+/– surrounding perineal/perianal regions). Seek immediate surgical review if any of the following are present:

- severe pain or tenderness (especially if disproportionate to skin appearances)
- dusky appearance of skin, fluctuation, crepitation or gangrene
- systemically unwell, e.g. sepsis (see Ch. 14), shock (see Ch. 30).

In the absence of these features, consider scrotal cellulitis but monitor frequently and have a very low threshold for surgical review, particularly in older or diabetic patients.

2 Isolated scrotal skin oedema?

In patients with scrotal wall oedema, look for evidence of generalized oedema, ascites, ↑JVP and/or pleural effusions. ↑JVP indicates systemic venous congestion and strongly suggests a cardiogenic cause, e.g. cardiac failure or severe pulmonary hypertension/cor pulmonale. Also consider a cardiac cause in patients with a significant cardiac history (e.g. previous myocardial infarction, valve disease, cardiomyopathy), severe chronic lung disease or exertional/nocturnal dyspnoea. Check U+E and serum albumin to exclude severe renal failure/hypoalbuminaemia and consider ECG and or cardiology review. Suspect filariasis if other causes are excluded and the clinical history is suggestive, e.g. from endemic area – seek expert advice.

3 Painful and/or inflamed scrotal contents?

Suspect a strangulated hernia if the swelling arises from the inguinal canal (see above), is not reducible (or severe pain persists despite reduction) and is tender, hot and red, or associated with systemic toxicity. Seek urgent surgical review, as there is a risk of bowel ischaemia.

If the swelling arises from the scrotum (or pain prohibits examination) and is painful, tender, inflamed and/or accompanied by acute severe unilateral scrotal pain, you MUST exclude testicular torsion. There may be associated features as below:

- nausea or vomiting
- pain duration <24 hours
- high position of the testis
- abnormal cremasteric reflex.

Consider initial investigation with scrotal USS if the clinical presentation suggests an alternative diagnosis such as epididymo-orchitis, e.g. urethral discharge, tenderness localized to epididymis, age >30 years and none of the above are present. In all other cases, arrange immediate surgical review without delay for imaging.

4 Unable to feel above swelling?

If it is not possible to palpate above the swelling, the swelling is likely to originate from outside the scrotum.

Suspect a varicocoele if it feels like a 'bag of worms'; confirm with scrotal USS and exclude underlying renal cell carcinoma if sudden onset, unilateral and left-sided or not reducible in supine position.

Otherwise, suspect an inguinal hernia – look for bowel obstruction (p. 32) and arrange urgent surgical review if it is non-reducible. If easily reducible, refer for outpatient surgical evaluation.

5 Transilluminates?

Suspect hydrocoele if there is a painless swelling of the scrotum that transilluminates. (Epididymal cyst and spermatocoeles also transilluminate and are part of the differential.) Consider USS to assess for testicular abnormality (e.g. tumour, inflammatory mass) if there is tenderness, systemic upset or difficulty in palpating the testicular structures.

6 Any palpable swelling?

USS is the investigation of choice in scrotal swelling and differentiates malignant tumours from other masses, e.g. spermatocoele, with a high degree of accuracy. Arrange scrotal USS in any patient with a detectable scrotal lump or swelling. Testicular tumours grow extremely rapidly so admit for urgent testicular USS and urology referral +/– tumour markers and CT staging if there is a high suspicion of malignancy, e.g. painless testicular lump in a young man. Refer to Urology in any case for further assessment/ treatment if the diagnosis remains uncertain.

29

Shock is a clinical syndrome characterized by inadequate systemic and specific organ perfusion. It is recognized by features of tissue hypoperfusion (Box 30.1), usually with hypotension; however, BP may be maintained until the advanced stages of shock, particularly in young, fit individuals.

Three processes may cause shock: hypovolaemia, pump failure (cardiogenic shock) and vasodilatation (distributive shock). These processes can be difficult to distinguish, as components of the circulation are interdependent and different mechanisms often coexist, e.g. vasodilatation, myocardial suppression and relative hypovolaemia may occur simultaneously in sepsis.

Many presentations in this book may be complicated by shock but here shock is considered as the primary presenting problem detected on routine observations or on targeted examination of a severely or non-specifically unwell patient.

Hypovolaemic shock

Decreased intravascular volume reduces cardiac filling pressures and cardiac output. A compensatory increase in heart rate and systemic vascular resistance occurs. Characteristic findings are ↓JVP, tachycardia, ↓pulse volume and cool, clammy peripheries. Tachycardia may be absent in patients on rate-limiting medications, e.g. beta-blockers, calcium channel antagonists.

Haemorrhage

Blood loss is not always visible; it may be left at the scene of an accident or concealed within surgical drains. The pelvis, retroperitoneum, peritoneum, thorax and thighs can accommodate several litres of extravascular blood. In addition to trauma, important causes include GI bleed (see Ch. 15), ruptured abdominal aortic aneurysm (AAA) and ectopic pregnancy.

Other fluid losses

Hypovolaemia may result from burns, diarrhoea, vomiting, polyuria or from prolonged dehydration, particularly in the elderly. Significant volumes of fluid may also be lost into the 'third space', e.g. in conditions such as bowel obstruction and acute pancreatitis.

Cardiogenic shock

Cardiac disorders may cause valvular or myocardial dysfunction, and extracardiac disorders may impede cardiac inflow or outflow (also known as 'obstructive' shock). Peripheral signs are similar to those of hypovolaemia but the JVP is usually raised (reflecting right heart failure) and there may be pulmonary oedema (reflecting left heart failure) as well as features specific to the underlying cause. ECG is often diagnostic.

Myocardial infarction

Shock may result from large infarcts, particularly in the anterior wall; from smaller infarcts in patients with pre-existing ventricular impairment; or from structural complications of myocardial infarction (MI), such as papillary muscle rupture, ventricular septal defect or tamponade.

Left ventricular dysfunction without infarction

This includes tachy- or bradyarrhythmias, acute myocarditis and end-stage cardiomyopathy.

Valve disorders

Examples of valve disorders include prosthetic valve dysfunction, endocarditis and critical aortic stenosis.

Tension pneumothorax

The urgency of treatment mandates a clinical diagnosis. Typical findings include increasing respiratory distress, ↓ipsilateral breath sounds, tachycardia and hypotension. Tracheal deviation is often absent. Immediate decompression is essential.

Cardiac tamponade

Accumulation of fluid in the pericardial space (pericardial effusion) impedes cardiac filling. As little as 200 mL of fluid may cause tamponade if accumulation is rapid, e.g. trauma, aortic dissection, myocardial rupture. Hypotension, tachycardia, ↑JVP and pulsus paradoxus are usually present. There may also be muffled heart sounds, Kussmaul's sign (a 'paradoxical' rise in JVP on inspiration) and small ECG complexes. ECG will confirm the presence of an effusion, provide evidence of cardiac compromise and guide therapeutic drainage.

Pulmonary embolism

Massive pulmonary embolism (PE) typically presents with sudden onset of chest pain, dyspnoea and hypoxia with shock. The JVP is usually elevated and the ECG may show features of right heart strain. In critically unwell patients, bedside echocardiography may assist the diagnosis.

Distributive shock

In distributive shock, peripheral vasodilatation causes a drop in systemic vascular resistance and 'relative hypovolaemia' (↑size of vascular space without corresponding increase in intravascular volume). A compensatory rise in cardiac output is insufficient to maintain blood pressure. Tachycardia and hypotension are often accompanied by warm peripheries and ↑pulse volume.

Systemic inflammatory response syndrome/sepsis

Distributive shock may complicate sepsis (p. 141) or non-infective conditions associated with a major systemic inflammatory response, e.g. acute pancreatitis. Features of relative hypovolaemia may predominate initially. An arterial or venous lactate of 4 mmol/L or greater has been associated with increased mortality in sepsis.

Anaphylaxis

This produces a very rapid onset of bronchoconstriction, widespread erythematous rash and severe distributive shock. A precipitant (foodstuffs, drugs – particularly antibiotics, insect stings) may be identified. A related problem is transfusion reaction; ABO incompatibility may present with shock as the only initial sign, particularly in unconscious or sedated patients. In severe anaphylaxis, severe shock or even cardiac arrest may occur without other symptoms or signs.

Drug causes

Antihypertensives and anaesthetic agents (particularly epidural and spinal anaesthesia) may cause distributive shock through excessive peripheral vasodilatation.

Adrenal crisis

Glucocorticoid deficiency may result in distributive shock, particularly during acute stress, e.g. infection, surgery.

Neurogenic shock

Neurogenic shock is a rare form of distributive shock associated with direct injury to the sympathetic fibres that control vascular tone from a traumatic spinal injury.

30

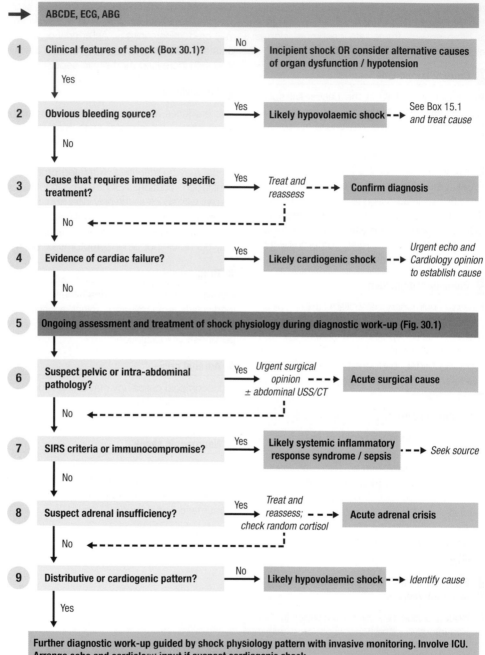

ABCDE, ECG, ABG

1 Clinical features of shock (Box 30.1)? — No → Incipient shock OR consider alternative causes of organ dysfunction / hypotension

Yes ↓

2 Obvious bleeding source? — Yes → Likely hypovolaemic shock - -▶ See Box 15.1 and treat cause

No ↓

3 Cause that requires immediate specific treatment? — Yes → *Treat and reassess* - - - ▶ Confirm diagnosis

No ↓

4 Evidence of cardiac failure? — Yes → Likely cardiogenic shock - -▶ *Urgent echo and Cardiology opinion to establish cause*

No ↓

5 Ongoing assessment and treatment of shock physiology during diagnostic work-up (Fig. 30.1)

↓

6 Suspect pelvic or intra-abdominal pathology? — Yes → *Urgent surgical opinion* - - -▶ Acute surgical cause *± abdominal USS/CT*

No ↓

7 SIRS criteria or immunocompromise? — Yes → Likely systemic inflammatory response syndrome / sepsis - - -▶ *Seek source*

No ↓

8 Suspect adrenal insufficiency? — Yes → *Treat and reassess;* - - -▶ Acute adrenal crisis *check random cortisol*

No ↓

9 Distributive or cardiogenic pattern? — No → Likely hypovolaemic shock - -▶ *Identify cause*

Yes ↓

Further diagnostic work-up guided by shock physiology pattern with invasive monitoring. Involve ICU.
Arrange echo and cardiology input if suspect cardiogenic shock
Maintain suspicion of sepsis; consider rarer causes, e.g. neurogenic shock

1 Clinical features of shock (see Box 30.1)?

Use the features in Box 30.1 to identify shock. Tissue hypoperfusion is the defining feature. Absolute values of HR and BP are less informative than monitoring of trends over time. Some patients may maintain BP within normal limits despite organ dysfunction, but consider local pathology if there is single organ dysfunction, e.g. oliguria, without clear evidence of haemodynamic compromise. If the patient falls short of the criteria in Box 30.1 but you suspect significant circulatory compromise, pursue a working diagnosis of 'incipient shock' and continue through the diagnostic pathway.

2 Obvious bleeding source?

Where shock arises from acute haemorrhage, the initial aims of treatment are to minimize further blood loss and restore adequate circulating volume. Assess resuscitation requirements and monitor response to treatment as described in Box 15.1, page 153. In patients with traumatic haemorrhage, always consider the possibility of an additional cause of shock, e.g. tamponade, tension pneumothorax.

3 Cause that requires immediate specific treatment?

In some cases, specific interventions to reverse the underlying cause of shock offer the only effective treatment (e.g. decompression of a tension pneumothorax) and take precedence over further investigation or supportive measures (Table 30.1). Most will be identified and treated

---

Box 30.1 Clinical features of shock

Haemodynamic

- Systolic BP <100 mmHg or a drop of >40 mmHg from baseline
- Pulse >100/min

Tissue hypoperfusion

- Skin: capillary refill time >2 sec or cold/pale/mottled extremities
- Renal: oliguria (<0.5 mL/kg/hr) or ↑serum creatinine (acute)
- CNS: GCS <15, confusion or agitation
- Global: ↑lactate (in the absence of hypoxaemia)

≥2 of the above indicate shock

---

as part of the ABCDE assessment (p. 8). If one of these disorders is suspected but the diagnosis remains uncertain, seek urgent expert assistance, e.g. Cardiology review.

4 Evidence of cardiac failure?

Pulmonary oedema suggests cardiogenic shock. The most common cause is severe left ventricular dysfunction from acute MI. Perform (serial) ECG to look for evidence of infarction or ischaemia (see Box 6.1, p. 51). Arrange bedside ECG to assess left ventricular function and exclude mechanical causes (especially acute mitral regurgitation).

Patients without pulmonary oedema but with ↑JVP ± peripheral oedema may have a cardiogenic component to shock. Those with right ventricular infarction (suspect with inferior or posterior MI in the previous 72 hours), chronic right heart failure or tricuspid regurgitation may be inadequately filled despite ↑JVP and will respond to fluid challenge. Otherwise, echocardiography is mandatory to look for evidence of right ventricular dysfunction, tamponade and PE.

Patients with cardiogenic shock require invasive monitoring and specialist interventions; if appropriate, urgent Cardiology and ICU referral is essential.

5 Ongoing assessment and treatment of shock physiology during diagnostic work-up (Fig. 30.1)

In the absence of obvious haemorrhage, major cardiac dysfunction or a rapidly reversible cause of shock, the next step is to initiate treatment and assess response. As shown in Fig. 30.1, the effect of repeated fluid challenge on haemodynamic variables and tissue perfusion helps to delineate the mechanism(s) of shock and guide further resuscitation and treatment. This process should be carried out in parallel with continued evaluation for a specific underlying cause. Beware concealed bleeding. Haemorrhagic shock is frequently missed in the early stages. Haemoglobin/haematocrit levels may be misleading as they are usually normal in acute haemorrhage, and only fall following fluid replacement. Lactate clearance (change in blood lactate levels over time) is a proxy for monitoring response to treatment. Bedside USS of the inferior vena cava (IVC) and its degree of collapsibility has also

30

Table 30.1 Rapidly reversible causes of shock			
Reversible cause	Suspect if	Test to confirm	Specific intervention
Tension pneumothorax	Respiratory distress/tracheal deviation/unilateral hyper-resonance, ↓breath sounds	Nil – treat immediately	Needle aspiration
Tachyarrhythmia	Ventricular tachycardia (VT) or supraventricular tachycardia (SVT) >150 bpm	Nil – treat immediately	DC cardioversion
Bradyarrhythmia	3rd degree atrioventricular block or HR <40 bpm	Nil – treat immediately	Atropine, adrenaline, external or transvenous pacing
Anaphylaxis	Respiratory distress, stridor, wheeze, angioedema, rash, precipitant	Nil – treat immediately	Adrenaline, IV fluid
ST elevation myocardial infarction (MI)	Chest pain, ECG criteria (see Box 6.1, p. 51)	Nil – treat immediately	Primary angioplasty or thrombolysis
Pulmonary embolism	Dyspnoea, hypoxia (especially with clear lung fields), chest pain, ↑JVP risk factors, ECG changes (p. 58)	CTPA if stable; urgent ECG if unstable; nil if peri-arrest	Thrombolysis
Cardiac tamponade	↑JVP, pulsus paradoxus, small QRS complexes on ECG	ECG	Pericardiocentesis

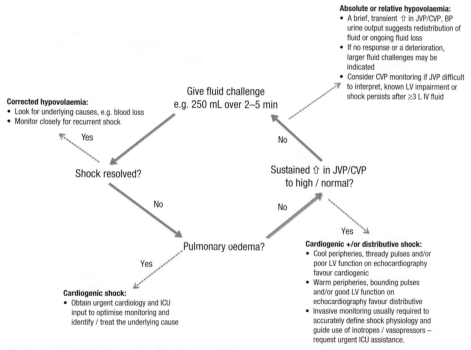

Fig. 30.1 Shock physiology: The cycle of assessment.

been shown to be useful in both diagnosing shock type and guiding response to treatment. In a spontaneously breathing, previously healthy person, variations in pleural cavity pressure with breathing are transmitted to the right atrium. This leads to a reduction of about 50% in IVC diameter on inspiration. Volume depleted spontaneously breathing patients will have a reduction of greater than 50% sometimes leading to complete collapse of the IVC on inspiration.

6 Suspect pelvic or intra-abdominal pathology?

Request urgent surgical review if you suspect acute abdominal or pelvic pathology. AAA or ruptured ectopic pregnancy require immediate intervention. Suspect ruptured AAA in patients >60 years, those with known AAA, a pulsatile abdominal mass or sudden-onset, severe abdominal/back; perform an immediate bedside USS, withhold fluid resuscitation if the patient is fully conscious and contact a vascular surgeon as an emergency.

Suspect ruptured ectopic pregnancy in any woman of child-bearing age with recent-onset lower abdominal pain, shoulder-tip pain or PV bleeding; perform an immediate bedside urine pregnancy test and consider bedside transabdominal USS to look for free fluid. A more extensive scan to locate a pregnancy can be performed by the Gynaecology team if the patient is stable. Other pointers to an underlying surgical cause include severe abdominal pain +/− tenderness/guarding/peritonism, air under the diaphragm on CXR or ↑amylase. Look for intestinal obstruction on abdominal X-ray in patients with abdominal pain/distension and repeated vomiting. Request an urgent surgical review. See Chapter 4 for further details.

7 Evidence of infection/inflammation or predisposition to infection?

Look for features of sepsis (p. 141). If present, perform a full septic screen, (Clinical tool, p. 142) to identify a likely source but do not delay antibiotics. Assume sepsis in any patient with immunocompromise until proven otherwise. See 'Surviving Sepsis' guidelines (http://www.survivingsepsis.org/GUIDELINES/Pages/default.aspx).

8 Suspect adrenal insufficiency?

Adrenal insufficiency is often overlooked, as many patients have fever and are assumed, at least initially, to have septic shock. Always consider the diagnosis and look for clinical/biochemical features. Useful indicators include prominent GI symptoms (almost always present but non-specific), pigmentation of recent scars, palmar creases and mucosal membranes, vitiligo, ↓Na^+, ↑K^+ and hypoglycaemia. Even a blood glucose at the low end of normal (3.5–4.5 mmol/L) suggests an inadequate 'stress response'. If you suspect adrenal insufficiency, send blood for a random cortisol level then treat with IV hydrocortisone without waiting for the results. A short ACTH (Synacthen) test may be helpful but takes 30 minutes to perform and should not delay empirical treatment in critically unwell patients. Remember that any patient taking systemic steroids for ≥3 months will have some adrenal suppression.

9 Distributive or cardiogenic pattern?

Identify the presence of relative or absolute hypovolaemia (see Fig. 30.1). Look for concealed sources of haemorrhage, dehydration (reduced skin turgor, dry mucous membranes) and causative/contributory factors, e.g. history of diarrhoea and vomiting, reduced intake, diuretics, antihypertensives.

Check for ketonuria and metabolic acidosis to exclude diabetic ketoacidosis. If the response to IV fluids suggests a distributive or cardiogenic element, involve ICU, institute appropriate (invasive) monitoring and consider urgent echocardiography.

30

Transient loss of consciousness (T-LOC) presents a particular diagnostic challenge. The event has usually resolved by the time of assessment and since critical elements of the history are unknown to the patient, witness accounts are crucial. Risk stratification of patients may identify those at risk of cardiac or arrhythmia-related syncope requiring admission for further investigation and those at low risk (often with a diagnosis of reflex or orthostatic syncope) who can be evaluated as outpatients.

Syncope

'Syncope' denotes T-LOC resulting from global cerebral hypoperfusion, typically associated with a BP <60 mmHg for ≥6 seconds. It is characterized by rapid onset, short duration and spontaneous complete recovery.

Syncope can be divided into four aetiological subtypes:

- Arrhythmia-related – due to transient compromise of cardiac output by a tachy- or bradyarrhythmia, e.g. ventricular tachycardia, complete heart block.
- Cardiac – due to structural heart disease, especially left ventricular outflow obstruction, e.g. severe aortic stenosis, hypertrophic obstructive cardiomyopathy. Acute pulmonary embolism (PE) or aortic dissection may also cause syncope.
- Orthostatic – due to failure of homeostatic maintenance of BP on standing, e.g. caused by antihypertensive medications or autonomic neuropathy.
- Reflex (neurally mediated) – reflex vasodilatation and/or bradycardia occurs in response to a particular 'trigger', e.g. 'vasovagal' or 'carotid sinus' syncope.

Seizure

Disordered electrical activity affecting the whole brain ('generalized' seizure) can lead to T-LOC. This may be primary or result from a focal (partial) seizure that spreads to the whole brain (secondary generalization). In the absence of secondary generalization, partial seizures may cause altered consciousness (complex partial seizures) without T-LOC. Epilepsy is the tendency to have recurrent seizures. Factors that may provoke seizures in patients with epilepsy are shown in Box 31.1.

Hypoglycaemia

Hypoglycaemia may cause impairment of consciousness that resolves with prompt correction of capillary blood glucose. Most cases are iatrogenic, from treatment of diabetes with insulin or sulphonylurea drugs. Causes of 'spontaneous' hypoglycaemia include alcohol, liver failure, insulinoma and adrenal insufficiency.

Functional disorders (apparent T-LOC)

'Pseudoseizure' and 'pseudosyncope' are terms used to describe episodes that resemble seizure and syncope respectively but do not

---

Box 31.1 Trigger factors for seizures

- Alcohol excess or withdrawal
- Recreational drug misuse
- Sleep deprivation
- Physical/mental exhaustion
- Intercurrent infection
- Metabolic disturbance ($\downarrow Na^+$, $\downarrow Mg^{2+}$, $\downarrow Ca^{2+}$, uraemia, liver failure)
- Non-compliance with medication or drug interaction
- Flickering lights

Box 31.2 Atypical features in apparent T-LOC

- Prolonged duration (>5 minutes) of episodes
- Eyes closed during episode
- Numerous attacks in single day
- Purposeful movements during apparent period of T-LOC
- Established diagnosis of other functional disorder, e.g. chronic fatigue syndrome

---

have an underlying somatic mechanism, i.e. no epileptiform activity or cerebral hypoperfusion. They can present major diagnostic difficulty and may require specialist assessment. Features that may raise suspicion of a functional aetiology for symptoms over true loss of consciousness are shown in Box 31.2.

Other causes

For clinical presentations not suggestive of either tonic-clonic seizure or syncope, consider rarer causes such as cataplexy, narcolepsy and atypical seizures, e.g. absence, as well as conditions which may mimic T-LOC, including falls, functional disorders, drug/alcohol intoxication. Transient ischaemic attacks present with focal neurological signs and symptoms and very rarely cause T-LOC. Concussion is a common cause of T-LOC associated with head trauma.

31

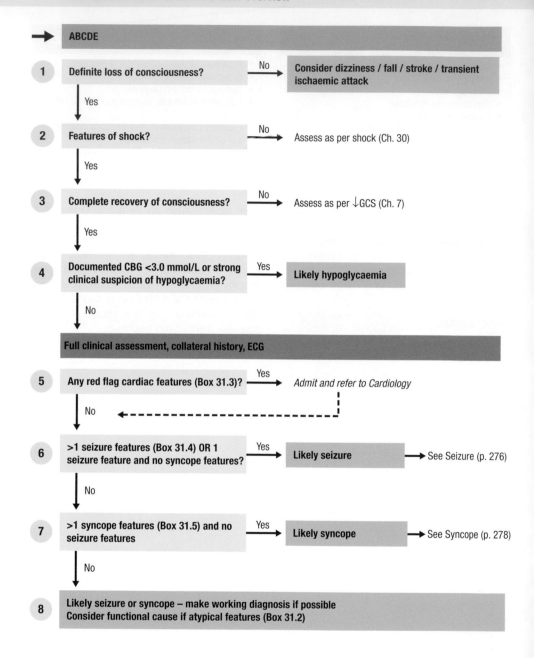

1   Definite loss of consciousness?

In the absence of a clear witness account this may be difficult to establish – ask the patient to recount the events in as much detail as possible.

Assume T-LOC if:

- a witness confirms a period of unresponsiveness
- the patient describes 'waking up' or 'coming to' on the ground, especially if there is no recollection of falling
- there are facial injuries (most conscious patients can protect their face as they fall).

T-LOC is unlikely if:

- there was no loss of postural tone
- the patient recalls landing on the ground
- a witness account suggests interaction with or awareness of the environment throughout the episode.

2   Features of shock?

Syncope may be a manifestation of major haemo-dynamic compromise, e.g. massive PE, severe GI bleed. If you find evidence of shock (see Box 30.1, p. 267) during the ABCDE assessment, evaluate further as per Chapter 30.

3   Complete recovery of consciousness?

The diagnostic pathway below is appropriate only for a transient episode of loss of consciousness. If there is evidence of persistently ↓GCS during the ABCDE assessment, evaluate in the first instance as described in Chapter 7.

4   Documented CBG <3.0 mmol/L or strong clinical suspicion of hypoglycaemia?

Attributing an episode of reduced consciousness to hypoglycaemia requires:

- demonstration of low blood glucose in association with T-LOC
- recovery with restoration of normoglycaemia.

Corroborate a low CBG with a formal lab glucose measurement whenever feasible but do not wait for the result to initiate treatment. Patients may have had corrective treatment prior to assessment without a CBG, e.g. from ambulance crew. In these circumstances, suspect hypoglycaemia if the episode resolved with administration of carbohydrate/glucagon and was preceded by symptoms of autonomic activation (sweating, trembling, hunger)/neuroglycopenia (poor concentration, confusion, incoordination) or occurred in a patient taking insulin or a sulphonylurea.

5   Any red flag cardiac features (see Box 31.3)?

Always exclude a serious underlying cardiac cause for T-LOC if any of the features in Box 31.3 is present. Continue through the diagnostic pathway but admit the patient to hospital and discuss with a cardiologist.

6   >1 seizure feature (see Box 31.4) OR 1 seizure feature and no syncope features?

Differentiating between seizure and syncope is a key step in the assessment process. Features that strongly suggest seizure are listed in Box 31.4. Descriptions of 'jerking', 'twitching' or 'fitting' are unhelpful since 'seizure-like' movements may occur in up to 90% of syncopal episodes. In contrast to seizure, the abnormal movements in syncope are usually non-rhythmic and brief (<15 seconds).

Box 31.3 Red flag cardiac features

- T-LOC during exertion
- Severe valvular heart disease, coronary artery disease or cardiomyopathy
- Family history of unexplained premature sudden death
- Previous ventricular arrhythmia or high risk for ventricular arrhythmia, e.g. prior MI or ventricular surgery
- Sustained or non-sustained ventricular tachycardia on telemetry
- High-risk ECG abnormality:
  - bifascicular or trifascicular block (see Fig. 31.3)
  - new T wave or ST segment changes (see Box 6.1, p. 51)
  - sinus bradycardia <50 bpm or sinus pause >3 seconds
  - second-degree AV block or complete heart block (see Figs 31.1 and 31.2)
  - evidence of pre-excitation (see Fig. 26.2, p. 233)
  - marked QT interval prolongation, e.g. QTc >500 milliseconds
  - Brugada pattern: RBBB with ST elevation in leads V_1–V_3 (see Fig. 31.5)

31

The episode of T-LOC is highly likely to have been a seizure if >1 of the features in Box 31.4 are present. Seizure is also likely if any of these features are present, and there are no specific pointers to syncope (Box 31.5). In both cases, proceed to 'Seizure' (p. 276).

7 **≥1 syncope features (see Box 31.5) and no seizure features**

Suspect syncope if any of the features in Box 31.5 and none of those in Box 31.4 are present – proceed to 'Syncope' (p. 278).

8 **Likely seizure or syncope – make working diagnosis if possible. Consider functional cause if atypical features (see Box 31.2)**

Where differentiation between seizure and syncope is not straightforward, other clinical features may be helpful: amnesia for events before and after the episode, and headache or aching muscles after the episode suggest a seizure diagnosis; previous episodes of pre-syncope, witnessed pallor during T-LOC, known cardiovascular disease and an abnormal ECG favour syncope. Urinary incontinence is not a useful discriminating feature. Consider a functional aetiology if atypical features are present (see Box 31.2). Have a low threshold for specialist input if the cause remains unclear.

Box 31.4 Clinical features strongly suggestive of seizure

- T-LOC preceded by typical aura, e.g. unusual smell, 'rising' sensation in abdomen, déjà vu
- A witness account of abnormal tonic-clonic limb movements that are:
  - coarse and rhythmic
  - maintained for >30 seconds (ask witness to demonstrate movements)
- A witness account of head-turning to one side, unusual posturing, cyanosis or automatisms such as chewing or lip-smacking during the episode
- Severely bitten, bleeding tongue or bitten lateral border of tongue
- A prolonged period (>5 minutes) of confusion or drowsiness after the episode

Box 31.5 Clinical features strongly suggestive of syncope

- T-LOC preceded by chest pain, palpitation, dyspnoea, light-headedness or typical 'pre-syncopal' prodrome, e.g. lightheadedness, warmth, nausea, vomiting
- T-LOC after standing up, after prolonged standing, during exertion or following a typical precipitant:
  - unpleasant sight, sound, smell or pain
  - venepuncture
  - micturition
  - cough
  - large meal
- Brief duration of T-LOC (<1 minute)
- Rapid return of clear-headedness after T-LOC

31

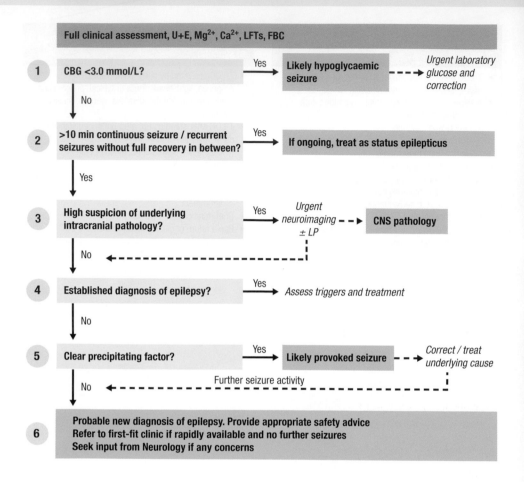

1   CBG <3.0 mmol/L?

Consider hypoglycaemia at the outset because it:

- is easily identified and corrected
- will cause permanent neurological damage if not corrected
- needs to be excluded prior to assessment for other causes.

If CBG <3.0 mmol/L, assess and treat as described above.

2   >10 min continuous seizure/recurrent seizures without full recovery in between?

Status epilepticus is a medical emergency requiring urgent intervention. Formal diagnosis requires >30 minutes of continuous seizure activity or repeated seizures without full recovery in between, but a lower time threshold facilitates early recognition and action.

Provide appropriate anticonvulsant therapy, e.g. IV diazepam, and supportive measures concurrently with clinical assessment. Rapidly exclude or correct reversible factors (see below) and seek urgent input from ICU ± the Neurology team.

3   High suspicion of underlying intracranial pathology?

Seizure may be a manifestation of important underlying intracranial pathology, such as

Box 31.6 Indications for urgent neuroimaging in seizure

- Status epilepticus
- Focal or partial onset seizure
- Confusion, $\downarrow$GCS or focal neurological signs >30 minutes post-fit
- Recent head injury
- Acute severe headache preceding seizure
- Known malignancy with potential for brain metastases
- Immunosuppression (especially HIV)
- Meningism, fever or persistent headache and suspicion of CNS infection
- Anticoagulated or bleeding disorder

haemorrhage, infarction, infection or space-occupying lesion.

Arrange urgent neuroimaging, usually CT, if the patient is at risk of these pathologies (Box 31.6). Consider neuroimaging to exclude new intracranial pathology in any patient with known epilepsy with a change in seizure type/pattern without an apparent precipitating factor.

Provided there are no contraindications, perform a lumbar puncture (p. 170), following CT, if any features suggest CNS infection, e.g. fever, meningism, rash.

4   Established diagnosis of epilepsy?

In patients with known epilepsy, address all factors that may have lowered seizure threshold (see Box 31.1) or triggered the event. Measurement of anticonvulsant drug levels is not routinely indicated but consider it if there has been a recent change in medication or you suspect non-compliance.

5   Clear precipitating factor?

Important causes of seizure in adults without epilepsy include: alcohol (excess or withdrawal), recreational drug misuse, e.g. cocaine, amphetamines, drug overdose, e.g. theophylline, tricyclic antidepressants, severe metabolic disturbance $\downarrow$Na$^+$, $\downarrow$Mg^{2+}, $\downarrow$Ca^{2+} and CNS infection. Look for all of these factors and refer for specialist neurological evaluation (see below) if none is evident.

6   Probable new diagnosis of epilepsy. Refer to a neurologist as inpatient or outpatient

Admit any patient with repeated seizures or a significant causative factor that requires inpatient treatment. Consider early discharge only if patients have fully recovered, exhibit no neurological abnormalities and have a responsible adult to accompany and stay with them. Seek advice from a neurologist if you have any concerns.

Arrange neuroimaging for all first-fit episodes in patients >20 years or with focal features. Depending on local resources, imaging may be performed as an outpatient – provided there are no indications for urgent imaging (see Box 31.6) and a 'first-fit' follow-up service is available. Further investigation may not be required in patients with a pre-existing diagnosis of epilepsy who have fully recovered following a typical, uncomplicated fit.

Prior to discharge, inform all patients of statutory driving regulations (in the UK see www.dft.gov.uk/dvla/medical/ataglance.aspx) and advise them to avoid activities where T-LOC may be dangerous, e.g. swimming, operating machinery, cycling, etc.

31

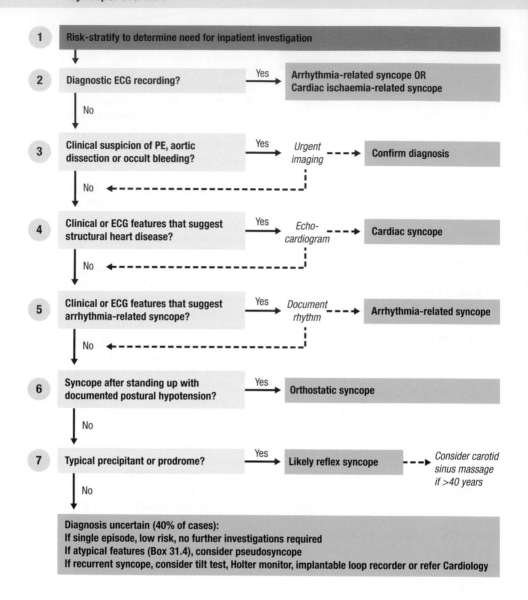

1 Risk-stratify to determine need for inpatient investigation

2 Diagnostic ECG recording? — Yes → Arrhythmia-related syncope OR Cardiac ischaemia-related syncope

No

3 Clinical suspicion of PE, aortic dissection or occult bleeding? — Yes → *Urgent imaging* ---→ Confirm diagnosis

No

4 Clinical or ECG features that suggest structural heart disease? — Yes → *Echo-cardiogram* ---→ Cardiac syncope

No

5 Clinical or ECG features that suggest arrhythmia-related syncope? — Yes → *Document rhythm* ---→ Arrhythmia-related syncope

No

6 Syncope after standing up with documented postural hypotension? — Yes → Orthostatic syncope

No

7 Typical precipitant or prodrome? — Yes → Likely reflex syncope ---→ *Consider carotid sinus massage if >40 years*

No

Diagnosis uncertain (40% of cases):
If single episode, low risk, no further investigations required
If atypical features (Box 31.4), consider pseudosyncope
If recurrent syncope, consider tilt test, Holter monitor, implantable loop recorder or refer Cardiology

1 Risk-stratify to determine need for inpatient investigation

Admit all syncopal patients with red flag cardiac features (see Box 31.3) and discuss promptly with the Cardiology team. Clinical decision rules and risk prediction tools, e.g. the San Francisco Syncope Rule may be useful, but lack sensitivity and specificity. Consider discharge with outpatient investigation (preferably in a syncope clinic if available) if the patient has recovered fully and has no other medical problems or no **red flag** features; otherwise, admit for a period of observation and investigation (monitoring +/− ambulatory monitoring and ECG). Syncope observation units, if available, facilitate rapid investigation while the patient is under observation for 6 to 24 hours.

2 Diagnostic ECG recording?

Mobitz type II 2nd degree atrioventricular (AV) block (Fig. 31.1), complete heart block (Fig. 31.2), prolonged pauses, ventricular tachycardia or very rapid supraventricular tachycardia (>180/min) on the presenting ECG or telemetry establish an arrhythmic cause of syncope. Arrhythmia-related syncope is also highly likely with persistent sinus bradycardia <40 bpm, alternating left and right bundle branch block (LBBB and RBBB) or pacemaker malfunction with pauses.

ECG evidence of acute ischaemia suggests an arrhythmia secondary to ischaemia, e.g. ventricular tachycardia, or cardiac ischaemia-related syncope. Acute coronary syndrome (ACS) is unlikely in the absence of chest pain or ECG evidence of ACS.

Discuss urgently with a cardiologist if any of the above features is present.

3 Clinical suspicion of PE, aortic dissection or occult bleeding?

These conditions may present with syncope, but this is rarely the predominant symptom. Exclude PE and aortic dissection if syncope occurs in the context of sudden-onset chest pain with no obvious alternative explanation. Also consider PE in syncopal patients with dyspnoea, hypoxia, evidence of DVT or major thromboembolic risk factors. Suspect aortic dissection if there is a new early diastolic murmur, pulse deficit or widened mediastinum on CXR (see Ch. 6). Consider subarachnoid haemorrhage if there is associated headache (see Ch. 18) and ruptured ectopic pregnancy or abdominal aortic aneurysm if there is abdominal pain (see Ch. 4).

4 Clinical or ECG features that suggest structural heart disease?

ECG may identify 'structural' causes of cardiac syncope, e.g. severe aortic stenosis, hypertrophic cardiomyopathy, prolapsing atrial myxoma or conditions that predispose to arrhythmia, e.g. severe left ventricular (LV) systolic impairment.

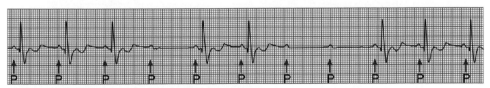

Fig. 31.1 Mobitz type II atrioventricular block. (From Boon NA, Colledge NR, Walker BR. Davidson's Principles & Practice of Medicine, 20th edn. Edinburgh: Churchill Livingstone, 2006.)

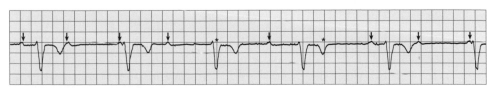

Fig. 31.2 Complete heart block. Arrows indicate P waves. (From Douglas G, Nicol F, Robertson C. Macleod's Clinical Examination, 12th edn. Edinburgh: Churchill Livingstone, 2009.)

31

Request an ECG if there is exertional syncope, a family history of sudden unexplained death (especially <40 years), a new murmur, clinical features of cardiac failure, or (unless performed recently) a history of myocardial infarction (MI), cardiomyopathy, valvular heart disease or congenital heart disease. Discuss with a cardiologist if any relevant abnormalities are detected.

5 Clinical or ECG features that suggest arrhythmia-related syncope?

Suspect an arrhythmic aetiology for syncope in the following circumstances:

- sudden-onset palpitation rapidly followed by syncope
- syncope during exertion or while supine
- previous MI or significant structural heart disease, e.g. cardiomyopathy, aortic stenosis
- any of the following ECG abnormalities:
  - LBBB (see Fig. 6.5, p. 55), bi- or trifascicular block (Fig. 31.3)
  - sinus bradycardia <50 bpm
  - Mobitz type I 2nd degree AV block (Fig. 31.4)
  - sinus pause >3 seconds

- evidence of pre-excitation (see Fig. 26.2, p. 233)
- prolonged QT interval (QTc >440 milliseconds in men or >460 milliseconds in women)
- Brugada pattern: RBBB with ST elevation in leads V_1–V_3 (Fig. 31.5)
- features of arrhythmogenic right ventricular cardiomyopathy: negative T waves in leads V_1–V_3 and epsilon waves
- pathological Q wave.

- any ECG abnormality or history of cardiovascular disorder in the absence of a typical prodrome or precipitant for reflex or orthostatic syncope.

The correlation of a syncopal episode with a documented rhythm disturbance is the gold standard for diagnosis of arrhythmia-mediated syncope. This is frequently challenging, particularly when syncopal episodes are infrequent. The choice of investigation and degree of persistence depend on the risk of life-threatening arrhythmia and frequency of syncope.

Admit patients with red flag cardiac features (see Box 31.3) immediately for continuous inpatient ECG monitoring. Arrange Holter (1 to 7 day

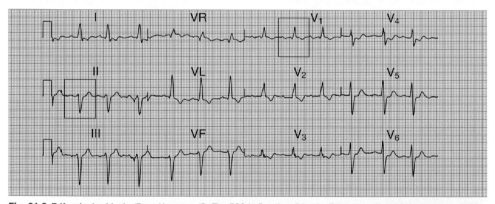

Fig. 31.3 Trifascicular block. (From Hampton JR. The ECG in Practice, 5th edn. Edinburgh: Churchill Livingstone, 2008.)

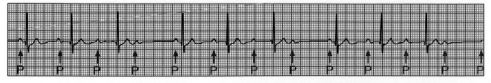

Fig. 31.4 Mobitz type I atrioventricular block. (From Boon NA, Colledge NR, Walker BR. Davidson's Principles & Practice of Medicine, 20th edn. Edinburgh: Churchill Livingstone, 2006.)

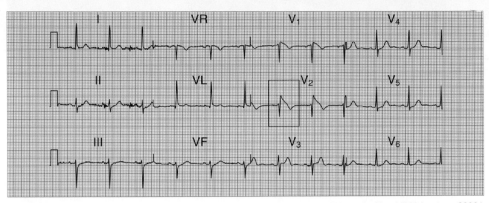

Fig. 31.5 Brugada syndrome. (From Hampton JR. The ECG in Practice, 5th edn. Edinburgh: Churchill Livingstone, 2008.)

tape) or ambulatory patch monitoring (14 days) if symptoms occur relatively frequently. Consider an event recorder (external or implanted) if there is a high suspicion of arrhythmia but episodes are infrequent or prove difficult to capture by other methods.

6 Syncope after standing up with documented postural hypotension?

Diagnose orthostatic syncope if there is:

- a history of light-headedness shortly after standing, followed by brief T-LOC
- a documented postural BP drop (of ≥20 mmHg in systolic BP or ≥10 mmHg in diastolic BP within 3 minutes of moving from lying to standing).

In other circumstances, it may be difficult to distinguish orthostatic from reflex syncope, e.g. when symptoms occur with prolonged standing.

Look for an underlying cause of postural hypotension. In severe form it may reflect fluid loss, e.g. major haemorrhage or severe dehydration. Other causes include Parkinson's syndromes, autonomic neuropathy and drugs, e.g. antihypertensives, vasodilators (especially sublingual nitroglycerine) and diuretics, particularly in the elderly.

7 Typical precipitant or prodrome?

A clear precipitating trigger, e.g. intense emotion, venepuncture or prolonged standing (vasovagal syncope) or coughing, sneezing or micturition (situational syncope), together with typical prodromal symptoms, strongly suggests reflex syncope, especially in patients with no ECG or clinical evidence to suggest structural heart disease or arrhythmia. Consider tilt-table testing in cases of diagnostic doubt. Carotid sinus hypersensitivity is a form of reflex syncope and is usually diagnosed with carotid sinus massage (CSM). CSM should be avoided in patients with a history of cerebrovascular accident/transient ischaemic attack or a carotid bruit, and requires continuous ECG monitoring; it is diagnostic if syncope is reproduced in the presence of asystole lasting >3 seconds.

31

Urinary incontinence (UI), the involuntary leakage of urine, affects 15% of women and 10% of men aged >65 years. Treatment or amelioration of UI can greatly enhance quality of life but it tends to be under-reported and under-recognized in clinical practice. UI is frequently multifactorial, particularly in frail elderly patients, so seek to identify all potentially modifiable contributing factors. Take care also to evaluate the impact of symptoms on daily activities and quality of life.

Stress incontinence

Urine leakage is provoked by an increase in intra-abdominal pressure, such as during coughing, sneezing, effort or exertion. It is usually due to insufficient urethral support from the pelvic floor muscles but can also be caused by intrinsic weakness of the urethral sphincter, e.g. post-pelvic surgery. Stress incontinence is far more common in females than males and most often relates to obstetric trauma. It frequently accompanies pelvic organ prolapse and may also occur with atrophic vaginitis. Stress incontinence in males is usually a complication of prostatectomy.

Urge incontinence

Urine leakage occurs due to intense bladder contraction and is preceded by the sensation of urgency. This can result from neurological disease, e.g. multiple sclerosis, spina bifida but is more often due to intrinsic bladder activity ('detrusor overactivity'). Lower UTI may produce acute transient urge incontinence.

Mixed incontinence

A combination of stress and urge incontinence; treatment should be aimed at the more dominant aspect.

Overflow incontinence

The involuntary passage of urine from an overfull bladder which may or may not be accompanied by a sensation of urgency. Incomplete bladder emptying may result from:

- bladder outflow obstruction: benign prostatic hyperplasia (BPH), prostate cancer, bladder tumour, urethral stenosis, severe constipation
- bladder atonia in neurological disease, e.g. cauda equina or conus medullaris compression, autonomic neuropathy
- drugs with anticholinergic effects such as antipsychotics or antidepressants.

Treatment of overflow incontinence is with relief of obstruction (e.g. resection of prostate cancer, medical treatment of BPH) or intermittent catheterization.

Box 32.1 Aggravating factors

- Polydipsia/polyuria including: poorly controlled diabetes mellitus, diabetes insipidus, hypercalcaemia, psychogenic polydipsia
- Caffeine
- Alcohol overuse/misuse
- Mobility problems (see Ch. 24)
- Visual impairment
- Obesity
- Respiratory disease
- Smoking
- Cognitive impairment, e.g. delirium or dementia (see Ch. 8)

Box 32.2 Medications potentially aggravating incontinence

- Diuretics
- Drugs with cholinergic effects[1]
- Drugs with anticholinergic effects[2]
- Alpha-agonists
- Calcium channel blockers
- Beta-agonists
- Sedatives
- Lithium

[1]May cause or aggravate urge incontinence.
[2]May cause or aggravate overflow incontinence.

Continuous incontinence

Constant leakage of urine throughout the day (and night) suggests the presence of a fistula between the bladder and the urethra or vagina. Underlying causes include urogynaecological cancer, previous pelvic surgery/radiotherapy or obstetric trauma.

Functional/multifactorial incontinence

This occurs when the person is aware of the need to urinate, but for one or more physical or cognitive reasons are unable to get to the toilet in time. Potential contributing factors are shown in Box 32.1 and aggravating medications in Box 32.2.

32

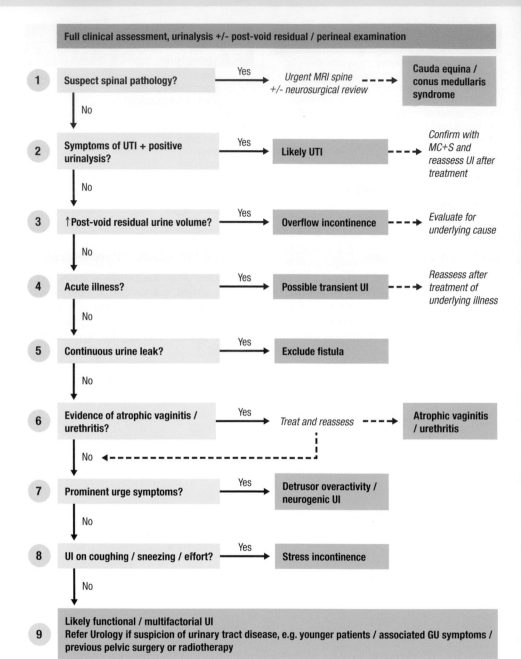

Full clinical assessment, urinalysis +/- post-void residual / perineal examination

1 Suspect spinal pathology? — Yes → *Urgent MRI spine +/- neurosurgical review* ---→ **Cauda equina / conus medullaris syndrome**

No ↓

2 Symptoms of UTI + positive urinalysis? — Yes → **Likely UTI** ---→ *Confirm with MC+S and reassess UI after treatment*

No ↓

3 ↑Post-void residual urine volume? — Yes → **Overflow incontinence** ---→ *Evaluate for underlying cause*

No ↓

4 Acute illness? — Yes → **Possible transient UI** ---→ *Reassess after treatment of underlying illness*

No ↓

5 Continuous urine leak? — Yes → **Exclude fistula**

No ↓

6 Evidence of atrophic vaginitis / urethritis? — Yes → *Treat and reassess* ---→ **Atrophic vaginitis / urethritis**

No ↓

7 Prominent urge symptoms? — Yes → **Detrusor overactivity / neurogenic UI**

No ↓

8 UI on coughing / sneezing / effort? — Yes → **Stress incontinence**

No ↓

9 **Likely functional / multifactorial UI**
Refer Urology if suspicion of urinary tract disease, e.g. younger patients / associated GU symptoms / previous pelvic surgery or radiotherapy

1 Suspect spinal pathology?

Arrange urgent spinal MRI to exclude cauda equina/conus medullaris syndrome in any patient with recent onset of UI associated with lower limb weakness, altered perianal/perineal sensation (does toilet paper feel normal when wiping?), faecal incontinence or new low back or leg pain. Seek immediate neurosurgical/neurology input if concerning imaging features or unexplained neurological findings.

2 Symptoms of UTI and positive urinalysis?

Suspect UTI if there is a short history of UI accompanied by fever, dysuria, frequency or malodourous urine; the absence of leucocytes and nitrites on dipstick makes UTI very unlikely. If dipstick testing is positive or there is strong clinical suspicion, send an MSU for culture; treat confirmed infection then re-evaluate to ensure that UI resolves. Evaluate for prostatic disease (see Step 3) in men with >1 UTI and arrange renal tract imaging (USS initially) in women with >2 UTI; in both cases consider referral to Urology for further specialist investigation.

3 ↑Post-void residual (PVR) urine volume?

Measure PVR in all patients with unexplained UI using a bladder USS scan (correlates well with urinary catheter volumes). Suspect overflow incontinence due to incomplete bladder emptying if the PVR is >100 mL (or >50 mL in younger patients). In men, ask about other symptoms of bladder outlet obstruction, e.g. hesitancy, poor stream, check a PSA (prior to rectal exam) and evaluate the prostate by rectal examination. Exclude constipation/faecal impaction as an underlying cause, particularly in frail elderly patients, with rectal exam +/– abdominal X-ray. Seek a neurological opinion if there is a history of neurological disorder or associated symptoms/signs of neurological disease, e.g. lower limb weakness. Otherwise, consider CT abdomen/pelvis and refer to Urology for further assessment and investigation, e.g. cystoscopy.

4 Acute illness?

Suspect transient UI as a non-specific manifestation of illness in elderly patients with frailty or multimorbidity who are acutely unwell, have experienced an abrupt decline in function, mobility or cognition or who have evidence of newly-deranged physiology. Seek and treat the underlying illness then re-evaluate continence once the patient has returned to baseline status.

5 Continuous urine leak?

Suspect a fistula between the bladder (or ureter) and the vagina/urethra if UI is continuous rather than intermittent – especially if there is a history of previous pelvic surgery/radiotherapy or a complex obstetric history. Request an IV urogram and refer to Urology for specialist assessment.

6 Evidence of atrophic vaginitis/urethritis?

Suspect this as a cause of UI (usually stress-type) in postmenopausal women with symptoms of urethral irritation (e.g. burning, frequency, painful intercourse) but negative urine dipstick and culture or with mucosal pallor or erythema on perineal examination. Reassess symptoms after treatment with topical oestrogen for at least 14 days. Continue to seek other causes of UI unless symptoms fully resolve.

32

Box 32.3 IQ questionnaire

1. During the past 3 months, have you leaked urine (even a small amount)?
   - Yes – move to question 2
   - No – stop questionnaire.
2. During the past 3 months did you leak urine:
   - when performing physical activity (coughing, sneezing, lifting, exercising)?
   - when felt urge to empty your bladder, but not able to get to the toilet in time?
   - neither of the above circumstances.
3. During the past 3 months did you leak urine MOST often:
   - when performing physical activity (coughing, sneezing, lifting, exercising)? **Stress incontinence predominant**
   - when felt urge to empty your bladder, but not able to get to the toilet in time? **Urge incontinence predominant**
   - neither of the above circumstances. **Other cause** (neither urge incontinence or stress incontinence)
   - both of the above circumstances equally as often. **Mixed urinary incontinence**.

---

7 Prominent urge symptoms?

Evaluate as urge incontinence if the patient reports a clear and consistent history of urgency to void prior to leakage of urine. Consider using the 3 IQ questionnaire (Box 32.3) or a voiding diary if the history is unclear or the pattern of UI is variable.

Ensure you have excluded urinary retention: repeat post-void bladder scan if initial results equivocal and perform post-void catheterization if there is a strong clinical suspicion. Consider a neurogenic aetiology and obtain specialist input in patients with a history of neurological disorder (e.g. multiple sclerosis, spina bifida) or associated neurological signs or symptoms.

In the absence of urinary retention or neurological features, assume detrusor overactivity as the likely diagnosis. Refer for specialist urological assessment, e.g. urodynamic studies if the diagnosis is uncertain or symptoms fail to respond to standard treatments.

8 UI on coughing/sneezing/effort?

Evaluate as stress incontinence if urine leakage consistently coincides with manoeuvres that increase intra-abdominal pressure, e.g. coughing, sneezing, laughing, sitting/standing-up – especially if there is no associated sensation of urgency. Where the history is unclear, inspect for leakage of urine while asking the patient to cough or, again, consider using the 3 IQ questionnaire (see Box 32.3) or a voiding diary.

Refer to Gynaecology if there is uterine/vaginal prolapse. Consider potentially aggravating factors such chronic lung disease (cough) or medications (see Box 32.2). In women with uncomplicated stress UI, reassess after simple measures such as pelvic muscle retraining but consider surgical evaluation if symptoms remain severe. Refer male patients with stress UI for Urology assessment.

9 Likely functional/multifactorial UI. Specialist urological assessment in selected cases

In frail or elderly patients UI is very often due to a constellation of factors that prevent timely toileting (functional incontinence) rather than a single specific urinary tract pathology. Consider specialist urological assessment/investigation if there are associated genitourinary (GU) symptoms such as haematuria or pelvic pain, a complex obstetric history, previous pelvic surgery or radiotherapy, or where functional incontinence seems unlikely, e.g. younger patients or those without significant comorbidity.

Otherwise, systematically address all factors that may be contributing to UI (see Box 32.1). Review medications (see Box 32.2) and amend where necessary. Establish whether the patient has awareness of the need to void. If not, try prompted toileting (particularly after diuretics). If the patient has awareness of the need to void but can't reach the toilet in time, assess mobility (see Ch. 24) and consider the need for walking aids, a downstairs toilet or commode. Evaluate the effectiveness of continence aids such as pads, urisheath or commode. Finally, determine the level of distress caused by symptoms and the overall impact on quality of life. Consider referral for comprehensive geriatric assessment.

Vaginal bleeding is a distressing symptom with a wide variety of potential causes. These may be categorized broadly according to the reproductive age of the patient, their pregnancy status, the duration of symptoms and any associated features. Examine the patient carefully to identify rectal, urethral, vaginal and cervical sources of blood; if necessary, place a urinary catheter to differentiate between vaginal bleeding and haematuria. Be sensitive and empathetic, but ensure that the assessment is thorough. Arrange urgent gynaecological/obstetric review in any patient with major PV bleeding.

Pregnancy-related bleeding

First trimester

Vaginal bleeding in the first trimester is very common. Bleeding may be due to miscarriage or ectopic pregnancy, or may have a benign explanation in the presence of an ongoing intrauterine pregnancy. Miscarriages may be threatened (the foetus is still viable), partial (non-viable products of conception remain in the uterus) or complete (products of conception have been passed). In miscarriage, patients may describe a loss of pregnancy-related symptoms. Miscarriages and ectopic pregnancies are often associated with abdominal pain. Miscarriages typically present with central, crampy, menstrual-like lower abdominal pain. In ectopic pregnancy, the pain is unilateral and constant since there may be bleeding into the peritoneal cavity causing peritoneal irritation. Unilateral lower abdominal pain in females of reproductive age (regardless of PV bleeding) should be assumed to be an ectopic pregnancy until ruled out.

Second and third trimester

Bleeding during the second and third trimesters is abnormal and must be investigated. Serious and potentially life-threatening causes include placenta praevia (a low-lying placenta with subsequent bleeding from the placental edge) and placental abruption (bleeding due to placental separation from the uterus; 1% pregnancies). Placenta praevia is diagnosed on USS and causes painless bleeding. Placental abruption is essentially a clinical diagnosis based on abdominal pain and vaginal bleeding, since the absence of a retro-placental haematoma on USS does not exclude the diagnosis. Be aware that placental abruption may be 'concealed' – with no/minimal visible PV bleeding. In this situation, blood loss may still be significant but remains contained within the uterine cavity. The patient will have haemodynamic instability out of keeping with the apparently absent/small volume PV bleeding together with a 'woody hard' uterus due to blood accumulation. The treatment for placental abruption is delivery of the baby and placenta.

Heavy menstrual bleeding

Heavy menstrual bleeding (HMB; previously known as menorrhagia) may be defined objectively or subjectively. The objective definition is blood loss greater than 80 mL in a cycle, but in practice diagnosis is based on women subjectively reporting using more tampons/pads than usual, using pads and tampons together or soaking through protection onto clothing.

Pathological causes of HMB may be structural or non-structural. Structural causes include fibroids (leiomyomas) (20–30%), endometrial and cervical polyps (5–10%), adenomyosis (5%) and malignancy or hyperplasia. Non-structural causes include coagulopathy (e.g. von Willebrand disease, anticoagulants), ovulatory dysfunction, endometrial disorders (e.g. endometritis), iatrogenic causes (e.g. contraceptives, tamoxifen). After investigation, approximately 40–60% of patients with HMB have no identifiable uterine, endocrine, haematological or infective pathology.

Intermenstrual bleeding

Intermenstrual bleeding is usually low volume. The pattern of bleeding may be related to contact such as postcoitus, or intermenstrual bleeding with no clear precipitants. Causes of contact bleeding are typically cervical, such as cervical ectropion, cervical cancer, cervical polyps or infections (typically chlamydia but also gonorrhoea). Non-contact, intermenstrual bleeding has a wide range of causes. There is a continuum between intermenstrual and irregular menstrual bleeding that can be difficult to differentiate. However, in many instances, the treatment is similar. Causes include endometrial lesions (cancer, polyps), fibroids (although more commonly cause HMB), contraceptives, sexually transmitted infections and, rarely, medical causes such as coagulopathies and hypothyroidism. Oral contraception and intrauterine device contraception may cause abnormal menstrual bleeding.

Uncommonly, low-volume mid-cycle bleeding may be due to ovulation (when the Graafian follicle ruptures and hormonal balance becomes predominantly progesterone-based, resulting in a shed of blood from the endometrium). This is associated with acute, unilateral, lower abdominal pain (mittelschmerz, 'middle pain') lasting hours to days, which is often the presenting problem.

Postmenopausal bleeding

Postmenopausal bleeding (PMB) is defined as vaginal bleeding >12 months after the last menstrual cycle. Up to 10% of women with PMB have endometrial cancer. Other malignant causes include cervical, vaginal, vulval and, rarely, ovarian cancer. Atrophic vaginitis with contact bleeding due to postmenopausal dryness, pessary devices or intercourse is a diagnosis of exclusion.

33

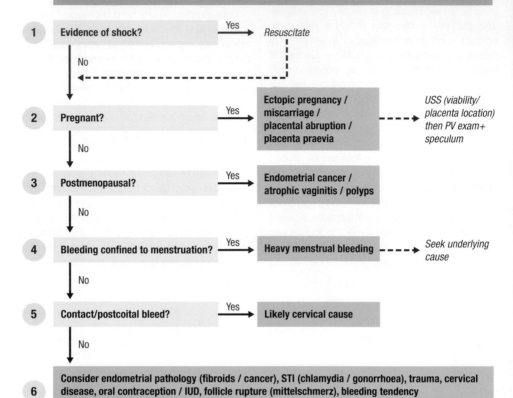

Full clinical assessment + vaginal examination (see Clinical tool)

1 Evidence of shock? — Yes → *Resuscitate*

No

2 Pregnant? — Yes → Ectopic pregnancy / miscarriage / placental abruption / placenta praevia ---- → *USS (viability/ placenta location) then PV exam+ speculum*

No

3 Postmenopausal? — Yes → Endometrial cancer / atrophic vaginitis / polyps

No

4 Bleeding confined to menstruation? — Yes → Heavy menstrual bleeding ---- → *Seek underlying cause*

No

5 Contact/postcoital bleed? — Yes → Likely cervical cause

No

6 Consider endometrial pathology (fibroids / cancer), STI (chlamydia / gonorrhoea), trauma, cervical disease, oral contraception / IUD, follicle rupture (mittelschmerz), bleeding tendency (e.g. coagulopathy)

Clinical tool
Examination of the female genitalia

Vaginal examination is not routine but is often indicated if inflammatory or neoplastic disease of the genitourinary organs is suspected (Fig. 33.1). Its intimate nature raises medicolegal considerations necessitating both informed consent and the presence of a chaperone throughout the examination.

The vaginal examination of females with an intact hymen should be avoided, particularly as the information required can often be obtained by digital examination of the rectum. Vaginal examination of minors requires the consent of a parent or guardian.

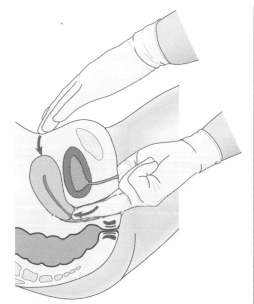

Fig. 33.1 Vaginal examination. (From Ford MJ, Hennessey I, Japp A. Introduction to Clinical Examination, 8th edn. Edinburgh: Churchill Livingstone, 2005.)

1   Evidence of shock?

Use Boxes 15.1 and 15.2 (p. 153 [GI haemorrhage]) as a framework for assessing resuscitation requirements in acute severe vaginal bleeding. Remember that young patients, especially pregnant women, may maintain relatively normal physiological parameters until shock is profound. Assume major blood loss if there are features of intraperitoneal bleeding, e.g. peritonism, shoulder-tip pain or cervical excitation. Arrange immediate gynaecological/obstetric review in any patient with major vaginal bleeding.

2   Pregnant?

Test for pregnancy by urine dipstick and/or serum β-HCG, which is quantitative and more sensitive in very early pregnancy, in all women of reproductive age with vaginal bleeding. Perform urgent USS in all first trimester patients (including newly diagnosed) as part of the initial assessment to determine foetal viability and location (intrauterine or ectopic) as well as the location of the placenta. For women in the second and third trimester, exclude placenta praevia by USS prior to bimanual examination or speculum to avoid disruption of the placenta–cervical junction and catastrophic bleeding. When performing bimanual and speculum examination, assess the volume of passed blood, check for adnexal tenderness (ectopic pregnancy) and identify products of conception at the cervix that require removal.

3   Postmenopausal?

Look for associated features of gynaecological cancer such as pelvic pain, pelvic mass, obstructive GI or urinary tract symptoms or weight loss, but exclude malignancy in all patients with PMB.

Identify sources of lower reproductive tract (endocervix, vagina, vulva) bleeding through careful examination and biopsy any visible lesions. Arrange transvaginal USS to image the ovaries and endometrium and proceed to endometrial biopsy if the endometrium is thickened (e.g. >3 mm). Even if the USS appears normal, consider hysteroscopy and biopsy to exclude endometrial cancer if bleeding persists. Arrange cervical smear cytology to rule out cervical cancer, especially if endometrial pathology is

33

excluded. Biopsy all visible cervical lesions even if the cytological smear is apparently normal. Do not rely on gynaecological tumour markers such as CA125 to rule in or rule out underlying malignancy in patients with PMB.

Consider other common causes of PMB such as atrophic vaginitis and polyps only once malignancy is excluded. Take vaginal/cervical swabs if the history raises suspicion of sexually transmitted infection.

4 Bleeding confined to menstruation?

Most patients are unable to quantify menstrual blood loss accurately so ask about the functional effect of menstruation to identify HMB: is the patient using more sanitary products (tampons, pads, etc.) than normal, do they require double protection (tampons and pads together), are they experiencing flooding (soiling of clothes through the sanitary products) or clots? Check FBC to exclude iron deficiency anaemia. Enquire carefully about associated postcoital or intermenstrual bleeding – if present assess as per step 5.

Ask specifically about contraceptive use – IUDs are associated with HMB; conversely recent discontinuation of an oral contraceptive may lead to increased menstrual blood loss.

Check thyroid function tests if there are clinical features of hypothyroidism (p. 133, Ch. 13) and prolactin levels if there is a history of galactorrhoea.

Screen for coagulopathy if the patient has had HMB since the onset of periods; has a family history of bleeding disorder; or reports spontaneous bruising, troublesome epistaxis or unexplained GI bleeding. Enquire about anticoagulant use but only attribute HMB to anticoagulation once other causes have been excluded.

Take high vaginal and endocervical swabs if there is any suspicion of infection. Consider gynaecological referral for further investigation including USS (pelvic +/– transvaginal) and/or hysteroscopy, especially if there is persistent/troublesome bleeding, associated pelvic pain or a palpable pelvic mass on abdominal/bimanual examination.

Remember that 40–60% of patients with HMB have no identifiable uterine, endocrine, haematological or infective pathology.

Establish the degree of distress caused by bleeding and the impact on quality of life as this may influence treatment options. Non-hormonal treatment comprises tranexamic acid (antifibrinolytic) or NSAIDs such as mefenamic acid (inhibit prostaglandin response) during menstruation. Hormonal treatment is progesterone (oral/IUD) or combined contraception. Surgical options include endometrial ablation, myomectomy (removal of fibroids), or, if all other avenues are unsuccessful and the patient wishes for no more children, hysterectomy.

5 Contact/postcoital bleed?

Examine carefully for vaginal and cervical pathology (see clinical toolkit – vaginal examination) and take high vaginal/endocervical swabs in any patient who reports postcoital or other contact bleeding. Arrange cervical smear cytology unless recently performed and biopsy any visible cervical lesion even if the cytological smear is apparently normal.

6 Consider other causes of intermenstrual bleeding

Establish the pattern and nature of symptoms – this may range from low-volume 'spotting' between defined periods to apparently totally irregular and excessively frequent periods of variable duration. Intermenstrual bleeding unrelated to intercourse/contact is more likely to have an endometrial or systemic cause. Enquire about contraception use and, in particular, any recent changes: the combined oral contraceptive pill typically causes breakthrough bleeding (small volume spotting between the monthly bleed when omitting the tablets for 7 days). Progesterone-based contraceptives (depot preparations such as Nexplanon, hormonal coil such as Mirena) typically result in an irregular pattern of bleeding. Consider screening for coagulopathy if there are suggestive features (see step 4). Refer any patient with persistent unexplained intermenstrual bleeding for gynaecology review and further investigation.

34 Weight loss

Unintentional weight loss of >5% body weight in ≤12 months requires investigation. Lesser degrees of weight loss may also signify underlying pathology, particularly in the frail elderly. Establish how much weight has been lost, and over what time frame; whether there has been a change in clothes size; and whether there has been a corresponding change in appetite. If present, use 'system-specific' symptoms or signs (e.g. haemoptysis, altered bowel habit) to narrow the differential diagnosis and guide appropriate investigation.

Malignancy

In observational studies, 16–36% of adult patients with unintentional weight loss have underlying malignancy. Of these, approximately 50% originate within the GI tract. Weight loss in non-GI cancers tends to be associated with more advanced disease.

Non-malignant GI disease

Weight loss is frequently observed in disorders that lead to swallowing difficulty (see Ch. 11), malabsorption (e.g. coeliac disease) or persistent inflammation (e.g. inflammatory bowel disease). In peptic ulcer disease, mesenteric ischaemia and chronic pancreatitis, the pain associated with eating may lead to weight loss through avoidance of food. However, weight loss is not an expected feature of functional GI disorders such as irritable bowel syndrome.

Endocrine disorders

Persistent hyperglycaemia due to uncontrolled or undiagnosed diabetes causes weight loss, alongside polydipsia and polyuria. In thyrotoxicosis weight loss occurs despite normal or increased appetite. Patients with hypercalcaemia may experience weight loss due to underlying malignant disease or the direct effects of ↑Ca^{2+}, e.g. osmotic diuresis, anorexia, nausea and vomiting. Weight loss is also one of several non-specific presenting symptoms in chronic adrenal insufficiency (Box 25.2, p. 223).

Chronic disease

In severe non-malignant disease such as advanced COPD, heart failure or chronic kidney disease, several mechanisms may contribute to weight loss including poor appetite, persistent catabolic state and polypharmacy. Prominent weight loss is also a feature of chronic infection, e.g. tuberculosis, infective endocarditis and HIV.

Neurological disorder

Motor neuron disease, Parkinson's disease, multiple sclerosis and stroke may lead to weight loss through dysphagia (see Ch. 11). Limb weakness and impaired functional abilities can present a significant barrier to food preparation and consumption. Multifactorial weight loss is also common in dementia, particularly in advanced stages.

Medication

Drug side effects such as anorexia, dry mouth, altered taste sensation, nausea, vomiting or sedation may result in reduced calorie intake (Box 34.1). Certain drugs are misused to facilitate weight loss, e.g. laxatives or thyroxine.

Psychiatric

Low mood can lead to low appetite, or lack of motivation to prepare meals, resulting in weight loss. This is a more common phenomenon in elderly people with mood disorders. The prevalence of depression in older adults (>65 years old) is estimated at around 35%, and higher still in those living in institutional settings. Addressing the underlying depressive illness can lead to improved oral intake and weight gain. Primary eating disorders (anorexia and bulimia) are most commonly identified in younger women, but are

Box 34.1 Drug causes of weight loss

Direct weight loss effect

Diuretics ('pseudo' weight loss)
Levothyroxine (if excessive dosage)
Topiramate (mechanism uncertain)
Appetite suppressants, e.g. Lorcaserin
Glucagon-like peptide-1 (GLP-1) analogues, e.g. Liraglutide
Sympathomimetic agents, e.g. methylphenidate, dextroamphetamine
Sodium-glucose Cotransporter-2 (SGLT2) inhibitors, e.g. Empagliflozin

Other drug-induced mechanisms of weight loss

Nausea and vomiting: see Box 25.1, p. 223
Altered sense of taste, e.g. Allopurinol, Zopiclone, Metronidazole
Dry mouth, e.g. anticholinergics, clonidine, diuretics
Sedation, e.g. opiates, benzodiazepines, antipsychotics

increasingly recognized in young men; the patient may deny that a problem exists and concerns are often raised by relatives and friends who have noticed a change in eating behaviour or physical appearance.

Other

Explore possible social causes for weight loss such as lack of money to buy food, social isolation and/or chronic alcohol excess. Poor dentition or ill-fitting dentures may also contribute to undernutrition.

Unintentional weight loss is a concerning but non-specific symptom. Refer, initially, to the relevant chapter if one of the following symptoms is present: Breast lump (Ch. 5), Dysphagia (Ch. 11), GI haemorrhage (Ch. 15), Haematuria (Ch. 16), Haemoptysis (Ch. 17), Jaundice (Ch. 19), Scrotal swelling (Ch. 29), Vaginal bleeding (Ch. 33). Return to this pathway if no cause for weight loss is identified.

34

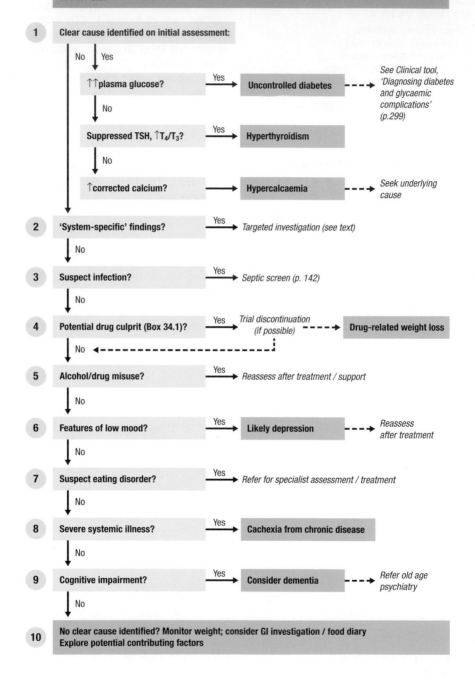

Full clinical assessment, breast, genital & rectal examination, FBC, U&E, LFT, calcium, glucose, TFT +/- CXR

1 Clear cause identified on initial assessment:

No → Yes

↑↑plasma glucose? — Yes → **Uncontrolled diabetes** ---→ *See Clinical tool, 'Diagnosing diabetes and glycaemic complications' (p.299)*

No ↓

Suppressed TSH, ↑T₄/T₃? — Yes → **Hyperthyroidism**

No ↓

↑corrected calcium? → **Hypercalcaemia** ---→ *Seek underlying cause*

2 'System-specific' findings? — Yes → *Targeted investigation (see text)*

No ↓

3 Suspect infection? — Yes → *Septic screen (p. 142)*

No ↓

4 Potential drug culprit (Box 34.1)? — Yes → *Trial discontinuation (if possible)* ---→ **Drug-related weight loss**

No ↓

5 Alcohol/drug misuse? — Yes → *Reassess after treatment / support*

No ↓

6 Features of low mood? — Yes → **Likely depression** ---→ *Reassess after treatment*

No ↓

7 Suspect eating disorder? — Yes → *Refer for specialist assessment / treatment*

No ↓

8 Severe systemic illness? — Yes → **Cachexia from chronic disease**

No ↓

9 Cognitive impairment? — Yes → **Consider dementia** ---→ *Refer old age psychiatry*

No ↓

10 No clear cause identified? Monitor weight; consider GI investigation / food diary
Explore potential contributing factors

1 Clear cause identified on initial screening?

Hyperglycaemia

Consider new-onset diabetes in patients without a pre-existing diagnosis (see Clinical tool, p. 299): check for ketoacidosis and, if present, admit for urgent treatment. In the absence of ketoacidosis, refer to your local diabetes service for treatment initiation. Remember that a mild, transient increase in blood glucose level may occur in any severe acute illness (stress hyperglycaemia). In older patients with new-onset diabetes and weight loss consider underlying pancreatic malignancy, especially if there is associated abdominal pain.

In patients with known diabetes, use plasma HbA1c to gauge the severity of recent hyperglycaemia; consider hyperglycaemia as a contributor to weight loss if control is suboptimal (especially in type 1 diabetes) but continue to search for alternative causes.

Thyrotoxicosis (TSH)

Suppressed TSH with $\uparrow T_4/T_3$ level is diagnostic of hyperthyroidism. Look for associated clinical features including tremor, poor sleep, heat intolerance and increased bowel activity +/– eye and skin changes in Graves' disease. Check thyroid receptor antibody (TRAB) levels to help identify the underlying aetiology and refer to Endocrinology.

Hypercalcaemia

Check plasma parathyroid hormone (PTH) levels to identify the likely cause. PTH should be suppressed by hypercalcaemia so $\uparrow$ or 'inappropriately normal' PTH suggests primary hyperparathyroidism. If $\downarrow$PTH, consider malignancy (e.g. skeletal metastases, multiple myeloma or tumour secretion of PTH-related peptide). Other causes, particularly if hypercalcaemia is mild, include sarcoidosis, thiazide diuretics and vitamin D analogues.

2 'System-specific' findings?

Consider underlying malignancy in any patient with unexplained weight loss. Look for clues in the history, physical examination and routine tests that may help to target further investigation.

Request an urgent CXR in patients with persistent respiratory symptoms (>3 weeks) or in those >40 years with a history of smoking or asbestos exposure. Refer for respiratory investigation (usually CT chest +/– bronchoscopy) in patients with an abnormal CXR (>95% of patients with symptomatic lung cancer) or respiratory symptoms for >6 weeks despite a normal CXR.

Refer patients with concerning GI symptoms or unexplained iron deficiency anaemia for urgent endoscopic evaluation: upper GI endoscopy if dysphagia, vomiting or upper abdominal pain/discomfort; colonoscopy if altered bowel habit, tenesmus or lower abdominal pain/discomfort; upper and lower GI endoscopy if iron-deficiency anaemia. CT colonogram provides a less-invasive alternative to colonoscopy and may be more appropriate in selected patients, e.g. frail or multimorbid.

Arrange appropriate imaging if you palpate an abdominal or pelvic mass. USS is often a helpful initial investigation, particularly for pelvic masses, but CT is frequently required for further characterisation +/– staging of malignant tumours.

Check a PSA level in males with prostatic symptoms. Measure PSA prior to the rectal exam to avoid false positive tests. Refer patients with a hard irregular prostate or $\uparrow$PSA ($\geq$3 ng/mL if <60 years; $\geq$4 ng/mL if 60–69 years; $\geq$5 ng/mL if $\geq$70 years) for urgent urological assessment. Bear in mind that localized prostate cancer is unlikely to account for significant weight loss so continue to seek alternative causes unless there are features of advanced disease, e.g. bone pain, biochemical evidence of skeletal metastases (e.g. $\uparrow$ALP) or a markedly $\uparrow$PSA, e.g. >20 ng/mL.

Lymphadenopathy, either local or generalized, may signify infection, inflammation, e.g. connective tissue disease, haematological malignancy or solid organ cancer with lymphatic involvement. Check LDH (often $\uparrow$ in haematological malignancy) and screen for infection and autoimmune disease. In persistent lymphadenopathy consider CT chest/abdomen/pelvis and arrange lymph node biopsy to establish a tissue diagnosis.

3 Suspect infection?

Perform a septic screen in patients with fever or elevated white cell count/inflammatory markers (see Clinical tool, p. 142). Ask about foreign travel, infectious contacts and risk factors for HIV. Examine carefully and repeatedly for murmurs and peripheral stigmata of endocarditis.

4 Potential drug culprit?

Review all medications, prescribed and non-prescribed, including any 'nutritional supplements'. In patients with reduced dietary intake ask about symptoms such as dry mouth, drowsiness, altered taste sensation or nausea and look for potential drug culprits (Box 34.1). If you suspect a drug cause, reassess weight and symptoms after trial discontinuation (if appropriate).

5 Alcohol/drug misuse?

Enquire about alcohol intake (Box 2.1, p. 11) and recreational drug use, e.g. cocaine, amphetamines in a non-judgmental manner. Where possible seek collateral history from friends or family (who may have raised the concerns re: weight loss). Explore associated factors that may be contributing to weight loss such as appetite suppression, replacement of meals with alcohol intake, lack of money to buy food or co-existent mood disorders.

6 Features of low mood?

Look for evidence of low mood such as anhedonia (loss of pleasure in life), undue pessimism or feelings of guilt/worthlessness pessimism as well as biological features of depression, e.g. lack of energy, poor sleep (early morning waking), reduced libido. Consider undertaking a depression score, such as the Geriatric Depression Scale in the elderly, or the PHQ-9 in younger adults. If you suspect depression as the cause of weight loss reassess weight and other symptoms after a period of treatment.

7 Suspect eating disorder?

Consider the possibility of an eating disorder particularly in younger women with amenorrhoea or a background of psychiatric or psychological problems. Be alert for important clues such as distorted attitudes to weight or body image (e.g. underplaying the seriousness of weight loss, fear of gaining weight, preoccupation with weight issues) or concerns raised by friends/family members, e.g. skipping meals, concealing food. Be sensitive and tactful but persistent in questioning and refer to specialist services if significant concern.

8 Severe systemic illness?

Assess the severity and trajectory of chronic disease, e.g. heart failure, COPD or renal failure using symptom status, functional performance, frequency of hospitalization and objective markers (e.g. GFR, FEV1). Weight loss and anorexia may occur in advanced disease. Seek specialist input to optimize management but consider the need for dietetic and/or palliative care input.

9 Cognitive impairment?

Assess cognition formally with a mini mental state examination or Addenbrooke's cognitive examination-III in patients with either established or suspected or cognitive impairment. Wherever possible, obtain a collateral history from friends, relatives or carers to evaluate the contribution from cognitive impairment to weight loss, e.g. forgetting meals, unable to prepare food, paranoid ideas about food. In patients with more advanced dementia enquire about the patient's ability to transfer food from plate to mouth and any swallowing problems. Refer patient for specialist evaluation, e.g. psychiatry of old age.

10 Consider further investigation and/or food diary. Explore factors contributing to reduced food intake

If weight loss persists with no clear cause, consider GI investigation/referral +/– CT if not already performed. Use a food diary to record calorie intake. Reconsider the possibility of a primary eating disorder or depression. Explore possible contributing factors to inadequate food intake including inadequate dentition, swallowing problems, lack of motivation (or money), impaired mobility (unable to get to shop) or subtle cognitive impairment. Refer frail, elderly patients for comprehensive geriatric assessment.

Clinical tool
Diagnosing diabetes and glycaemic complications

Diagnosis of diabetes

(Definition and diagnosis of diabetes mellitus and intermediate hyperglycaemia. WHO 2006; update 2011.)

Typical presenting symptoms of diabetes include thirst, polyuria and unexplained weight loss. These will be more prominent, with a shorter history, in type 1 diabetes, due to absolute insulin deficiency. In type 2 diabetes, there may be little in the way of symptoms, or they may go unnoticed due to their insidious onset. Biochemical cut-offs to clinch the diagnosis are described in Table 34.1. In symptomatic patients, one laboratory measure is required to confirm hyperglycaemia. In asymptomatic people, two confirmatory tests at separate times are needed.

Assessment of long-term glycaemic control

The target HbA1c in the ongoing management of diabetes, to avoid the development of long-term complications, is widely accepted as <58 mmol/mol (<7.5%). There has been a recent move in updated NICE guidance (2015) to a tighter target of 48 mmol/mol (6.5%), if able to achieve this without unacceptable hypoglycaemia or impact on co-morbidities. American Diabetes Association guidance recommends a target of <53 mmol/mol (7.0%). These targets should, of course, be individualized in consultation with the person with diabetes.

Acute complications of diabetes

Hyperglycaemic crises

Diabetic ketoacidosis (DKA) is a medical emergency, and involves a triad of diabetes, ketosis and acidosis. It is the result of insulin deficiency (absolute – type 1 diabetes/pancreatic disease; or relative – poorly controlled type 2

diabetes). It develops rapidly over hours. Severity can be graded as mild/moderate/severe depending on the degree of biochemical abnormality and presence of altered mental status (Table 34.2). Mortality is 0.2–2% (with higher rates in developing countries).

Hyperosmolar hyperglycaemic state (HHS) is usually a complication of poorly controlled type 2 diabetes, often with insidious onset over days to weeks. Blood glucose is very high, with high osmolality and hypercoagulability. It is life threatening, with a 15–20% mortality rate. The frail elderly are most at risk. It can be complicated by myocardial infarction, stroke or peripheral arterial thrombosis. In addition, overly rapid correction of metabolic abnormalities can lead to complications such as seizures, cerebral oedema and central pontine myelinolysis. It is, therefore, vital to correct abnormalities gradually and to carefully monitor the plasma osmolality ([2 × Na] + urea + glucose) during treatment.

Hypoglycaemia

Whilst there is no clear consensus on the biochemical definition of hypoglycaemia, it is largely accepted that a blood glucose <4 mmol/L (72 mg/dL) would be an appropriate level to trigger treatment in a person with diabetes. Severe hypoglycaemia is defined by the requirement for external assistance to restore normal blood glucose (whether relatives or emergency services). Symptoms (Table 34.3) will usually alert a person with diabetes to the development of hypoglycaemia, but it is important to be aware that some people lose their hypoglycaemia warning symptoms, known as impaired hypoglycaemia awareness, and they are at high risk of severe hypoglycaemia as a result.

34

Table 34.1 Biochemical criteria for diagnosis of diabetes mellitus

Diabetes

Fasting plasma glucose	≥7.0 mmol/L (126 mg/dL)
Random plasma glucose	≥11.1 mmol/L (200 mg/dL)
2-hour plasma glucose on OGTT[1]	≥11.1 mmol/L (200 mg/dL)
HbA1c[2]	≥48 mmol/mol (6.5%)

Impaired fasting glycaemia

Fasting plasma glucose	6.1–6.9 mmol/L (110–125 mg/dL)

Impaired glucose tolerance

2-hour plasma glucose on OGTT	7.8–11.0 mmol/L (140–200 mg/dL)

[1]OGTT – Oral glucose tolerance test: venous plasma glucose in fasting state, administer 75 g oral glucose load, repeat venous plasma glucose at 2 hours.
[2]Not suitable as a diagnostic test in children and young people or in the context of: suspected type 1 diabetes, symptoms for <2 months, acute illness, pregnancy, treatment with medications that cause rapid glucose rise (e.g. steroids, antipsychotics) or acute pancreatic damage/surgery.

Table 34.3 Symptoms of hypoglycaemia

Autonomic	Neuroglycopenic	Non-specific
Palpitation	Confusion	Tiredness
Sweating	Weakness	Nausea
Tremor	Dizziness	Headache
Hunger	Reduced concentration	
Anxiety	Incoordination	
	Drowsiness	
	Speech difficulty	

Table 34.2 Criteria for diagnosis of DKA and HHS

	DKA	Severe DKA	HHS
Plasma glucose[1]	>13.9 mmol/L (>250 mg/dL)	–	>33.3 mmol/L (>600 mg/dL)
Osmolality			>320 mOsm/kg
Arterial pH	<7.3	<7.0	>7.3
Serum bicarbonate	<18 mmol/L	<10 mmol/L	>18 mmol/L[2]
Blood ketones (capillary sample)	>1.5 mmol/L	–	Negative/small
Urine ketones	Positive	–	Negative/small
Mental status	Alert or drowsy	Stupor/coma	Stupor/coma

[1]If a patient with DKA has started treatment with supplementary insulin, they may present with a normal blood glucose, but still have ketosis and acidosis and be at risk of clinical deterioration.
[2]In some patients metabolic acidosis may be present due either to relative insulin deficiency (check ketones) or to intercurrent acute illness (lactic acidosis or AKI).
Adapted from Kitabchi AE et al. 2006. Hyperglycemic crises in adult patients with diabetes: a consensus statement from the American Diabetes Association. Diabetes Care. 29(12):2739–2748.

Appendix

Normal values for biochemical tests in venous blood

Analyte	Reference range[1] SI units	Non-SI units
Alanine amino-transferase (ALT)	10–50 U/L	–
Albumin	35–50 g/L	3.5–5.0 g/dL
Alkaline phosphatase (ALP)	40–125 U/L	–
Aspartate amino-transferase (AST)	10–45 U/L	–
Bilirubin (total)	2–17 μmol/L	0.12–1.0 mg/dL
Calcium (total)	2.12–2.62 mmol/L	4.24–5.24 meq/L or 8.50–10.50 mg/dL
Chloride	95–107 mmol/L	95–107 meq/L
Cholesterol (total)	Mild increase 5.2–6.5 mmol/L Moderate increase 6.5–7.8 mmol/L Severe increase >7.8 mmol/L	200–250 mg/dL 250–300 mg/dL >300 mg/dL
C-reactive protein (CRP)	<5 mg/L Highly sensitive CRP assays also exist which may be useful in estimating cardiovascular risk	

Creatine kinase (CK) (total)
  Male
  Female
	
	55–170 U/L
	30–135 U/L
		
		–
		–

Creatine kinase MB isoenzyme	<6% of total CK	–
Creatinine	60–120 μmol/L	0.68–1.36 mg/dL
Gamma-glutamyl transferase (GGT)	5–55 U/L	–
Glucose (fasting)	3.6–5.8 mmol/L	65–104 mg/dL
Glycated haemoglobin (HbA$_{1c}$)	5.0–6.5%	–
Lactate	0.6–2.4 mmol/L	5.40–21.6 mg/dL
Lactate dehydrogenase (LDH) (total)	208–460 U/L	–
Phosphate (fasting)	0.8–1.4 mmol/L	2.48–4.34 mg/dL
Potassium (plasma)	3.3–4.7 mmol/L	3.3–4.7 meq/L
Potassium (serum)	3.6–5.1 mmol/L	3.6–5.1 meq/L
Protein (total)	60–80 g/L	6–8 g/dL
Sodium	135–145 mmol/L	135–145 meq/L
Triglycerides (fasting)	0.6–1.7 mmol/L	53–150 mg/dL

Urate
  Male
  Female
	
	0.12–0.42 mmol/L
	0.12–0.36 mmol/L
		
		2.0–7.0 mg/dL
		2.0–6.0 mg/dL

Urea	2.5–6.6 μmol/L	15–40 mg/dL

[1]Note these values may vary according to local laboratory calibration.

Arterial blood analysis

Analysis	Reference range SI units	Non-SI units
Bicarbonate (HCO₃)	21–29 mmol/L	21–29 meq/L
Hydrogen ion (H⁺)	37–45 nmol/L	pH 7.35–7.43
PaCO₂	4.5–6.0 kPa	34–45 mmHg
PaO₂	12–15 kPa	90–113 mmHg
Oxygen saturation (SpO₂)	>97%[1,2]	

[1]Breathing room air.
[2]Varies with age.

Haematological values

Analysis	Reference range SI units	Non-SI units
Bleeding time (Ivy)	<8 min	–
Blood volume Male Female	75 ± 10 mL/kg 70 ± 10 mL/kg	–
Coagulation screen Prothrombin time Activated partial thromboplastin time	10.5–13.5 sec 26–36 sec	– –
D-dimer Routine Sensitive (for venous thromboembolism)	<0.2 mg/L Variable threshold (dependent on method)	–
Erythrocyte sedimentation rate (ESR) Adult male Adult female	Higher values may be normal in older patients 0–10 mm/hr 3–15 mm/hr	– –
Ferritin Male Premenopausal female Postmenopausal female	17–300 μg/L 7–280 μg/L 4–233 μg/L	17–300 ng/mL 7–280 ng/mL 4–233 ng/mL
Fibrinogen	1.5–4.0 g/L	0.15–0.4 g/dL
Folate Serum Red cell	2.0–13.5 μg/L 95–570 μg/L	2.0–13.5 ng/mL 95–570 ng/mL
Haemoglobin Male Female	130–180 g/L 115–165 g/L	13–18 g/dL 11.5–16.5 g/dL
Haptoglobin	0.4–2.4 g/L	0.04–0.24 g/dL
Iron Male Female	14–32 μmol/L 10–28 μmol/L	78–178 μg/dL 56–156 μg/dL
Leukocytes (adults)	4.0–11.0 × 10⁹/L	4.0–11.0 × 10³/mm³

Haematological values—cont'd

Analysis	Reference range SI units	Non-SI units
Differential white cell count		
Neutrophil granulocytes	$2.0–7.5 \times 10^9$/L	$2.0–7.5 \times 10^3$/mm^3
Lymphocytes	$1.5–4.0 \times 10^9$/L	$1.5–4.0 \times 10^3$/mm^3
Monocytes	$0.2–0.8 \times 10^9$/L	$0.2–0.8 \times 10^3$/mm^3
Eosinophil granulocytes	$0.04–0.4 \times 10^9$/L	$0.04–0.4 \times 10^3$/mm^3
Basophil granulocytes	$0.01–0.1 \times 10^9$/L	$0.01–0.1 \times 10^3$/mm^3
Mean cell haemoglobin (MCH)	27–32 pg	–
Mean cell volume (MCV)	78–98 fL	
Packed cell volume (PCV) or haematocrit		
Male	0.40–0.54	–
Female	0.37–0.47	–
Platelets	$150–350 \times 10^9$/L	$150–350 \times 10^3$/mm^3
Red cell count		
Male	$4.5–6.5 \times 10^{12}$/L	$4.5–6.5 \times 10^6$/mm^3
Female	$3.8–5.8 \times 10^{12}$/L	$3.8–5.8 \times 10^6$/mm^3
Red cell lifespan		
Mean	120 days	–
Half-life (^{51}Cr)	25–35 days	–
Reticulocytes (adults)	$25–85 \times 10^9$/L	$25–85 \times 10^3$/mm^3
Transferrin	2.0–4.0 g/L	0.2–0.4 g/dL
Transferrin saturation		
Male	25–56%	–
Female	14–51%	–
Vitamin B$_{12}$	130–770 pg/mL	

Source: Reproduced with permission from Innes JA. Davidson's Essentials of Medicine. Edinburgh: Churchill Livingstone, 2009.

Index

Page numbers followed by '*f*' indicate figures, '*t*' indicate tables, and '*b*' indicate boxes.